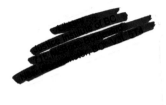

COGNITIVE PROCESSING THERAPY FOR PTSD

Cognitive Processing Therapy for PTSD

A Comprehensive Manual

Patricia A. Resick

Candice M. Monson

Kathleen M. Chard

THE GUILFORD PRESS
New York   London

The authors have checked with sources believed to be reliable in their efforts to provide
information that is complete and generally in accord with the standards of practice that are
accepted at the time of publication. However, in view of the possibility of human error or
changes in behavioral, mental health, or medical sciences, neither the authors, nor the editor
and publisher, nor any other party who has been involved in the preparation or publication
of this work warrants that the information contained herein is in every respect accurate or
complete, and they are not responsible for any errors or omissions or the results obtained from
the use of such information. Readers are encouraged to confirm the information contained in
this book with other sources.

Library of Congress Cataloging-in-Publication Data

Names: Resick, Patricia A., author. | Monson, Candice M., author. | Chard, Kathleen M.,
    author.
Title: Cognitive processing therapy for PTSD : a comprehensive manual / Patricia A. Resick,
    Candice M. Monson, and Kathleen M. Chard.
Description: New York, NY : Guilford Press, [2017] | Includes bibliographical references and
    index.
Identifiers: LCCN 2016035960 | ISBN 9781462528646 (pbk. : alk. paper)
Subjects: | MESH: Stress Disorders, Post-Traumatic—therapy | Cognitive Therapy—methods
Classification: LCC RC552.P67 | NLM WM 172.5 | DDC 616.85/21—dc23
LC record available at *https://lccn.loc.gov/2016035960*

To our loved ones, who were so supportive of our work and lives:

For my sister—P. A. R.

For my mother—C. M. M.

For my father—K. M. C.

About the Authors

Patricia A. Resick, PhD, ABPP, is Professor of Psychiatry and Behavioral Sciences at Duke University. She originally developed cognitive processing therapy (CPT) in 1988 at the University of Missouri–St. Louis, where she founded the Center for Trauma Recovery and was an Endowed Professor. Dr. Resick has served as president of the International Society for Traumatic Stress Studies (ISTSS) and the Association for Behavioral and Cognitive Therapies (ABCT). She is a recipient of the Robert S. Laufer Memorial Award for Outstanding Scientific Achievement in the field of traumatic stress from the ISTSS, the Leadership Award from the Association of VA Psychologist Leaders, the Outstanding Contribution by an Individual for Education/Training Award from the ABCT, and the Lifetime Achievement Award from Division 56 (Trauma Psychology) of the American Psychological Association.

Candice M. Monson, PhD, is Professor of Psychology at Ryerson University in Toronto, Ontario, Canada. A Fellow of both the American and Canadian Psychological Associations, she is a recipient of the Traumatic Stress Psychologist of the Year Award from the Canadian Psychological Association, the Distinguished Mentorship Award from the ISTSS, and the Award for Excellence in Professional Training from the Canadian Council of Professional Psychology Programs. Dr. Monson is well known for her research on interpersonal factors in traumatization and the development, testing, and dissemination of treatments for posttraumatic stress disorder (PTSD), including CPT and cognitive-behavioral conjoint therapy for PTSD.

Kathleen M. Chard, PhD, is Associate Chief of Staff for Research at the Cincinnati Veterans Affairs (VA) Medical Center and Professor of Psychiatry and Behavioral Neuroscience at the University of Cincinnati. As the VA CPT Implementation Director, Dr. Chard oversees the dissemination of CPT to VA clinicians across the United

States. She is an associate editor of the *Journal of Traumatic Stress* and a board member of the ISTSS. Dr. Chard is a recipient of the Mark Wolcott Award for Excellence in Clinical Care Leadership from the VA and the Heroes of Military Medicine Award from the United Service Organization. Known for her research on dissemination and clinical implementation of evidence-based treatments for civilians and veterans, she is the creator of the CPT for Sexual Abuse manual.

Acknowledgments

This book is the culmination of over 25 years of clinical work and research by many people who have made suggestions, tested cognitive processing therapy (CPT), and helped us add and revise handouts and modules based on their experiences. We believe that those readers who have seen earlier versions will find that we have made significant revisions while writing this book over the past 4 years.

We would like to thank Jim Nageotte, Senior Editor at The Guilford Press, who has been asking for this book for over 15 years. He has been very patient and supportive. We are grateful to our families and friends, who have been on this long journey with us, cheering from the sidelines. We acknowledge all the CPT trainers and providers who have enthusiastically adopted CPT and have helped shape it along the way. Finally, we thank the many clients who have received CPT and taught us so much about how to help them recover. It is most gratifying when a therapist passes along a note from a client who has appreciated the help received both from the therapist and from CPT. We hope that you, our readers, find implementing CPT as rewarding for you and your clients as we have all these years.

Contents

PART IV

Alternatives in Delivery and Special Considerations

> Purchasers of this book can download and print the handouts at
> *www.guilford.com/resick-forms* for personal use or use with individual
> clients (see copyright page for details).

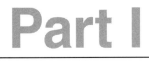

Part I

Background on Posttraumatic Stress Disorder and Cognitive Processing Therapy

1

The Origins of Cognitive Processing Therapy

Rather than writing a review chapter on theories of posttraumatic stress disorder (PTSD)—which have evolved from early learning theory to cognitive and constructivist theories as described elsewhere (Chard, Schuster, & Resick, 2012; Resick, Monson, & Rizvi, 2013; Monson, Friedman, & La Bash, 2014), and which may or may not have influenced the development of cognitive processing therapy (CPT)—I (Patricia A. Resick) have chosen to write this chapter in the first person and make it a little more autobiographical. I have done this so that readers can see how I first developed CPT, what the influences on it were, and how it has evolved into its present form through the engagement of my coauthors and of many others. This chapter also emphasizes the importance of theory: Theory guides therapists in explaining to their clients why they have PTSD, what has maintained it, and how to get over it, as well as in staying within the CPT protocol. It also guides particular ways of thinking about trauma recovery when therapists encounter challenges in treatment delivery. We address the theoretical underpinnings of CPT at several other points in this book as well.

The Origins of CPT

I started my career in the field of trauma during my internship at the Medical University of South Carolina (MUSC) and the Charleston Veterans Administration (VA; now Veterans Affairs) Medical Center. Specifically, I became one of the first cohort of rape crisis counselors at one of the few rape crisis centers in the United States in the mid-1970s. The very first night I was on call, I went to the hospital in the middle of the night to meet a woman who was nearly speechless in shock at what had happened to her. I was mostly just sitting with her silently, waiting for a nurse or doctor, when her husband came barreling through the doors of the emergency room yelling, "What have they done to me?" Aside from being flabbergasted at his response, I realized that I was clueless about what this woman was going through and how to help her. As advocates, my fellow counselors and I stayed with women in the emergency room (many times for numerous hours), and accompanied them into the exam rooms if they wished, while some (usually male) physician or resident performed an often rough medical examination and collected evidence, while clearly wanting to get back to the "real patients."

Some rape crisis advocates focused their efforts on more humane treatment of rape victims in emergency rooms and on the education of the medical community. Being a clinical psychology graduate student, I went to the literature in my field, which back then meant physically going to the library and reading through every index of *Psychological Abstracts*. A fellow student, Joan Jackson, and I did a volume-by-volume search and found only five articles, which were essentially useless. Other, more sociological articles focused on victims' precipitation of rape, and thus engaged in victim blaming.

However, at about that time, a number of things happened. Susan Brownmiller (1975) wrote *Against Our Will*, which chronicled the history of rape as a political and power weapon. In addition, women who had been raped were conducting "speakouts" through the National Organization for Women, and it soon became very clear to many how common the problem of rape was and how profound its effects were. Burgess and Holmstrom (1976) published an important article in the *American Journal of Psychiatry*, one of a series of articles on the reactions they observed from conducting interviews with 92 rape victims in an emergency room. Finally, the National Institute of Mental Health (NIMH) set aside $3 million for studies on rape, and I became involved in writing two grant applications—one with Dean Kilpatrick at MUSC, and one with Karen Calhoun when I went back to the University of Georgia to complete my graduate degree. Both grants were funded.

The first studies at MUSC included a prospective longitudinal study of fear and anxiety among victims, as well as an attempt to develop a brief behavioral intervention and then the use of stress inoculation training, based on Meichenbaum's work on coping skills training (Meichenbaum & Cameron, 1983, which was an unpublished 1972 manual at the time we used it). The University of Georgia study was conducted in Atlanta at Grady Memorial Hospital, where about 1,000 women a year who had been raped were being seen in the emergency room. The focus of the prospective longitudinal study was on depression. Our goals were simple: to see whether rape produced fear or depressive reactions (a question that had never been studied), and, if so, how long-lasting they might be. We also wanted to see whether we could develop treatments that could be used in rape crisis centers.

While those studies were being reviewed and conducted, I took a faculty position at the University of South Dakota and commuted to either Charleston or Atlanta once a month. After 4 years there and 1 year back in Charleston, I assumed a faculty position at the University of Missouri–St. Louis. Although I had been offered positions at better-known universities, I needed to be in a city that was large enough to allow me to continue my work, and St. Louis fit the bill.

My first grant, funded by both NIMH and the National Institute of Justice, was another prospective longitudinal study—this time comparing female rape or robbery victims with male robbery victims. In the meantime, I was trying to conduct treatment outcome research with small university grants. The first study I conducted, still within the anxiety perspective, was a comparison of group stress inoculation, assertiveness training (because assertiveness was thought to counter fear), and supportive psychotherapy. By then the *Diagnostic and Statistical Manual of Mental Disorders, Third Edition* (DSM-III; American Psychiatric Association, 1980) had been published, with a new diagnosis in the anxiety disorders category: PTSD. The DSM-III definition of a traumatic stressor used rape as an example, but there were as yet no measures of PTSD. My colleagues and I used the Impact of Event Scale (Horowitz, Wilner, & Alvarez, 1979) and the Derogatis Symptom Checklist–90 (Derogatis, 1977), among other measures. This small study found posttreatment improvements, but there were no differences among the three conditions (Resick, Jordan, Girelli, Hutter, & Marhoeder-Dvorak, 1988). Because we did not know how long it would take to fill a group, we could not use random assignment; however, we predetermined the order of groups, so the assignment was unbiased. Later I realized that the lack of differences was probably at least partially due to the small sample size and lack of power, but in the discussion of the study, I focused on the commonalities of the treatments, expectancy theory, psychoeducation, and cognitive change.

The prevailing theory about rape responses at the time was that they consisted of first-order classical conditioning of the fear reaction, along with second-order conditioning that generalized the reaction to other triggers (Kilpatrick, Resick, & Veronen, 1981; Kilpatrick, Veronen, & Resick, 1979). Later, once the PTSD diagnosis was introduced, came awareness of the importance of escape and avoidance learning in maintaining the primary symptoms of PTSD. If someone is experiencing strong conditioned emotional reactions, this person is likely to avoid or escape reminders of the trauma that have spread to nondangerous situations. Mowrer's (1960) two-factor theory of classical conditioning and operant avoidance became more commonly discussed, along with Foa and Kozak's (1986) emotional processing theory of PTSD, which in turn was based on Lang's (1977) theory that people develop fear networks with stimulus, response, and meaning elements. Because there were enough women who said to me, "I knew he wasn't going to kill me, but it was such a huge betrayal, and I feel so much shame and disgust at what he did to me," I began to have doubts that PTSD after rape was just a fear/anxiety disorder. One exception to a theory means that the theory needs to be revised. I began to look toward cognitive theories of PTSD.

Theoretical Influences

In our earliest conceptualizations of depression among rape victims (Kilpatrick, Veronen, & Resick, 1982), we viewed the development of such depression within several extant theories: lowered levels of positive reinforcement (Lewinsohn, 1974), and learned helplessness resulting from the unpredictable and uncontrollable nature of the victimization experience (Seligman, 1971). Paykel (1974) proposed that depression occurs following negative interpersonal events, threatening events, or blows to self-esteem. Of course, rape victims experience all of these.

In the 1960s and 1970s, Aaron T. Beck studied the causes of depression and developed his cognitive theory, which focuses on how people absorb negative and erroneous beliefs from society that leave them feeling ashamed and depressed. He and his colleagues produced a treatment manual for cognitive therapy of depression (Beck, Rush, Shaw, & Emery, 1979). Although this was one of the first manualized treatments, I wanted something more specific and progressive that would tell therapists how to proceed session by session. I was hoping that clinicians could pick up the manual and conduct the therapy. I also wanted to help clients to become their own therapists by teaching them new, more balanced ways to cope and think, much as we had done with stress inoculation. I liked the Socratic style of therapy that Beck and colleagues proposed, in which therapists asked clients questions so that they could figure out the answers for themselves. However, Beck et al.'s cognitive therapy for depression focused on current thoughts, and I believed that in treating PTSD, we first needed to go back to revisit the traumatic events to see where clients' thinking developed and whether they had emotionally processed the traumatic events at the time. I started conceptualizing that those who hadn't been able to recover had been "stuck" in their thinking since the time of the traumatic events, and I began to call such clients' thoughts "Stuck Points."

Additional inspiration came from an article and book by McCann and colleagues (McCann, Sakheim, & Abrahamson, 1988; McCann & Pearlman, 1990), who developed the constructivist self-development theory of traumatic victimization. This theory was based on Mahoney's (1981) constructivist perspective, in which humans actively create their personal realities, such that new experiences are constrained to fit people's determinations of what "reality" is (Mahoney & Lyddon, 1988). McCann et al. proposed a constructivist theory of trauma in which people construct meaning from events. They theorized that aside from frame of reference (the need for a stable and coherent framework for understanding experiences), the schemas (mental structures and needs) that are likely to be affected by trauma are those regarding safety, trust, power/control, esteem, and intimacy. These constructs can be self- or other-directed. Because these constructs appeared so frequently in our discussions with clients, my colleagues and I also began to think that we could use the work of McCann and colleagues in a briefer cognitive-behavioral therapy.

I was also influenced by a chapter by Hollon and Garber (1988), in which they proposed that when someone is exposed to schema-discrepant information, one of two things happens. The information may be altered so that it can be assimilated into the person's existing beliefs/schemas without changing the prior beliefs (e.g., "It wasn't a rape, it was a misunderstanding; I must have done something for him to think it was OK"). The other alternative is that existing beliefs (e.g., "Only strangers rape") are changed to incorporate the new, discrepant information (e.g., "It is possible to be raped by someone you know"). This new learning represents accommodation and is the goal for therapy. Hollon and Garber's proposal, of course, was based on the work of Piaget (1971), but I had not thought about it in the context of therapy or trauma before.

I realized further in working with trauma survivors that sometimes people changed their beliefs too much, even while they were distorting and attempting to assimilate the traumatic events. They overgeneralized their beliefs to whole classes of schemas (e.g., "I always make bad decisions," "No one can be trusted," "I must control everyone around me"). We called this "overaccommodation" (Resick & Schnicke, 1992, 1993). As we (my graduate student Monica Schnicke and I) were in the early stages of developing CPT, we realized that it was important to work on assimilation of the trauma first and not move to the overaccommodated beliefs until the index trauma was resolved. For example, once clients stop blaming themselves for the occurrence of the traumatic event, then it is easier to tackle the idea that they can't make good decisions. Accordingly, we placed the work with overaccommodated themes later in the therapy.

Early Development of CPT

My first study of CPT was again funded with small grants from the University of Missouri–St. Louis. I conducted CPT in groups for the very practical reason that I could collect more data on clients in groups than on those receiving individual therapy. However, by the time I was funded by NIMH to conduct a randomized controlled trial (RCT), I had conducted 84 pilot cases and the first CPT manual was published, which included the results of the first 35 participants in group treatment and the first 9 clients in individual treatment (Resick & Schnicke, 1993).

In 1994, while she was a graduate student, Kathleen M. Chard (my first postdoctoral fellow) created a version of CPT for individuals with childhood sexual abuse histories that combined group and individual sessions of CPT. While working as a therapist on the study comparing CPT with prolonged exposure and a wait-list control (see Chapter 2 for a discussion of this study), she submitted a grant application for research on her adaptation of CPT (CPT-SA). In addition to combining group and individual treatment, CPT-SA included several sessions to cover these topics: family "rules" (e.g., "If anything goes wrong, it is your fault"); what children are developmentally capable of (e.g., telling a 4-year-old to come home at 5:00 is expecting too much of the child); assertive communication; ways of giving and taking power; and social support.

In the process of developing CPT-SA, Chard noted that not everyone's beliefs were shattered by trauma (Janoff-Bulman, 1992), and it soon became obvious as we continued to study and treat PTSD that sometimes trauma was schema-congruent. We observed that if clients had been abused as children (emotionally, physically, or sexually), or had other prior traumas, they might already have (and perhaps had always had) negative beliefs about themselves and about their roles in the traumatic events (e.g. "I must deserve bad things to happen to me"). Any new trauma would be assimilated without alteration because it was not schema-discrepant, but schema-congruent. The question then arose: Why would such people have PTSD, if their beliefs were already matching the new events? It is possible that these individuals did not get *new* PTSD; they might have already had it. However, the new events might have strengthened their distorted beliefs about themselves and others and about their roles in traumatic events. In other words, they might be using the new events as "proof" that their prior beliefs were accurate. Their PTSD would worsen, and their beliefs would become more entrenched (Resick, 2001; Resick, Monson, & Chard, 2007). On the other hand, even with prior negative schemas about themselves or others, people might still ask, "Why me?" or "Why again?" They might still find new traumatic events to be schema-discrepant, because they had done everything they could to change what they perceived to be the cause of prior trauma ("I try to be perfect"), or they could see how members of other families behaved toward one another and couldn't figure out what they were doing wrong.

Another difference between the theoretical approach that led to CPT and the theories on which other therapies are based lies in the range and type of emotions addressed in CPT. Because PTSD was classified as an anxiety disorder until the publication of DSM-5 (American Psychiatric Association, 2013), most of the extant theories on PTSD focused on fear and anxiety. Because I did not come from an academic background of work in the anxiety disorders, I was impressed by the amount of "erroneous" guilt, shame, disgust, sadness, and so forth that we were finding among the clients. In the longitudinal studies we conducted, nearly everyone said that they were afraid during the event—but most people recovered from their fear, and fear did not always seem to be the driving force behind the flashbacks, intrusive memories, nightmares, and avoidance we observed. Furthermore, if PTSD were only about fear conditioning, then it wouldn't matter what the trauma was; the rates of PTSD should be equal. The epidemiological studies of PTSD (e.g., Kessler, Sonnega, Bromet, Hughes, & Nelson, 1995) made it clear that all traumas did not have the same effects: Rape and other interpersonal traumas produced greater rates of PTSD than impersonal traumas such as natural disasters and accidents. Something else was going on besides fear conditioning, because the persons who had experienced these traumatic events evaluated it in relation to their beliefs and prior experiences.

In addition, self-blame and/or erroneous other-blame, leading to guilt or shame, were almost universal among those with PTSD. By the time I wrote an unpublished manual for a generic version of CPT (Resick, 2001), after the September 11 attacks, I was differentiating "natural" emotions from "manufactured" emotions. The "natural" emotions are those we humans are hard-wired with and do not need to think about (e.g., fight–flight leads to fear or anger; losses elicit sadness). The emotions referred to as "manufactured" result from faulty cognitions about the traumatic event. While natural emotions may take a while to dissipate, if not avoided, emotions that are generated by thoughts ("It must have been my fault, because things like this don't happen to good people") will disappear immediately if the thought is changed with more accurate information.

As discussed in more detail in Chapter 2, the first RCT of CPT compared it with prolonged exposure and a minimal-attention wait list among women who had been raped. The large majority of the participants (85%) had experienced other interpersonal traumas, and 41% had experienced childhood sexual abuse (Resick, Nishith, Weaver, Astin, & Feuer, 2002). The second RCT included women who had experienced any kind of interpersonal violence in adulthood or childhood as their primary (index) trauma to begin treatment (Resick et al., 2008). While we were conducting that study, Candice M. Monson received a grant from the VA to conduct the first study of CPT with veterans. The majority of participants were male veterans of the Vietnam War (Monson et al., 2006). Given that most of them had received treatment for years, and that all had a history of substance abuse, the loss of a PTSD diagnosis in 12 sessions among 40% of these veterans had an immediate impact on the field. Monson also noted that there were more commonalities than differences among trauma survivors, and that the veterans' interpretations of their traumas were very similar to those of the interpersonal violence victims in the earlier studies.

In 2003, I moved from St. Louis and academia to a job with the VA's National Center for PTSD as the director of the Women's Health Sciences Division. The following year, Monson moved to Boston to become my deputy director, and Chard moved from the University of Kentucky to the Cincinnati VA Medical Center to become the director of the PTSD programs there. Over the next few years, Chard not only expanded the outpatient clinic in Cincinnati, but developed three residential programs for PTSD: one for men, one for women, and one for those suffering from the aftermath of traumatic brain injury. She also adapted the individual and group protocols for veterans receiving treatment in residential centers. Monson continued her work on a couple therapy for PTSD that incorporated aspects of CPT.

Dissemination of CPT

In 2006, the three of us received funding from the VA Central Office to begin developing materials for disseminating CPT throughout the VA system. We wrote a treatment manual for active-duty military personnel and veterans; developed training materials (slides with notes, videos, trainers' manual, consultants' manual); and then trained a first group of national trainers. Because there were so few people in the VA system who had conducted CPT, many of the trainers were from St. Louis (former faculty colleagues, postdoctoral fellows, or graduate students of mine). Up until then I had only conducted 1-day workshops, with no follow-through with case consultation. Monson rightly suggested that we emphasize the teaching of the Socratic method as the most difficult part of the therapy, but we had to think through what we were doing naturally at that point to teach it to other therapists, who might have been taught never to ask a question or to let thoughts go rather than changing them. We also had to teach the reasoning behind the approach of asking questions that would help clients examine their Stuck Points, (erroneous thoughts and beliefs dating from the time of the trauma, as explained earlier), to put them back into the context of what they actually knew at the time, what choices they really had, and (if they had choices) why they made the ones they did. We also had to help clients differentiate among intentionality, responsibility, and the unforeseeable. Finally, Chard noted that we needed to include a Stuck Point Log that would serve as a "living" document throughout the therapy. This log would help to keep both a client and a therapist focused on the unhealthy cognitions and not get derailed into more supportive forms of therapy.

The first 2 years of the dissemination project included 22 workshops each year, and then the project was cut back slowly, as more VA therapists completed training that included workshops and case consultation. Along the way, we received good feedback from the trainers about ways to streamline the handouts and make them more accessible to people with lower education levels or with traumatic brain injuries. We also developed "help sheets" for understanding Stuck Points and for answering challenging questions. Beyond the VA context, CPT is now being disseminated through mental health centers in the United States, as well as in different countries.

The CPT manuals have been translated into 12 languages thus far, and the therapy appears to work rather well across cultures (see Chapter 14). Because the cognitive impact of a traumatic event is very individualized, clients across cultures can describe why they think their events happened and what the events mean to them. Even though there may be differences in some concepts, many of them translate well—and even in very strict traditional cultures, it can be pointed out that not all people believe identically and that there is some flexibility in beliefs. People can change their minds.

A Biological Model of PTSD and CPT

The most recent additions to our training and conceptualization involve the connections between the biological underpinnings of PTSD and the reasons why CPT works. Most of this new material reflects research on activation of the amygdala, which triggers strong emotions and sends neurotransmitters throughout the brain to activate the emergency response. Additional factors that were not noticed immediately, but are actually found more frequently in research, are the diminished responsivity and smaller size of the prefrontal cortex (Shin, Rauch, & Pitman, 2006) among those with PTSD.

In a normal fight–flight response, activity in the prefrontal cortex (which is the seat of decision making and control over the amygdala) decreases, along with other immune functions and normal physical processes like digesting food, in order to free all available resources for either running or fighting. The natural emotions accompanying flight and fight are fear and anger. During a life-threatening emergency, it is more important to activate the brain stem and neurotransmitters to aid in the fight–flight response than to think about what to have for dinner or whether to change jobs. However, in a well-modulated emergency response (see Figure 1.1), the prefrontal cortex is activated enough to notice when the danger is over, and to send messages out to

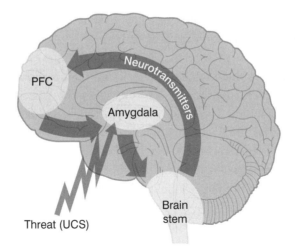

FIGURE 1.1. Well-modulated emergency response. UCS, unconditioned stimulus; PFC, prefrontal cortex.

the amygdala to stop the fight–flight response and return to normal parasympathetic functioning. In other words, there is a reciprocal relationship between the prefrontal cortex and the amygdala.

In studies of people with PTSD, by contrast, researchers have found that the amygdala shows heightened responsivity while the prefrontal cortex shows greatly decreased activity, and that there is a functional relationship between the two (Shin et al., 2004). Because the amygdala is too highly activated and the activity in the prefrontal cortex is diminished (see Figure 1.2), it takes a person with PTSD much longer to recognize that the perceived danger has ended and to calm down.

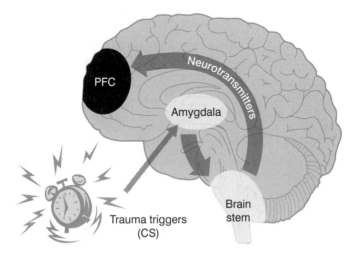

FIGURE 1.2. Emergency response in PTSD. CS, conditioned stimulus. Data from Liberzon and Sripada (2008), Milad et al. (2009), Rauch et al. (2000), and Shin et al. (2001).

In imaging studies, Hariri and colleagues (Hariri, Bookheimer, & Mazziotta, 2000; Hariri, Mattay, Tessitore, Fera, & Weinberger, 2003) found that when participants were shown pictures of emotional faces or dangerous objects, and were asked either (1) to pick pictures that matched the original pictures, or (2) to label the emotions or objects, in the first case there was no change in the activation of the amygdala. However, when participants were asked to label the objects or to describe whether each picture was of a natural or an artificially created danger, the instruction to use words resulted in the activation of the prefrontal cortex (including Broca's area, which is the speech area), while the amygdala quieted.

It occurred to us that if merely labeling objects or pictures was sufficient to activate the prefrontal cortex and quiet the amygdala, we could accomplish much more with regard to affect regulation through cognitive therapy—specifically, having clients talk *about* and answer question about the trauma—than through having clients reexperience the images of the traumatic events. In other words, these findings reinforced the idea that cognitive therapy could be a more direct route to change than having clients imagine the traumatic events repeatedly (see Figure 1.3). It also reminded me that day care teachers know this intuitively: When dealing with small children who are upset, they remind them, "Use your words." They may not know about the reciprocal relationship between the prefrontal cortex and the amygdala, but they know that if children are talking about what is upsetting them, they can calm down.

Neurobiology also helps us to understand why younger people are more likely to develop PTSD, aside from the fact that physical and sexual abuse, rapes, assaults, car accidents, and combat are all more likely to occur to those who have not reached full adulthood. The prefrontal cortex is not fully developed until humans are well into their 20s, so not only are young people likely to be traumatized, but they have fewer

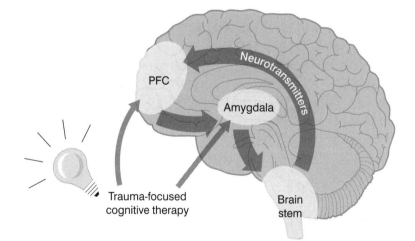

FIGURE 1.3. How cognitive therapy may work: It may force the frontal lobe online, which inhibits the amygdala and prevents extreme emotional responses, even while the trauma circuit is simultaneously and sufficiently activated.

resources to deal with trauma once it occurs (Johnson, Blum, & Giedd, 2009). According to the Johnson et al. (2009) review article,

> The prefrontal cortex coordinates higher-order cognitive processes and executive functioning. Executive functions are a set of supervisory cognitive skills needed for goal-directed behavior, including planning, response inhibition, working memory, and attention. These skills allow an individual to pause long enough to take stock of a situation, assess his or her options, plan a course of action, and execute it. Poor executive functioning leads to difficulty with planning, attention, using feedback, and mental inflexibility, all of which could undermine judgment and decision making. (p. 218)

By the time child and adolescent trauma victims receive therapy as adults, they may have settled on cognitions that were constructed at a time when their executive functions were not fully developed. This is probably the reason why so many clients with PTSD have extreme beliefs and have been traumatized repeatedly. CPT may well assist such clients in developing affect regulation, increasing their cognitive flexibility, and changing many assumptions and beliefs that were developed at a period of cognitive immaturity and that were never reexamined because of avoidance symptoms. One of the goals of CPT is to teach these clients greater flexibility in thinking—specifically, to teach them how to think critically about what they have been saying to themselves regarding the reasons why the traumatic events happened and the events' implications about themselves and others.

A Change in Name and a Note on Terminology

Since 1988, CPT has been referred to as a 12-session therapy that included cognitive therapy and, at first, "written exposures." However, because the initial "written exposures" did not meet the standards of exposure interventions at the time (i.e., repetitions of the trauma for 45–60 minutes to encourage strong emotions, with ratings of distress to monitor habituation within and between sessions), this term was changed to the more precise description of the technique as "written accounts." This part of the protocol is described in Chapter 11.

When the CPT dismantling study was conducted (Resick et al., 2008; see Chapter 2), the version of CPT without written accounts was referred to as CPT-C, meaning CPT with cognitive therapy only. The dismantling study found that CPT-C was as effective as CPT and that the written accounts did not add to the outcomes; in fact, CPT-C had a faster trajectory of improvements and had a 22% dropout rate compared with a 34% dropout rate for CPT. Also, Walter, Dickstein, Barnes, and Chard (2014) examined program evaluation data in a U.S. VA hospital and found that the outcomes for CPT and CPT-C were not statistically different from each other. Although the label CPT-C was perhaps appropriate for a single study, we realized that it was rather redundant. Because of these findings and factors, and the positive results of other CPT-C studies, we have decided to give the cognitive version of CPT primacy. In this book, therefore, we call the cognitive-therapy-only version CPT, and the version with written accounts CPT+A. The main description of the therapy in Part III (Chapters 5–10) is a description of CPT. Chapter 11 covers CPT+A. The written-account-only protocol that was implemented in the Resick et al. (2008) dismantling study is not described in this book, but I can provide a manual of this protocol for interested readers.

A note on the use of two terms in this book is also in order here. We have used both the terms "victims" and "survivors" to refer to CPT clients, with "victims" used more often. On the one hand, many people with PTSD who seek or are referred for CPT are still "victims" and have not yet become "survivors"; also, the term "survivor" may connote that a person could have died as a result of a traumatic event, and this is not always the case (though it often is). On the other hand, the term "survivors" may be more empowering in some contexts.

2

Research on CPT

There are strong empirical data supporting the efficacy and effectiveness of CPT in its various forms and with various populations. In fact, two recent meta-analyses of PTSD treatments (Haagen, Smid, Knipscheer, & Kleber, 2015; Watts et al., 2013), comparing various evidence-based cognitive-behavioral therapies and medications, found that CPT+A had the highest average effect sizes of all interventions examined.

In this chapter, we review the empirical basis of CPT. To date, there have been 14 published RCTs testing CPT, and many more are currently being conducted. In addition, there have been large uncontrolled studies testing the effectiveness of CPT in real-world clinical settings. Given the state of the literature on CPT, we limit this chapter to a review of these two types of studies, although there have been important case studies and smaller uncontrolled trials initially documenting the efficacy of CPT and application to unique traumas and comorbidities. We first review the primary outcomes of the RCTs, followed by studies emanating from these RCTs that document the efficacy of CPT for secondary outcomes and their potential influence in treatment. We then examine cognitive change studies and discuss how change in cognition is a mechanism of change for PTSD, and we conclude with a review of the effectiveness studies.

Randomized Controlled Trials

The first RCT compared CPT+A with prolonged exposure (PE; Foa, Rothbaum, Riggs, & Murdock, 1991) and a wait-list control condition for female rape victims (Resick et al., 2002). PE is a therapy involving two types of exposure to trauma. A client engages in imaginal exposures (i.e., the client repeatedly recounts aloud his or her index trauma to the therapist, in the first person and the present tense) in sessions; each imaginal exposure is followed by emotional processing of the recounting with the therapist. The client is assigned to listen to the recordings of the imaginal exposures every day at home. In addition, the client is assigned 45 minutes of daily *in vivo* exposure to increasingly distressing trauma-related cues in his or her daily life between sessions.

Both treatments were highly efficacious in improving PTSD and depression at posttreatment compared with the wait-list control, although there were no statistical differences between the active treatments at any assessment. In fact, there were very few differences of any kind between the two active treatments, except that participants receiving CPT+A reported significantly more improvement in guilt (Resick et al., 2002), health-related concerns (Galovski, Monson, Bruce, & Resick, 2009), hopelessness (Gallagher & Resick, 2012), and suicidal ideation (Gradus, Suvak, Wisco, Marx, & Resick, 2013). These improvements were sustained at the 3-month and 9-month follow-up points. Following the waitlist, participants were offered one of the randomized treatments. They responded the same as the first samples did to CPT+A and PE.

A long-term follow-up of participants in this study was conducted (Resick, Williams, Suvak, Monson, & Gradus, 2012). An attempt was made to reach everyone randomly assigned to one of the three conditions in the study (i.e., the intention-to-treat sample) with the assigned waitlist/treatment groups folded into the two-group sample for follow-up assessment 5–10 years after treatment. Of those located (144/171), 88% ($n = 126$) were reassessed. Again, there were no differences between CPT+A and PE on PTSD and depression outcomes, and participants in both treatments continued to maintain their improvements gained at posttreatment. Moreover, neither further treatment nor subsequent traumatization was significantly associated with the maintained improvements.

Chard (2005) conducted a wait-list-controlled trial of CPT with adult survivors of child sexual abuse. She expanded CPT+A to include a combination of group and individual treatment, in order to allow individual processing of trauma, but also the experience of group cohesion and normalization of typical problems following child sexual abuse. She found statistically significant differences between those receiving her adapted version of CPT and those in the wait-list group on clinician-rated PTSD symptoms, depression, and dissociation. In addition, the rate of dropout from treatment was quite low (only 18% did not attend all sessions). Of those receiving CPT, only 7% met diagnosis for PTSD at posttreatment, 3% at the 3-month follow-up, and 6% at the 1-year follow-up.

Monson et al. (2006) conducted the first CPT+A study with military veterans who were recruited through a U.S. VA hospital. Sixty veterans (80% Vietnam veterans) were randomly assigned to CPT+A or to treatment as usual. There were significant improvements in chronic PTSD and a range of comorbidities at posttreatment and 1-month follow-up for those receiving CPT+A versus the treatment-as-usual condition. At posttreatment, 40% of the sample receiving CPT+A had a remission in their PTSD diagnosis. Moreover, service-connected disability status was not associated with treatment outcomes or PTSD diagnostic status.

Resick et al. (2008) conducted a dismantling study of CPT+A with female victims of sexual and physical assault. In this study, CPT+A, CPT, and written accounts only (abbreviated here as WA) were compared; the researchers controlled for time spent in the therapy sessions. There was an overall group difference between CPT and WA, but all participants were significantly improved at posttreatment and follow-up periods. However, according to clients' self-report, CPT led to faster symptom reduction during treatment than WA did, and participants in CPT achieved clinically significant improvements two sessions faster than those in CPT+A and four sessions faster than those in WA (see Figure 2.1). Although the differences were not statistically significant, it is clinically meaningful that 22% of CPT participants dropped out of treatment, compared with 34% of CPT+A participants and 26% receiving WA. Although CPT and CPT+A are described in this book, WA is not. As noted in Chapter 1, the WA manual is available from one of us (Patricia A. Resick).

Forbes et al. (2012) conducted an RCT of CPT+A with veterans served within the Australian veterans' health care system. They trained clinicians within this system to provide the therapy, versus using expert therapists to deliver CPT+A, increasing the generalizability of the findings. As in Monson et al.'s (2006) study, CPT+A was compared with treatment as usual. Forbes and colleagues found CPT+A to be superior to usual care with regard to PTSD, anxiety, depression, social relationships, and dyadic relationships, even when delivered by clinicians with varying experience levels, treatment orientations, and disciplines.

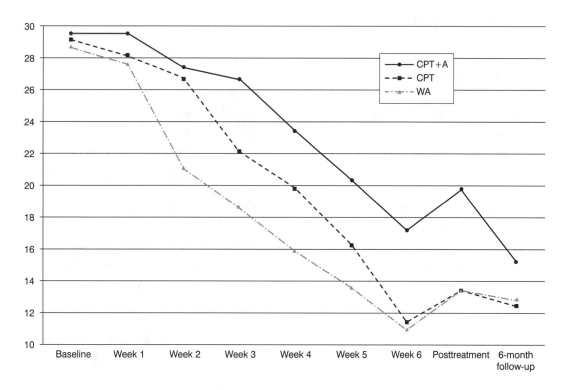

FIGURE 2.1. Change in client's self-reported PTSD symptoms on the Posttraumatic Diagnostic Scale across treatment and follow-up by treatment condition. Data from Resick et al. (2008).

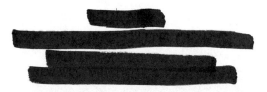

Galovski, Blain, Mott, Elwood, and Houle (2012) conducted an important study of CPT+A aimed at determining treatment completion based on outcome criteria versus a fixed 12-session protocol. In this study (an RCT with delayed symptom monitoring as a control condition), a "treatment completer" was defined not as someone who attended all 12 sessions of the CPT+A protocol, but as someone who met the definition of "good end-state functioning," whether this criterion was met before or after 12 sessions of therapy. Good end-state functioning was defined as a Posttraumatic Diagnostic Scale (PDS; Foa, Cashman, Jaycox, & Perry, 1997) score at or below 20; a Beck Depression Inventory–II (BDI-II; Beck, Steer, & Brown, 1996) score at or below 18; agreement between the client and therapist that treatment goals had been reached; and an assessment by an independent evaluator that the client no longer met criteria for a PTSD diagnosis. Clients could be evaluated for stopping treatment as early as Session 4, and if they agreed to stop earlier than Session 12, they completed the final CPT Impact Statement and were delivered the interventions included in the final CPT+A session. At the end of Session 12, if it was determined that clients still had PTSD and higher scores on the self-report measures, they could receive up to a total of 18 sessions. At that point, if they had still not reached good end-state functioning, they were considered "treatment nonresponders."

In this study, 27% of participants dropped out of treatment. Of the 50 who remained, only 8% completed treatment exactly at 12 sessions, 58% completed it earlier than 12 sessions, 26% needed more than 12 sessions, and 8% were deemed nonresponders at posttreatment. However, by the 3-month follow-up, only 1 participant still had a diagnosis of PTSD.

Recruiting a sample of male and female veterans with PTSD secondary to military sexual trauma from a U.S. VA hospital, Suris, Link-Malcolm, Chard, Ahn, and North (2013) compared CPT+A to present-centered therapy (PCT; Schnurr et al., 2007), which focuses on current symptoms and problem solving. As in the Forbes et al. (2012) study, clinicians not previously trained in CPT+A provided the treatment. PTSD and depressive symptoms were decreased with both therapies at posttreatment, but veterans who received CPT+A had a significantly larger reduction in their self-reported PTSD symptoms, compared with those receiving PCT. Improvements were maintained in both conditions up to the 6-month follow-up. Although the difference in dropout rate was not statistically different in this relatively small sample, the rate for PCT was 18% versus 35% for CPT. The authors noted that the study was affected by treatment fidelity issues: One therapist had below-satisfactory competency ratings in the delivery of CPT, leading to the removal of data for that therapist's clients. This study thus emphasizes the importance of clinicians' fidelity to treatment.

Bass et al. (2013) conducted an RCT of CPT in the Democratic Republic of Congo—a country with not only low resources, but high levels of ongoing violence. The authors randomly assigned participants to treatments by village, with women in 7 villages receiving group CPT (n = 157) and women in 8 villages (n = 248) receiving individual support and resources. The therapists had high school educations at most,

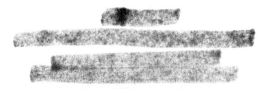

and a majority of the clients were illiterate. Bass et al. found that CPT was superior to support and resources in reducing PTSD, anxiety, and depression, and improving functional impairment. At 6-month follow-up, only 9% of the CPT participants met criteria for probable PTSD, anxiety, or depression, as opposed to 42% of the supportive therapy participants. When the study was released, Bass was quoted in *The New York Times* as saying, "'If you can do this in Congo, you can do it anywhere'" (Grady, 2013).

Morland and colleagues (Morland, Hynes, Mackintosh, Resick, & Chard, 2011; Morland et al., 2015) conducted two RCTs, one with male veterans and one with female veterans and civilians. In the study with male veterans, CPT+A was delivered in face-to-face groups versus videoconferencing. These two delivery methods were tested with a "noninferiority" design, meaning that delivering group CPT+A by videoconference would not be inferior to delivering it face-to-face. Both methods of delivery resulted in significant reductions in PTSD that were maintained at follow-up assessments, with no differences between them. In addition, there were high levels of therapeutic alliance, treatment compliance, and satisfaction, with no differences between the two formats of delivery. In the study with women, Morland et al. (2015) compared individual in-person delivery with telehealth delivery, but they were also able to compare veteran women with civilian women. They found that both formats of treatment were equivalent, but that the civilian women had better results than the veterans.

A third study of telehealth versus in-person therapy was conducted by Maieritsch et al. (2016), except that this one focused on veterans of the recent wars in Iraq and Afghanistan. They too found that the two formats appeared to be equivalent, but they also found that with this younger cohort, the dropout rate was quite high in both conditions (43% instead of the expected 20%). They suggested that, as in other studies of this younger cohort, the emphasis on future research should be placed on engagement and retention in therapy. Because of the developmental stage of recent veterans, their attention may be more focused on jobs, relationships, and children.

Bolton et al. (2014) conducted an RCT with community mental health workers working in rural health clinics in Kurdistan, northern Iraq. They were trained in behavioral activation treatment for depression (BATD; Lejuez, Hopko, & Hopko, 2001; Lejuez, Hopko, Acierno, Daughters, & Pagoto, 2011) and CPT; a wait-list condition was also included. All participants had experienced systematic violence and were enrolled according to the severity of their depression symptoms. They were randomly assigned to one of the three conditions. BATD had significant effects on depression and functional impairments, while CPT had a significant effect on functional impairments only. These findings may be attributable to the inclusion criterion focused on depression versus PTSD, because prior studies with torture survivors and refugees recruited specifically for PTSD have found significant effects for PTSD and other comorbid conditions (e.g., Hinton et al., 2004; Schulz, Resick, Huber, & Griffin, 2006).

An RCT conducted in Germany by Butollo, Karl, König, and Rosner (2015) compared CPT with dialogical exposure therapy (DET), which is based on gestalt therapy. The trial included 141 male and female clients with PTSD; the types of traumas were mixed. Both conditions were variable in length, with up to 24 sessions. The dropout rate was very low for both conditions (12.2% in DET and 14.95% in CPT, including those who never started treatment; 8% of DET and 9% of CPT participants dropped out after starting therapy). Both types of treatment showed large reductions in PTSD symptoms, but CPT had significantly better results at posttreatment and had a larger effect size ($g = 1.14$ for DET and 1.57 for CPT).

Recently, Resick et al. (2015) compared CPT in a group format among U.S. active-duty military service members with PCT. Both treatments led to improvements in PTSD symptoms, but CPT led to significantly more improvements in PTSD. Moreover, CPT yielded significant improvements in depression that were maintained at a follow-up assessment. The PCT group only evidenced improvements from baseline to before the first session in depression symptoms, probably due to expectancy effects.

Secondary Conditions and Potential Moderators of Treatment

History of Child Maltreatment

Because some clinicians and researchers are concerned that people with a history of child maltreatment may need more than a short course of CPT or CPT+A, a follow-up study of the head-to-head study of CPT+A and PE examined more extensive symptoms by using the Trauma Symptom Inventory (TSI; Briere, 1995), which includes PTSD symptoms and other symptoms, such as dissociation, dysfunctional sexual behavior, impaired self-reference, and tension reduction behavior. The treatment sample was divided, not by type of treatment received, but by those who had a history of child sexual abuse (41%) in addition to adult rape, versus adult rape without child sexual abuse. Both groups had significant improvements (with large effect sizes) in PTSD, depression, and all of the problems measured on the TSI subscales. These improvements were maintained at a 9-month follow-up. Moreover, there were no differences in these outcomes between those who had a child sexual abuse history and those who did not.

Resick, Suvak, and Wells (2014) also conducted secondary analyses of data from both the head-to-head study of CPT+A versus PE and the dismantling study, to examine whether there were differences in outcomes for those with and without a history of child sexual abuse or child physical abuse. In the head-to-head study, they found that frequency of child sexual abuse predicted dropout from both treatments; however, severity of child physical abuse was associated with greater dropout from PE than from CPT+A. Regarding treatment outcomes, no form or amount of childhood abuse affected PTSD treatment outcomes. In the dismantling study, there were no differences in dropout by childhood abuse history for the three conditions. However, those patients without a childhood abuse history did better with CPT than with CPT+A or WA. Moreover, those with more frequent childhood abuse responded better to CPT and CPT+A than to WA.

Using data from the dismantling trial, Resick, Suvak, Johnides, Mitchell, and Iverson (2012) examined whether those with high levels of dissociation responded differently to CPT, CPT+A, and WA. There were significant decreases in dissociation symptoms across all three therapies, with no statistical differences among them. However, pretreatment levels of dissociation were associated with different PTSD outcomes: Those women with low pretreatment levels of dissociation responded best to CPT, while those with the highest levels of dissociation benefited more from CPT+A. Because they did not respond better to just the repetitions of writing accounts in the WA condition, the authors concluded that those with high levels of dissociation needed to write trauma accounts to facilitate making their traumatic memories into a coherent narrative before they could benefit from cognitive therapy.

These findings were further supported by a study of 110 female veterans reporting a history of military sexual trauma (61 with an additional history of child sexual abuse and 49 without), who were compared on pretreatment demographic and symptom measures, as well as outcome after CPT (Walter, Buckley, Simpson, & Chard, 2014). Study findings showed that these two groups did not significantly differ on pretreatment variables or treatment outcome. Results suggest that CPT delivered in a residential treatment program was effective for female veterans with PTSD related to military sexual trauma, with and without a history of child sexual abuse.

Borderline and Other Personality Disorder Characteristics

Clarke, Rizvi, and Resick (2008) examined the effects of borderline personality characteristics on treatment outcomes in the head-to-head trial of CPT+A and PE. They divided the sample into those with high or low borderline characteristics as measured by the Schedule for Nonadaptive and Adaptive Personality (Clark, 1993). They found that those with high versus low borderline personality traits had higher PTSD and depressive symptoms at baseline assessment, but were no more likely to drop out of treatment. Importantly, level of pretreatment borderline personality characteristics did not predict treatment outcomes. In fact, the group high in these traits, with more severe PTSD and depressive symptoms before treatment, had more improvements over the course of therapy and ended at similar levels of PTSD as the group low in borderline traits.

This finding was replicated for borderline as well as other personality disorders by Walter, Bolte, Owens, and Chard (2012), who looked at clients with and without personality disorders seeking treatment in a residential treatment program for veterans that combined group and individual CPT+A. They found no statistically significant differences in PTSD treatment gains between the two groups; in fact, those with personality disorders experienced greater improvement in pre- to posttreatment depression than those without a personality disorder.

Suicidality

Gradus et al. (2013) examined the effects of PTSD treatment on suicidal ideation, which is very common among those with PTSD, in the head-to-head trial of CPT+A versus PE. They found that suicidal ideation decreased sharply during both treatments, with continued but subtler decreases during the follow-up period. However, CPT resulted in larger reductions in suicidal ideation than PE did. Decreases in suicidal ideation were associated with improvements in PTSD symptoms over the course of both treatments, with some evidence of a stronger association for CPT+A than for PE. These associations were not accounted for by depression diagnosis at the start of the study or by changes in hopelessness over the course of treatment.

Bryan et al. (2016) examined whether CPT was associated with iatrogenic suicide risk among active military members, as a secondary analysis of the Resick et al. (2015) study of group CPT versus PCT. They found that rates of suicidal ideation decreased across both types of treatment. Among soldiers with pretreatment suicide ideation, severity of suicide ideation significantly decreased across both treatments and was maintained for up to 12 months after treatment. Exacerbation of preexisting suicide ideation was less common in group CPT (9%) than in group PCT (37.5%).

Health-Related Conditions and Sleep

Galovski et al. (2009) examined the effects of CPT+A and PE in the head-to-head trial on perceived health concerns and sleep impairments, given the high co-occurrence of these comorbid conditions in those who suffer from PTSD. Both treatments yielded improvements in health-related concerns, but there were more improvements in these concerns with CPT+A than with PE. With regard to sleep impairments, both treatments yielded improvements across treatment and follow-up, with no significant differences between them. However, sleep impairment did not improve to such an extent that the majority of the participants became "good sleepers." The authors note that the advantage of CPT+A over PE in terms of physical health complaints may be explained by the cognitive interventions employed in CPT+A, which may generalize to interpretation of a range of experiences, including perceived health status.

With data from the dismantling trial, Mitchell, Wells, Mendes, and Resick (2012) examined whether the three therapies improved symptoms of disordered eating. The Eating Disorders Inventory–2 (Garner, 1991) was used to measure problematic eating behavior in a subsample of the study. This inventory includes subscales of drive for thinness, bulimia, body dissatisfaction, ineffectiveness, perfectionism, interpersonal distrust, interoceptive awareness, maturity fears, impulse regulation, asceticism, and social insecurity. They found that some eating disorder symptoms (i.e., body dissatisfaction, interoceptive awareness, interpersonal distrust, impulse regulation, ineffectiveness, maturity) improved over the course of the three therapies. Moreover, these symptom improvements, with the exception of body dissatisfaction, were associated with changes in PTSD symptoms over the course of therapy. The authors note that the most closely overlapping symptoms of eating disorders and PTSD may be most responsive to the various components of CPT+A.

Psychophysiological Functioning

A follow-up study of the dismantling study examined changes in physiological reactivity, and specifically in startle response to loud tones, as results of treatment (Griffin, Resick, & Galovski, 2012). Participants who completed treatment were grouped into "responders" (72%) and "nonresponders" (28%), based on PTSD diagnosis and severity of symptoms. Responders and nonresponders did not differ on the physiological measures of eyeblink electromyogram, heart rate, or skin conductance before treatment. With treatment, responders demonstrated a significant reduction in startle according to all three measures. In addition, electromyographic and heart rate responses to the loud tones were significantly smaller among responders than nonresponders at post-treatment. Because of the study's size, the authors were unable to examine potential differences by treatment type. This study demonstrates that various forms of CPT, when completed, are effective in reducing startle generally (not just to trauma-related cues); the study thus provides more objective data about the effects of treatment.

Psychosocial Functioning

Extending research beyond individual mental health symptoms and physiology, Galovski, Sobel, Phipps, and Resick (2005) evaluated changes in psychosocial functioning as a result of CPT+A and PE within the head-to-head trial among participants who completed treatment. They found that every type of psychosocial functioning that was measured improved after these treatments, including improvements in occupational, social–leisure, extended family, family unit, fear of intimacy, sexual concerns, and dysfunctional sexual behavior domains across a range of measures.

Wachen, Jimenez, Smith, and Resick (2014) examined the social functioning of 154 participants in the study comparing CPT+A and PE. Using the Social Adjustment Scale—Self-Report (Weissman & Paykel, 1974), they examined overall social functioning, social and leisure, work, relationships within family unit, and economic status from pretreatment through the long-term follow-up with hierarchical linear modeling. They found large improvements on all measures, but no differences between the two treatment types.

Monson and colleagues (Monson et al., 2012) conducted follow-up analyses of Monson et al.'s (2006) wait-list study of CPT+A with U.S. veterans. They examined different spheres of social functioning that improved after a course of CPT+A, and how these changes were associated with changes in PTSD symptoms with treatment. Overall social adjustment, extended-family relationship functioning, and housework completion improved with CPT+A compared to the wait-list condition. In addition, improvements in emotional numbing were specifically associated with improvements in all of these spheres. Similarly, improvements in avoidance symptoms were associated with improvements in housework; however, improved avoidance symptoms were associated with declines in extended family adjustment. With regard to the latter finding, the authors suggest that increased contact with family members due to decreased avoidance, unaccompanied by improved interpersonal skills for interacting in these relationships, may lead to lower reported extended-family adjustment.

Similarly, Shnaider et al. (2014) examined domains of psychosocial functioning (i.e., daily living, household tasks, work, leisure/recreational, family relationships, and nonfamily relationships) following treatment within the dismantling study, as well as the associations between changes in functioning and changes in PTSD symptoms. They found improvements in psychosocial functioning for all three treatments, with no differences between the treatments at posttreatment or follow-up. Because there were no differences based on treatment, they then combined the sample to examine associations between changes in psychosocial functioning and four PTSD symptom clusters (i.e., reexperiencing, avoidance, numbing, and hyperarousal). They found that improvements in numbing symptoms were more specifically associated with improvements in nonfamily relationships; improvements in hyperarousal symptoms were associated with improvements in overall functioning, daily living, and household tasks.

Related to social functioning, Iverson et al. (2011) examined intimate-partner violence (IPV) in the dismantling study (Resick et al., 2008). Of the 150 intention-to-treat participants, 61% reported a lifetime history of IPV; 16% reported IPV perpetrated by their current partners within the year prior to the baseline assessment and reported the IPV as their index event. At the 6-month follow-up, 22% reported experiencing new IPV victimization in the period following treatment. Iverson et al. found that those who had a stronger response to treatment with regard to PTSD and/or depression were much less likely to experience IPV following treatment. These findings held for the women who were currently in relationships with partners committing IPV, as well as for those who had experienced IPV at some point during their lifetimes.

Sex Differences

Unfortunately, most CPT studies have been conducted with either female survivors of interpersonal violence or male combat veterans. However, in secondary analyses of Galovski et al.'s (2012) variable-length study of people with PTSD who had experienced interpersonal trauma, Galovski, Blain, Chappuis, and Fletcher (2013) examined potential sex differences in outcomes of CPT+A. They found few sex differences in trauma history or symptoms before therapy, except that women were more likely to be sexually assaulted and men were more likely to have anger directed inward. There were no differences between men and women with regard to the total number of sessions provided or the degree of changes in PTSD or depressive symptoms with treatment. However, at the 3-month follow-up, women were found to have lower levels of PTSD, depressive, guilt, anger/irritability, and dissociative symptoms, compared with men. The authors concluded that we may need to alter our existing treatments or develop new ones to serve men with PTSD more effectively.

Cognitions

Cognitions as Outcomes

Different types of cognitions have been examined as outcomes, because, as a cognitive therapy, CPT should have an effect on clients' beliefs. Changes in cognitions have also been studied with respect to improvements in PTSD symptoms, to see whether these changes serve as a potential mechanism of such improvements. As mentioned above, the RCT comparing CPT+A with PE included guilt cognitions as outcomes measured at pretreatment, posttreatment, and a 9-month follow-up (Resick et al., 2002). Compared with the wait-list condition, CPT+A showed large effect size differences and PE showed small to medium effect size differences from pre- to posttreatment. The two active treatments differed significantly from each other on two guilt subscales (hindsight bias and lack of justification), and there were small to medium effect size differences at the follow-up time points between CPT+A and PE on all four guilt measures.

Using data from Chard's (2005) study of adult survivors of child sexual abuse, Owens, Pike, and Chard (2001) examined the Personal Beliefs and Reactions Scale (PBRS; Resick, Schnicke, & Markway, 1991) and the World Assumptions Scale (WAS; Janoff-Bulman, 1989), which were both developed to examine cognitive distortions related to trauma and PTSD. Although none of the WAS subscales were correlated with PTSD symptoms at any time point (pretreatment, posttreatment, 3-month follow-up, and 1-year follow-up), PBRS safety, trust, power/control, esteem, and intimacy were correlated with PTSD at one or more time points, and all were strongly correlated at the follow-up assessments. Significant differences from pretreatment to posttreatment were found for the following PBRS subscales: undoing, self-blame, safety, trust, power/control, esteem, and intimacy. There were no further changes from posttreatment to the two follow-up assessments. Although they were not correlated with PTSD, there were significant differences on the WAS from pre- to posttreatment, which were maintained on two of the three subscales: benevolence of the world and self-worth.

Several studies have examined one cognitive component of CPT+A and CPT, the Impact Statement. After the first treatment session in either form of CPT, the first practice assignment is to write at least one page on the causes and consequences of the index traumatic event. This assignment is used to determine how the client views the index event and to define the Stuck Points that the client and therapist will work on during therapy. For the last session, the client is assigned to write another Impact Statement regarding what he or she now believes about the index event. (For more details, see Chapters 5, 6, and 10.)

Several groups of researchers have coded these Impact Statements to determine whether clients' beliefs have changed and whether they are associated with improvement in PTSD. The first study was by Sobel, Resick, and Rabalais (2009), who coded the Impact Statements with regard to thought clauses in one of four categories: assimilation, accommodation, overaccommodation, and information. Because Impact Statements varied in length, the authors analyzed percentage of total statements as well as total frequency. They found that from the beginning of treatment to the end, clients showed significant increases in accommodation and decreases in overaccommodation and assimilation.

Iverson, King, Cunningham, and Resick (2015) followed up this study by examining cognitions 5–10 years after treatment. In addition to conducting a long-term follow-up that included the same baseline measures, Iverson et al. asked participants to write yet another Impact Statement. Also, instead of just examining PTSD, this study examined depressive symptoms to see whether cognitions predicted maintenance or increase in symptoms. Fifty women completed the first and final treatment Impact Statements, as well as the long-term Impact Statement. Although overall PTSD and depression scores were maintained at low levels at the long-term follow-up (Resick, Williams, et al. 2012), changes in trauma-related beliefs between the end of treatment and long-term follow-up were significantly associated with changes in PTSD and depression symptoms. Improvement in accommodated thinking and declines in overaccommodated thinking were associated with lower PTSD and depression symptoms during this time period. Iverson et al. concluded that clients should be strongly encouraged to continue to practice balanced, accommodated thinking following the termination of treatment.

With a sample of active-duty military personnel, Dondanville et al. (2016) also coded Impact Statements, but this was conducted in the context of group or individual CPT. There were 63 participants who had written Impact Statements at the beginning and end of treatment. These investigators, too, found a decrease in assimilated and overaccommodated thought units and an increase in accommodated thoughts with treatment. There was the expected inverse relationship of PTSD and depression with accommodated thoughts, and positive relationship of overaccommodated thoughts with PTSD and depression scores. Those participants who did well with CPT had fewer overaccommodated and more accommodated thoughts by the end of treatment. Assimilated thoughts were not associated with PTSD and depression, even though they decreased over therapy, probably because there were so few assimilated statements in the Impact Statements at the beginning of treatment. It is possible that some clients may have a single assimilated thought (e.g., "It is all my fault") that keeps them stuck in their PTSD but results statistically in floor effects.

Price, Macdonald, Adair, Koerner, and Monson (2016) conducted a qualitative study (thematic analysis) of Impact Statements produced by 15 veterans who had completed both Impact Statements in the RCT with veterans described above (Monson et al., 2006), The themes that emerged were safety, trust, power/control, esteem, intimacy, emotions/symptoms, perspective, education/work, and positive statements about therapy (which occurred at posttreatment). For the most part, all of the themes showed improvement by the last Impact Statement, but some still expressed caution or described continuing struggles with Stuck Points on specific themes (e.g., safety, trust) or with emotions (e.g., sadness) that might have been avoided before treatment.

Cognitions as Mediators of Change

Using the study data from Resick et al. (2002), Gallagher and Resick (2012) examined hopelessness as both an outcome and a mediator of change in PTSD among women who had experienced rape as their index event. Participants assigned to CPT+A had larger pre–post reductions in hopelessness than those assigned to PE, and changes in hopelessness predicted changes in PTSD symptoms in the CPT+A participants to a greater extent than in the PE participants. Gilman, Schumm, and Chard (2011) also examined hope (rather than hopelessness, with a different measure from that used by Gallagher and Resick) with veterans seeking treatment for PTSD. Measures of PTSD symptoms, depression, and hope were gathered across the course of treatment in a residential program. Gilman et al. found that higher levels of hope at midtreatment were associated with reductions in PTSD and depression from mid- to posttreatment, and not the other way around; this finding thus supports the idea that hope is a change mechanism in symptom reduction.

Schumm, Dickstein, Walter, Owens, and Chard (2015) conducted a cross-lagged panel analysis from pretreatment to midtreatment to posttreatment among male and female veterans receiving CPT, to determine the longitudinal relationship among cognitions (negative beliefs about self, negative beliefs about the world, and self-blame), PTSD, and depression. They found significant improvements in scores on all scales over the course of treatment. They also found that pre- to midtreatment changes in self-blame and in negative beliefs about the self positively predicted and temporally preceded mid- to posttreatment changes in PTSD symptomatology. They also found that changes in negative beliefs about the self preceded changes in depression, but that pre- to midtreatment changes in depression preceded changes in self-blame and PTSD. These findings support the idea that improvement in negative cognitions is an important mechanism of change in PTSD.

Program Evaluation/Effectiveness Studies

Although it is important to conduct RCTs to determine whether a therapy is efficacious compared to a wait-list condition and other therapies, and whether the therapy only affects PTSD or is helpful for other symptoms and functioning, whether the therapy actually works in the community and is adopted is its ultimate test. There have been several studies that did not randomly assign participants to conditions, but examined program evaluation data on the implementation of CPT+A in clinical settings, particularly VA hospitals. CPT+A and CPT have been disseminated to thousands of therapists since 1987, and the implementation program has been keeping track of clients' scores on the PTSD Checklist (PCL; Weathers, Litz, Herman, Huska, & Keane, 1993; see

Handout 3.1). In an examination of the first therapy cases using CPT+A (Chard, Ricksecker, Healy, Karlin, & Resick, 2012), 327 therapists provided pre- and posttreatment PCL scores for 374 veterans. Following the 12-session protocol, veterans reported an average 19-point change on the PCL (10 points is clinically significant).

Kaysen et al. (2014) examined the VA records of 536 veterans from a Midwestern VA hospital who had attended at least one session of CPT+A or CPT, to determine the effect of alcohol use disorders on PTSD. They found that 49% reported a current or past diagnosis of such a disorder. The veterans had an average of 9 sessions of CPT+A, and there were no differences in treatment results among three groups: those without an alcohol use disorder history, those with such a history, and those with current alcohol use disorders. All groups showed significant reductions in both PTSD and depression.

In an implementation study in Australia, Lloyd et al. (2015) studied 100 cases in the National Veterans Treatment Service among therapists who were trained in CPT+A. The CPT+A therapists showed good fidelity to the treatment, and their results showed large effect sizes, comparable to those obtained in these researchers' RCT. They reported that 63% of cases showed clinically meaningful improvement in an average of 8 sessions. These studies demonstrate that CPT+A translates well into routine clinical care.

Dickstein, Walter, Schumm, and Chard (2013) found that veterans with subthreshold PTSD did as well as those who met full criteria for PTSD when these groups received CPT in a VA outpatient clinic. Very few studies have examined participants who do not meet full criteria for PTSD, and such participants are generally excluded from RCTs. However, Dickstein et al.'s findings help clinicians understand that clients who have partial PTSD may also benefit from CPT.

Walter, Dickstein, et al. (2014) compared those who received CPT or CPT+A in a VA residential program for those with traumatic brain injury and PTSD; this program combines group and individual therapy. They found no difference in PTSD outcomes or dropout rates, but a possible difference in depression, with the CPT+A participants showing more improvement. However, when an alpha correction was applied, the finding disappeared, so it is not clear that whether similar findings might emerge in an outpatient setting. Chard, Schumm, Owens, and Cottingham (2010) compared over 100 recent veterans of Iraq and Afghanistan with those from the Vietnam War who were treated in an outpatient VA PTSD clinic. They found that the recent veterans, who did not differ from the Vietnam veterans in any demographics (except for age) or service-connected disability, were likely to attend fewer sessions than the older veterans. They did not differ on their pretreatment scores, however, and among those who completed treatment, they improved more at posttreatment. Interestingly, those who attended more sessions were more likely to have higher PTSD scores at both pretreatment and posttreatment. Those who attended fewer sessions might have dropped out when they had achieved their goals.

Voelkel, Pukay-Martin, Walter, and Chard (2015) examined the effectiveness of CPT in male and female veterans with PTSD due to military sexual trauma compared to those without a history of such trauma. Of 481 veterans, 41% endorsed a history of military sexual trauma as their primary trauma, and scores at posttreatment showed that both groups improved significantly after receiving CPT, suggesting that CPT can be an effective treatment for this type of trauma regardless of veterans' gender.

In another study of veterans, Asamsama, Dickstein, and Chard (2015) evaluated the impact of depression on CPT results for 757 veterans. They found that 60.7% of participants met criteria for major depression at pretreatment, and that 75% showed a clinically significant reduction in symptoms after receiving CPT. There was no difference in treatment response based on BDI-II groupings, suggesting that CPT is an effective treatment even in case of severe co-occurring depression.

In a study of nonveterans, Schulz, Huber, and Resick (2006) found that CPT+A was effective in treating PTSD in foreign-born refugees to the United States when it was delivered in their native language (either by a native-language-speaking therapist or through an interpreter). Because this study was a report of program outcomes rather than an RCT, the number of sessions was not controlled. The refugees averaged 17 sessions, including several assessment sessions before treatment started. The effect sizes from pre- to posttreatment on PTSD symptoms were $d = 2.0$ for those with an interpreter and $d = 3.4$ for those with a native-language-speaking therapist. Both of these effect sizes are quite large, indicating a great deal of improvement in the refugees' self-reported PTSD symptoms.

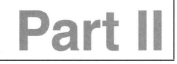

Part II

Setting the
Stage Clinically

3

Treatment Considerations

This chapter addresses the questions therapists often ask about when to start CPT and with which types of clients; how to assess PTSD and comorbid conditions; and how to conceptualize individual cases in CPT. In the recent past, many clinicians and researchers proposed that trauma-focused therapy could not begin without extensive rapport building and development of coping skills, even though there was no evidence that this was necessary. Furthermore, trauma-focused therapies were often not offered to clients with comorbid conditions, including substance misuse, personality disorder characteristics, and psychotic or bipolar symptoms. As reviewed in Chapter 2, our studies on CPT have included individuals with diverse trauma histories and varied symptom presentations, and clients have often begun treatment immediately after completion of their intake assessment. The following guidance is based on our various controlled and program evaluation studies, as well as our clinical experience in providing CPT.

For Which Clients Is CPT Appropriate?

CPT was originally developed for people not just with PTSD, but with additional disorders and conditions. It is helpful to remember that CPT is heavily grounded in Beck's cognitive therapy (Beck et al., 1979; Beck & Greenberg, 1984), which has been found to be effective for a number of disorders, including depressive, anxiety, and psychotic conditions. In both research and clinical practice, we have successfully used CPT with individuals at any time from 3 months to 60 years after their traumas, and some clinicians are using it even earlier in crisis situations such as combat, domestic violence, refugee work, and sexual assault (Nixon, 2012). In addition, CPT can be used for individuals with minimal formal education (e.g., fourth grade) and for people with

IQs as low as 75. (Note: We have now created modified/simplified versions of a few worksheets for individuals who find the original worksheets too complex; see Chapter 13.)

In addition to PTSD, most of our clients meet criteria for multiple comorbid diagnoses, such as depressive disorders, anxiety disorders, personality disorders, and substance use disorders. Moreover, CPT can be implemented with persons who do not meet full criteria for a PTSD diagnosis (Dickstein et al., 2013). The only caution in these latter cases is that if individuals do not meet at least subthreshold criteria for PTSD, but instead have other diagnoses such as major depression or panic disorder, they should not be offered CPT, but instead should receive a treatment designed for those disorders. One common misconception is that PTSD is the only disorder that follows traumatic events; in fact, a proportion of individuals never develop PTSD, and some may in fact develop another disorder.

Therapists often ask whether there are any hard-and-fast rules about excluding clients from CPT. We recommend that clinicians follow the same criteria that we use in our clinical studies to decide when it may be best to delay offering CPT or not to offer it at all. One of the most important things to consider is whether a person poses any imminent danger to self or others, in which case safety planning should precede CPT. The key is to differentiate between a client's thinking about death (i.e., ideation) and a firm intention or plan to commit suicide. A majority of our clients have suicidal or homicidal ideation, and they do very well in CPT. This ideation is best conceptualized as passive avoidance behavior, wherein clients want to escape their distress.

With regard to potential danger for further traumatization, we have many therapists providing CPT in the military, including those deployed to combat situations, and we are often asked to provide CPT for stateside service members prior to their next deployment. Similarly, CPT is commonly used in shelters for individuals experiencing intimate partner violence, after initial safety planning has been completed. In addition, recent international studies support the use of CPT with individuals in the midst of war and genocide (e.g., residents of the Democratic Republic of Congo). In these cases, it is important to carefully identify Stuck Points and to differentiate these from beliefs and threat appraisals that may be objectively true. For example, a client living in a war zone may have the belief that "I can be killed at any time," which is potentially true; therefore, a therapist would go deeper with the client to find out what this means to him or her and whether there are any situations that are relatively safer for the client. The therapist may uncover the Stuck Point "There is no point in living, since I am dying soon." This latter belief can be challenged to help the person resume fuller functioning, albeit with risk.

Other potential contraindications to CPT are other mental health conditions that can interfere with clients' successfully completing treatment. Two of the most significant concerns are unmedicated mania or psychosis. Once these conditions are stabilized on effective medication regimens, it will be easier for such clients to complete psychotherapy. Similarly, individuals with depressive disorders that prevent them from leaving the house or taking care of their basic needs may need medication or behavioral activation strategies before starting CPT. Individuals with substance use disorders that require inpatient or outpatient detoxification to prevent withdrawal symptoms should delay starting CPT until the initial detoxification process has been completed (often 7–10 days). Likewise, clients with such severe panic disorder that they cannot talk about even their thoughts about the trauma might do better to receive panic control treatment while receiving CPT. Multiple-channel exposure therapy (Falsetti, Resnick, & Davis, 2008) was developed as a combined treatment for PTSD and panic disorder that includes CPT components, as well as interoceptive treatment for panic (Barlow & Craske, 1994).

Similar points may be made about individuals who cannot engage in treatment because their dissociation is so extreme. Typically, when clients present for treatment and indicate that they dissociate, we ask them how often and how long the episodes occur. Is the dissociation caused by cues, and do the clients have enough control over the dissociation to stop it from happening before, during, or after a session? If the clients indicate that they are putting themselves or others at risk when they dissociate, then we typically recommend a brief course of training in grounding skills before CPT begins (Kennerley, 1996). Conversely, if the clients are not putting themselves or others at risk and seem to have some skill in focusing themselves, then we typically recommend that the clients initiate CPT without delay. Incidentally, one of our CPT studies described in Chapter 2 found that clients who had higher levels of dissociation at pretreatment did better with CPT+A than with CPT. This could be because of the need to process the trauma in more detail and put fragmented memories back into a narrative for those who dissociated a great deal during the traumatic event(s) (Resick, Suvak, et al., 2012).

In the end, the clients' motivation to address their PTSD symptoms is probably the most important factor to consider in deciding to proceed with CPT. Even clients with few coping skills, significant trauma histories, and various comorbid conditions have done very well in the different versions of CPT. Thus, in summary, the only reasons for not beginning CPT right after an intake session are suicidal or homicidal intent, severe self-harm for which immediate intervention is needed, severe dissociation in which a client cannot stay in the present during sessions, unmedicated psychosis or mania, and substance use requiring detoxification. In fact, we often find that therapists' readiness to engage their clients in trauma-focused treatment is as important as the clients' readiness. We discuss this later.

When Should the CPT Protocol Begin?

The next questions we are frequently asked are how many treatment sessions should occur before the CPT protocol begins, and whether it is important to spend time developing a trusting relationship with a client prior to starting trauma processing. Our answer to both questions is that sessions devoted exclusively to trust building are not needed, even if a clinician other than the CPT therapist has completed the assessment and psychosocial intake process. As highlighted above, if the therapist waits for weeks or months before starting the trauma processing, the client may infer that the therapist does not believe the client is ready or able to handle CPT. In fact, reluctance on the therapist's part may actually reinforce the client's natural desire to avoid doing trauma work, due to the PTSD avoidance symptoms. We argue that there is even an ethical issue in forestalling trauma-focused treatment, in that the client is being delayed in working toward improvement in PTSD and any comorbid symptoms.

We have found both in our clinical work and in our research studies that the therapeutic alliance can develop very quickly when the therapist uses a Socratic style of interacting with the client. This type of dialogue allows the therapist to convey a focused interest in understanding how the client thinks and feels about his or her world in general, and about the traumatic event in particular. Many clients who have been in other types of therapy before receiving CPT tell us that they have never felt so "heard" or "listened to" before. Finally, if the therapist engages in pretreatment sessions that are managed in a more open-ended, supportive counseling mode, the client will come to believe that this is what therapy should be like, and it may be difficult to reshape the treatment interactions to fit those required in a manualized treatment such as CPT.

If a therapist is engaging in CPT with a new client, we recommend that before CPT begins, the client should first be given one to three sessions of assessment and information gathering (depending on the length of the sessions and the assessment approaches used). These sessions may be conducted by the therapist who will be implementing CPT or by another clinician who performs intake assessments in that clinic. The assessment should focus on determining what the client's strengths and possible coping deficits are; what the client's trauma history is like; picking out an index event to assess for PTSD, whether the client actually has PTSD, according to a standardized assessment measure; and whether the client has any comorbid disorders (particularly ones with symptoms that may complicate or interfere with treatment; see the preceding section). Once it is determined that the client has PTSD and is ready to start treatment, the treating clinician can start CPT at the very next session.

If a therapist is starting CPT with an established client, it can be somewhat difficult to make the transition from other forms of therapy to a manualized treatment, as indicated above. We have found in these situations that it is best for the therapist to be very transparent with the client in discussing the option of initiating CPT. When a therapist has seen a client for months or even years, it is often easiest to start this conversation by discussing treatment goals and noting that there has been little to no progress toward those goals in some time. This provides a good opportunity to reassess the client's symptoms and gently offer a new approach. The therapist can provide information on how effective CPT has been with a wide variety of people suffering from various types of traumatic events. The therapist can then note that he or she has received training in this treatment and believes that the treatment would be very helpful, given the symptom presentation. Clients appreciate hearing that their therapists are acquiring new training and are interested in continually learning new approaches to facilitate providing the best care to their clients. At the same time, it is important for a therapist to avoid unintentionally undermining CPT by referring to it as a "new therapy" that "might work" with a client. Instead, the therapist should "sell" CPT by highlighting that CPT has been around for more than 25 years and that there are extensive data on its efficacy with a wide variety of client groups. It might even help to show some of the graphs from studies of CPT with traumas similar to the client's (for example, see Figure 2.1; others are available at *www.guilford.com/cpt-ptsd* and the PILOTS database at *www.ptsd.va.gov*).

The conversation with the client should not only include the reasons for trying something different, but also an explanation of how a course of CPT will differ from other types of therapy in terms of session structure and out-of-session assignment expectations. If the therapist has not been using cognitive-behavioral interventions, following an agenda during sessions, assigning homework, or focusing on a specific traumatic event during treatment, the change to CPT can be quite dramatic, and the therapist will want to make sure that the client is aware of and comfortable with the changes. We have found that when therapists are frank and clear with their clients, very few individuals have had difficulty with the change; indeed, many clients are very excited about trying something new that may help them recover further from their PTSD. Once the decision to start CPT has been made, it is very important that the therapist strives to stay consistent with the new therapy process. The avoidance symptoms of PTSD will continually push the client to want to revert to a non-trauma-focused treatment, so reminding the client of the rationale for the change to CPT can be important throughout the initial sessions of treatment.

If either the therapist or the client does not believe that they can manage the change to CPT together, another option is to refer the client to another therapist who has learned CPT. The referring therapist can highlight that the client has made excellent progress with him or her, but that sometimes a new perspective or new intervention can be what is needed to facilitate recovery. A client who is very attached to the original therapist may feel safer knowing that the relationship with this therapist is still available as a backup if needed, although we have found that most of the time, the client finishes CPT with the new therapist and is ready to terminate therapy altogether at that point. Regardless of whether a therapist is starting CPT with a new or long-term client, we find that the CPT treatment contract (discussed later) is a helpful tool in outlining the expectations for both the therapist and the client and in facilitating adherence to the protocol.

Choosing a Format for CPT

CPT can be offered in nine different formats: individual, group, or group + individual treatment, using CPT, CPT+A, or variable-length CPT. (As noted in Chapters 1 and 2, treatment with individual written accounts only is also available, but we do not discuss that format in this book.) When a therapist is deciding which treatment format to use with a particular client, perhaps the most important piece of information to consider is the client's own preference. In situations or clinics where therapists are not able to offer all the various formats of CPT, being able to offer at least CPT and CPT+A in group or individual formats is most advantageous. These options allow clients who are unable or unwilling to write trauma accounts the option of participating in CPT. For those clients who express a desire to go into detail about their traumas through written accounts, the CPT+A protocol gives them this possibility. Some clients prefer group treatment, while others refuse it. Some clinics only have group treatment as an option.

Pretreatment Assessment

Gathering the Client's Trauma History

Before CPT begins, several things must occur. First, the therapist (or intake assessor) must establish that the client has PTSD. A complete history of traumatic events should be part of any intake procedure, along with determination of the "index trauma." Throughout this book, when we refer to the "index trauma," this means the traumatic event for which the client is experiencing the most PTSD symptoms. Most individuals presenting for PTSD treatment have multiple traumas. In CPT, we advise working on the index trauma first, because therapeutic gains on that trauma are likely to lead to faster improvements in PTSD symptoms and to generalize to other traumas, especially those that are thematically similar (e.g., interpersonal traumas in adulthood and childhood). In determining the index trauma, the clinician is encouraged to pay attention to these clues: the specific content of intrusions; negative cognitions about the trauma; and the people, places, and events that are avoided. These are the symptoms of PTSD that differentiate it from anxiety and depressive disorders. As discussed throughout the CPT protocol (see Chapters 5–10), if there are assimilated Stuck Points about other traumas, these should be addressed after sufficient progress on the cognitions surrounding the index trauma has been made.

Determining the index event is not necessarily always easy. Sometimes abuse has occurred as long as the client remembers, or the client has trouble pinpointing one event that is most distressing because the events were serial. Sometimes clients focus on the most recent event and do not realize that they might not have developed PTSD after that event if earlier traumatic events had not set the stage for symptoms following the more recent event. If the therapist just asks, "What event bothers you the most?", clients may indicate a natural bereavement, divorce, or some other recent negative life event that is currently on their minds. Therapists should refer to DSM-5 (American Psychiatric Association, 2013) or the 10th revision of the *International Classification of Diseases* (ICD-10; World Health Organization, 1992) for help with determination of Criterion A events. If a client reports that the event that haunts him or her the most is not a Criterion A event, but that the client has other Criterion A events, the client should be reassured that this "most haunting" event can be covered during treatment, but that CPT should start with a PTSD-qualifying event.

A solution to this problem is to review the client's timeline of traumatic events. One way to do this is to develop a written timeline of the person's life, with the significant events marked on it. The therapist can determine whether a specific event meets the criterion for a traumatic event, but, in any case, constructing the timeline will inform the therapist about significant stressors that have occurred. If traumatic events are serial in nature, meaning that they occurred repeatedly over a period of time (e.g., child abuse, IPV, combat), the timeline can include the onset and end of that type of trauma and can delineate any particularly bad events within that. Figure 3.1 gives an example of a timeline.

When initially interviewing clients about their traumatic events, therapists must make sure not to use terms that clients may not have applied to themselves ("rape," "child abuse," etc.). Instead, questions should use behavioral descriptors: "Were you ever forced to have sexual contact with someone when you didn't want to?", "Did you ever have any kind of sexual contact as a child with an adult (or someone who was at least 5 years older than you?)", "How were you punished as a child? Were you ever injured?" (On the timeline and later in therapy, the accurate terms can be used.) These types of questions should be followed up with questions calling for more details about what occurred and when it occurred; whether there was a perpetrator (and, if so, what the client's relationship with the perpetrator was); whether the trauma occurred in a series of events; how long it lasted; and whether there was one occasion that stood out more than others. Instead of "Which one bothers you the most?", questions to identify the index trauma might include these: "Which one do you have the most intrusive memories or nightmares about?", "When you are tired or sick, or your defenses are down, which event pops into your mind?", "Which event are you hoping that you won't have to talk about in therapy or don't want to tell me about?", or "Which event do you avoid thinking about at all costs?" In the example shown in Figure 3.1, the client reported that the rape was the index event because she thought she was going to be killed, but during the therapy it became apparent that many of her Stuck Points were core beliefs she had developed earlier in childhood as a result of being abused by her father.

If none of those questions produce the index event, then the therapist should go for the event that elicited the first episode of PTSD. It is probable that once people have developed PTSD, their thoughts and assumptions about themselves and the world that are applied to that situation will be applied to future traumatic events. For example,

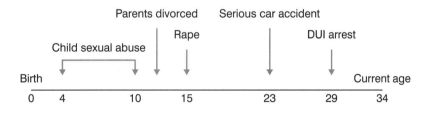

FIGURE 3.1. Example of a timeline of significant life events.

clients who were abused by a parent in childhood often develop such thoughts as "It's all my fault; I'm being punished," or "I can't trust anyone." Then, following another trauma, even if there is no way it could be their fault or there was nothing about trust in the traumatic situation, they may still focus on how it must be their fault, flash on the moment that they perceive they lost control over the situation, or reactivate the thought that no one can be trusted.

Assessing for PTSD

Once the index event is selected, the therapist should assess for PTSD with an interview and a self-report scale. The Clinician-Administered PTSD Scale (Weathers, Marx, Friedman, & Schnurr, 2014) has been updated and tested for DSM-5, and this new version is a bit quicker to complete than older versions of the scale (it can be ordered through the National Center for PTSD website, *www.va.ptsd.gov*). Using an interview is an important way to begin, because a therapist can refocus a client on the index event if the client tends to drift into using it as a measure of general distress or starts mixing up traumas and their effects. Therapists can also ask probing questions to ascertain whether clients actually meet the diagnostic criterion for a single item, and can ask for examples. They can then pinpoint whether clients meet all the criteria for PTSD for at least a month and thereby currently have the disorder. It is possible that clinicians may have to assess another event if it becomes apparent that clients do not have PTSD for the initial index event specified. An interview may not need to be used if formal diagnosis is not needed, but going over the PCL-5, monthly version (see below), orally to clarify what the items mean and how they refer to the index event may clarify whether the client has PTSD.

The purpose of using a self-report scale is so that clients can be trained to answer the questions focusing the same way on the index traumatic event rather than general life stressors. Self-report scales are used throughout therapy in order to assess the progress of it, much as a physician would assess blood pressure or take a temperature if one were physically ill.

There are a number of self-report PTSD scales. The PTSD Checklist (PCL) is a recommended scale that is in the public domain. It too has been updated for DSM-5 (PCL-5; Weathers et al., 2013, 2014). The PCL-5 consists of 20 items scored from 0 (not at all) to 4 (extremely). There are versions of the PCL-5 that ask clients to report the severity of their symptoms over the past month versus the past week; we provide both of these in Handout 3.1.* We recommend using the monthly version at initial assessment to correspond with the period of time for DSM-5 diagnosis and the weekly version over the course of therapy.

Although it is possible to score the individual symptom clusters, it is most common to use a total score over the course of treatment. One caveat about the PCL-5 relates to item 10, about blame of self or others. In the DSM-5, the item about erroneous

---

*All handouts are located at the ends of chapters.

or distorted self-blame was designed to look for the common tendency for people to blame themselves for events that they did not intend, did not cause, and could not have prevented. Such self-blame is often obvious to the therapist in statements like "I should have been able to fight off my father," or "If I had broken protocol, I would have saved my buddy." The definitive (e.g., "should have," "would have") nature of the statements is an indicator of the unlikelihood that they are true.

On the other hand, erroneous other-blame is a bit harder to detect with a self-report measure. Erroneous other-blame occurs when a client blames someone in proximity to the traumatic event, rather than the person who actually intended the harm and committed the event. For example, instead of blaming the person who buried a mine that blew up a truck, a soldier with PTSD may blame the commander who sent the troops down the road, as if the commander knew what was going to happen. It is not uncommon to blame one's mother as much or more for sexual abuse by a male relative, even if she did not know about it (e.g., "She should have known, even if she was at work"). Blaming someone in proximity to the event or victim allows the client to maintain the illusion that the event was preventable and brings the focus to someone who in fact did not intend harm. If therapists do not explain item 10 on the PCL-5 carefully, therefore, it is possible that there will be no change in clients' scores if they move from blaming an innocent bystander to blaming the actual perpetrator. The administrator of the self-report measure may need to check to see if there is a change in whom a client is blaming for the event over the course of treatment.

Assessing for Comorbid Conditions and Other Clinical Considerations

Most individuals with PTSD present with at least one comorbid condition or clinical problem (Kessler et al., 1995). As described in Chapter 2, CPT has been tested with a wide range of individuals with these co-occurring issues. That said, it is important for a therapist to consider these other conditions in a given client's individual case conceptualization, and to help the client manage them in order to profit most fully from CPT. For the most part, these problems improve along with successful amelioration of PTSD, but the symptoms of these conditions may need to be addressed during the course of treatment in order not to interfere with treatment success. A client may also have psychosocial strengths or limitations that the therapist can help the client leverage or address to get maximum benefit from CPT (e.g., family functioning). Moreover, the therapist should consider lifespan developmental issues when working with individual clients. These issues are addressed later in the chapter.

Depression

Depressive disorders are the most common comorbid disorders with PTSD. Not only is depression not a rule-out for CPT; as noted in Chapter 2, treatment outcome studies on CPT have found substantial and lasting changes in depressive symptoms, along with PTSD symptom improvement. The Patient Health Questionnaire-9 (PHQ-9; Kroenke, Spitzer, & Williams, 2001), a module of the longer Patient Health Questionnaire (PHQ), is a brief instrument for screening and monitoring depression; it should be used if a client has depression as well as PTSD. The PHQ-9 is provided in Handout 3.2.

Some clients who are struggling with even the smallest activities of daily living may require antidepressant medications and/or behavioral activation before starting trauma treatment, as noted above. However, the majority of clients with PTSD and depression can start CPT right after their initial assessment. For some clients and therapists, it can be tempting to start antidepressants at the same time as CPT, embracing the adage that "more is better." However, if a client is beginning or increasing a medication while starting psychotherapy, neither the client nor the clinician will know which element of treatment is more effective. Thus, when the client begins to feel better, the client may attribute the change to the medication even if this is not the case, and may not attribute the change to his or her own efforts in CPT. This can lead the client to decide to drop out of treatment, believing that he or she only needs the medications to manage the symptoms. We have found it helpful to caution clients when starting CPT at the same time as medications that they should not assume all gains are due to the medications and cease treatment. Instead, they should complete the CPT protocol and then have their PTSD and depressive symptoms formally assessed at the end of the treatment.

It is also helpful to collaborate with clients' prescribers if the clients begin to show an increase in symptoms during CPT. Some prescribers will assume that such clients are in need of a higher dose and automatically make that change if they are not informed of the potential for some clients to experience symptom worsening (e.g., more nightmares or ruminating about the traumatic event) during treatment. Unfortunately, we do not have a great deal of literature on the combination or sequencing of medication and psychotherapy for PTSD to guide us at this point, but we do know that psychotherapy is considered more effective than medication for the treatment of PTSD (e.g., Watts et al., 2013). Open communication between providers can assist with decision making on the appropriateness and sequencing of medication with CPT.

Substance Use Disorders

We have found that substance-using clients can do very well in CPT, especially if steps are taken to help increase the likelihood of their success. First, a thorough assessment of their substance use should be conducted to determine whether the clients are in need of medical detoxification before starting treatment. Second, therapists may want to employ motivational interviewing techniques to help the clients commit to not using substances before, during, or after therapy sessions or the times they allocate for their practice assignment completion. That said, we have treated clients with significant substance use (including alcohol, heroin, cocaine, and marijuana use) quite successfully by not entirely restricting use and not punishing the clients or stopping treatment if they binge or lapse between sessions. Instead, we typically label the substance use as a form of avoidance and work with the clients to identify the Stuck Points that led to their use, as well as specific Stuck Points about using that are making it difficult for the clients to recover. Furthermore, we do not rule out starting CPT right after completion of a substance use treatment program; in fact, many substance use clinics are adopting CPT as part of their treatment programs. Frequently, when clients decrease or stop their use of substances, they experience an increase in nightmares, flashbacks, and painful emotions that are no longer being medicated by the drugs. This may be an ideal time to start treatment, while the clients are motivated and before the PTSD symptoms cause a relapse or a shift to another unhealthy avoidance behavior.

Psychotic and Bipolar Disorders

Individuals with well-managed psychotic and bipolar disorders have successfully engaged in CPT. It is important for a therapist to consult with such a client's psychopharmacologist and other treatment providers, to make them aware of the initiation of CPT and to enlist them in monitoring for the unlikely event that the client experiences a change in his or her mental status. The therapist will also likely need to reassure other providers of the safety of CPT for clients with serious and persistent psychological disorders, citing the outcome research on CPT. It is important to highlight that decreasing the PTSD symptom burden in these clients may make them less susceptible to relapses of their other serious mental health conditions.

It is our experience that clients with psychotic disorders can be more rigid than other clients in their thinking. Moreover, the hypervigilance symptoms of PTSD can overlap with, or exacerbate, the paranoia experienced by these clients. Thus a therapist should take care in the use of Socratic dialogue to minimize defensiveness. If a client's symptoms begin to escalate in the face of challenges to his or her thinking, the therapist should immediately back off, to avoid the possibility that the client's thinking may become more entrenched. Encouraging the client to challenge his or her own thinking with the cognitive worksheets may be most beneficial; during this process, the therapist should be especially attuned to joining with the client and developing a strong working alliance to navigate the client's paranoia.

Risk for Harm to Self and Others

Many clients with PTSD who engage in CPT report suicidal and homicidal ideation. As noted above, it is appropriate for such a client to pursue CPT, as long as there is no imminent plan or intention to harm self or others. The therapist should consistently monitor for any changes in risk in these areas, and should set up a safety plan that is kept in the front of the client's therapy materials binder. (Note that each client should have a binder or workbook in which to keep worksheets, informational handouts, and other materials used during therapy.) Similarly, clients may have a history of self-injurious behavior. Controlled trials have generally required that clients have a 3-month period in which they have not self-harmed. In clinical practice, we have treated clients with more recent histories of self-harm, and we have had clients in research studies who had not self-harmed in the prior 3 months, but who engaged in such behavior during treatment. One of us also treated a woman with severe trichotillomania dating back to her childhood; for her, the hair pulling served as an anxiety management/distraction strategy. As long as a self-injurious client is not engaging in potentially *lethal* self-harm, we believe that it is safe (and ultimately better for the client) to attempt a course of CPT to decrease the need for such escape behavior. Of course, the self-harm should be directly addressed and monitored.

With the new criteria for PTSD in DSM-5 (American Psychiatric Association, 2013), reckless and aggressive behavior toward others has been recognized as a potential symptom of the disorder. This represents greater recognition of the "fight" aspect of the fight–flight–freeze response of the sympathetic nervous system. Reckless behavior may be seen in adolescent and young adult clients who drive too fast, engage in reckless sexual behavior, or have other impulsive behaviors. We have extensive experience in treating male veterans who have presented with such behavior. Like self-harm behavior, aggressive behavior toward others can serve as a dysfunctional emotion regulation strategy. The likelihood of aggressive behavior can also be potentiated by substance use, which is often comorbid with PTSD (see above). Thus, CPT clinicians should carefully assess and monitor substance use and the potential for aggression against others or other reckless behavior. One of us had a client who had a history of substance use, an extensive history of fighting with others, and a history of violence against his wife and children. This client found his aggressive behavior inconsistent with his desired self-image, and was willing to engage in CPT with the goal of decreasing his PTSD, substance use, and aggressive behavior.

It is important for the therapist, as well as the client, to understand that suicidal/aggressive/homicidal ideation, as well as self- and other-harm, represents efforts to avoid and escape emotions. In reaction to emotional distress, clients may engage in such ideation and/or behavior in an effort to escape psychological pain. Doing so serves to reinforce avoidance of emotions, and consequently maintains the clients' perception that they cannot tolerate either their natural or their manufactured emotions. Clients should be encouraged to embrace and immerse themselves in the natural emotions emanating from their traumatic events, because these emotions will run their natural course and abate if they are experienced rather than avoided. Manufactured emotions, which are products of the clients' assimilation of the trauma and overaccommodated beliefs resulting from the trauma, should be directly addressed with the use of cognitive worksheets.

CPT therapists should use Socratic dialogue and assign cognitive worksheets to address clients' concerns that their emotions will overwhelm them and heighten their risk for ideation and destructive behavior against themselves or others. Examples of Stuck Points that might be challenged include "I will be overwhelmed by my emotions if I feel them," "I will become suicidal if I think about my trauma," or "Someone will get hurt if I get in touch with my feelings." An important part of a successful course of CPT is increasing clients' tolerance and mastery of feeling the natural emotions that were encoded with their trauma memories, as well as those generated by the clients' thinking about the trauma and its consequences.

Personality Disorder Traits

As described in Chapter 2, individuals with comorbid personality disorders have never been excluded from trials or from the clinical practice of CPT; indeed, there is evidence that these characteristics improve with a course of CPT. That said, individuals with personality disorders or traits of these disorders are likely to require more work on the part of their therapists to manage their characteristic thoughts, emotions, and behaviors.

The most typical personality disorder traits that clinicians anticipate or find difficult to manage in CPT are borderline personality disorder traits. More specifically, difficulties with emotion regulation and related impulsive behaviors (e.g., self-harm, suicidality) can be treatment-interfering. We find that the structure and clear expectations of the CPT protocol are emotionally containing for these clients. If such clients are prone to crises, we recommend that clinicians contract with clients to have a certain number of nonprotocol or "urgent" sessions (usually, two sessions) that the clients can choose to use over the course of the treatment. When presenting with an urgent issue, clients are asked whether they want to use one of their contracted nonprotocol sessions to discuss the issue. If the clients know ahead of time that they have a limited number of these nonprotocol sessions, and have control over when they use them, it tends to decrease their tendency to present chronically with urgent issues. If a client chooses not to utilize a contracted session, a therapist can still address the issue at the end of the session to reinforce completion of the trauma-focused work, or can incorporate the issue into the skill being taught in a certain session (e.g., the therapist can identify a Stuck Point related to the issue and assign this as the topic of a Challenging Questions Worksheet). Regardless of the topic, the therapist should stay within the cognitive framework and use CPT materials that are appropriate to the stage of treatment of the client.

Therapists should be aware of other personality disorder traits that can affect the therapeutic process. For example, those with traits of avoidant personality disorder may be particularly resistant to approaching versus avoiding. Individuals with narcissistic personality disorder traits may find it more difficult to develop the requisite nonspecific elements of any psychotherapy (e.g., a working alliance, empathy), or may be relatively more defensive than other clients when engaging in Socratic dialogue. Those with traits of obsessive–compulsive personality disorder may be relatively more rigid in their thinking and get caught up in the process of doing the cognitive worksheets precisely, rather than (in the spirit in which the worksheets were written and are presented) using them to help develop alternative thoughts about either traumatic or day-to-day events. It is not unusual to see dependent personality traits in women who have been abused by partners and whose self-worth has been so damaged that they don't believe they can make decisions or survive on their own.

As discussed below in the section on case conceptualization, clinicians are encouraged to think about personality disorder traits as the results of schemas/core beliefs developed in early life that guide how people process information about themselves, others, and the world. When they are considered in this way, personality traits are modifiable; they do not constitute a life sentence of impaired functioning. It also explains why CPT results in personality trait changes. Although therapists may need to work harder with such clients to maintain fidelity to the CPT protocol, we have seen significant improvements in PTSD, comorbid conditions, and overall functioning in these clients.

Sleep Disruptions

The CPT protocol does not include specific interventions to address sleep disturbances (e.g., sleep hygiene, sleep restriction). As reviewed in Chapter 2, CPT has been found to improve sleep, but not necessarily to a point at which clients become "good sleepers" (Galovski, Monson, Bruce, & Resick, 2009; Pruiksma et al., in press), and the addition of self-hypnosis prior to CPT has not augmented treatment gains (Galovski et al., 2016). Consequently, we do not currently recommend integrating specific sleep interventions into CPT, although research is underway examining whether a short course of cognitive-behavioral therapy for insomnia (Edinger & Carney, 2008; Taylor & Pruiksma, 2014) before or after CPT may improve both sleep and PTSD symptoms (Taylor, personal communication, 2016).

Cognitions related to sleep disturbance may be challenged with the practice assignments. For example, those with sleep disturbance often catastrophize about their loss of sleep (e.g., "If I don't get at least 7 hours of sleep, I won't be able to function tomorrow," or "My body is being permanently damaged by my insomnia"). Therapists should bear in mind that a focus on sleep disturbance can serve as a strategy to avoid trauma-related material, and therefore we recommend that this challenging occur through the use of worksheets outside sessions. If a client completes a successful course of CPT and sleep disturbance remains, we recommend contracting with the client for a course of cognitive-behavioral therapy for insomnia or referring the client to a clinician with expertise in these specific interventions. One case study (Pruiksma, Molino, Taylor, Resick, & Peterson, 2016) demonstrated further improvement in nightmares, insomnia, PTSD, and depression with four sessions of sleep treatment, even though he no longer had PTSD at the end of CPT.

Medications

In clinical trials, clients are required to maintain their psychopharmacological regimen, in order to rule out the possibility that initiation of or changes in medications might account for changes in PTSD or comorbid conditions. In clinical practice, we encourage clinicians to contract with their clients and consult with the clients' prescribers to maintain any medication regimen during the course of CPT. As suggested earlier, when medication changes are made during psychotherapy, clients are prone to attribute any changes in their symptomatology to the medication changes rather than the psychotherapy, which can undermine the clients' self-efficacy and sense of accomplishment in the therapy. In general, it is important to instill in clients that changes are the results of their hard work and are not attributable to their medications, prescribers, or CPT therapists. On the other hand, it is important for clients not to stop taking medications "cold turkey." This can produce rebound effects, which can also disrupt treatment and be misinterpreted. Finally, clients and (whenever possible) CPT therapists should confer with prescribers about the use of medications, especially antianxiety agents, that may be prescribed as needed. Such medications can prevent natural emotions from emerging, and can become addictive and a means of avoidance if taken just before a therapy session or when clients are doing practice assignments.

Family Involvement

By now, several studies document the importance of interpersonal factors, including family functioning, in individual treatment outcomes for PTSD. In an early study comparing individual imaginal exposure and cognitive therapy for PTSD, Tarrier, Sommerfield, and Pilgrim (1999) found that patients whose relatives displayed high levels of criticism or hostility (i.e., high "expressed emotion") exhibited significantly less improvement in PTSD symptoms, depressive symptoms, and general anxiety following treatment than did patients with relatives who expressed low levels of these behaviors. Similarly, Monson, Rodriguez, and Warner (2005) studied the role of interpersonal relationship variables in two forms of group cognitive-behavioral therapy for veterans with PTSD. The two forms were trauma-focused cognitive-behavioral therapy (i.e., exposure to trauma memories and cognitive restructuring of trauma-related beliefs) and skills-focused treatment (i.e., symptom management skills without focus on traumatic memories and reminders). Although there were no differences in the PTSD outcomes of the two forms of treatment, pretreatment intimate relationship functioning was more strongly associated with treatment outcomes in the trauma-focused therapy than in the skills-focused treatment. In the trauma-focused group, there was a stronger relationship between pretreatment intimate relationship functioning and IPV perpetration outcomes. Better intimate relationship adjustment at pretreatment was associated with lower levels of IPV perpetration at follow-up for veterans who received trauma-focused versus skills-focused treatment.

In a related vein, two studies have investigated the role of pretreatment social support in PTSD treatment outcomes (Price, Gros, Strachan, Ruggiero, & Acierno, 2013; Thrasher, Power, Morant, Marks, & Dalgleish, 2010). Using data from an RCT comparing exposure and/or cognitive restructuring to relaxation for civilians with chronic PTSD, Thrasher and colleagues investigated the effects of perceived social support specific to coping with the effects of trauma, averaged across two close significant others nominated by each participant (most of these others were family members). Pretreatment social support was positively associated with PTSD treatment outcomes across conditions. However, the effect of pretreatment social support was stronger among those receiving exposure and/or cognitive restructuring than among those in the relaxation condition. Similarly, in a sample of veterans with PTSD or subthreshold PTSD receiving exposure therapy, Price et al. (2013) investigated the associations between each of four domains of perceived social support (i.e., positive social interactions, emotional/informational support, tangible support, and affectionate support) and pretreatment PTSD symptom severity, as well as the effects of social support on treatment response. Greater pretreatment emotional/informational support was associated with better response to treatment.

In summary, these studies suggest that family members can play an important role in the success of CPT with clients. As a result, we suggest that clinicians at least consider including family members or close significant others in the assessment of clients. Some clients may not have good insight into their PTSD symptoms; collateral reports on these symptoms may thus be helpful in getting a full picture of their type and severity. In addition, collateral assessment can be extremely important in various possible comorbid conditions. For example, clients may not report or may minimize impulse-related disorders or symptoms (substance use, eating disorder symptoms, pornography use, etc.). Clients with dissociative symptoms may also be less cognizant of the extent of their symptoms.

Including significant others as collateral informants in the assessment process can serve as a gateway to incorporating these others into the provision of CPT. We recommend, if possible, that significant others hear the rationale and overview of treatment from clinicians; if this is not possible, clients should be encouraged to share their understanding of this material with their significant others. The National Center for PTSD website (*www.ptsd.va.gov*) has very good information about PTSD for families, as well as information about CPT. In addition, clients should be aware of ways in which loved ones may be interfering with treatment, knowingly or unknowingly. For example, one of us had a client who indicated that his wife was being "helpful" to him in doing trauma accounts by offering him a glass of wine before he began writing these accounts.

Some significant others, such as spouses or partners, may collude with avoidance by offering to do all the shopping in crowded stores or to do all the driving (or, conversely, never to do the driving so that the clients can have control). They may try to talk the clients into quitting therapy early if the clients decrease their avoidance and subsequently have more nightmares or flashbacks. They may perceive that therapy is making the clients worse, and may not notice that the clients are finally processing their natural emotions and thinking about the meaning of the traumatic events. Some spouses/partners or other family members may feel threatened that they are losing important roles in their relationships with the clients, and may fear that they are not needed any more. Therapists should address these issues early in treatment, preferably before beginning CPT. The significant others can be support persons, not by nagging clients to do their practice assignments, but perhaps by giving them the space and time to do them. The family members or friends do not need to hear the gory details about the trauma, but can show interest in the clients' completion of the worksheets and can see how the questions the clients are asking themselves can be used in other everyday situations, as well as with regard to the traumatic events.

Ongoing Assessment

Assessment is not just for initial determination of whether clients meet criteria for PTSD and comorbid disorders. Assessment should occur throughout treatment. If clients are seen twice per week, the PCL-5 (or other PTSD self-report measure) should be given once a week. If the clients are seen once a week, it should still be given once a week. The PCL-5 should be administered regularly to determine whether clients are recovering or not and which symptoms have improved or not. If a client's PTSD scores have not decreased at all after six or seven sessions (i.e., by the time the client has processed the index event for several sessions), the therapist should question whether the client has Stuck Points related to another traumatic event that has not been identified; whether the client, in discussions with the therapist, has left out a crucial part of the incident that is maintaining PTSD; or whether the client is holding on to beliefs in protection of scarier ideas to maintain a core belief (e.g., "The world is predictable and controllable"). These issues are discussed again in Chapter 7.

Case Conceptualization

Although CPT is a protocol-based therapy, with prescribed session content and out-of-session assignments, this does not mean that a CPT therapist is a mere technician who does not have to conceptualize each client's case in order to understand the client's possible impediments to recovery. Clinicians have told us that they appreciate that the cognitive theory underlying CPT takes into account each client's developmental history and the intersections of traumatic experiences with that history of learning.

We consider the most important case conceptualization skill for clinicians to be differentiating between assimilated and overaccommodated beliefs, because this differentiation guides the prioritization of Stuck Points to be targeted over the course of therapy. In CPT, assimilated Stuck Points are negative trauma-related appraisals that impede recovery. In other words, these are the problematic ways that clients look "backward" about the index event. These thoughts generally involve hindsight bias and efforts to "undo" the event. It may include the attempt to wonder "why" the event happened to them, indicating an attempt to return to the "just-world belief" (i.e., the belief that the world should be fundamentally fair and just) and to a sense that the world is predictable and controllable.

A key to discovering these Stuck Points is figuring out how a client believes that he or she should have been omniscient or omnipotent to predict and control the index event. For example, one of us treated a police officer who witnessed two children drowning. Her assimilated beliefs were that she should have acted differently to prevent the children from drowning. Specifically, she appraised that the children would not have drowned if the reservoir ice had not broken because of the weight of her police belt; that her fear got in the way of responding (even though, as a "rookie," she responded when others did not know what to do); and that if she had gotten there seconds earlier, the children would not have died. She held to these beliefs in spite of realistic evidence that her police partner (who was about the same size as the client) broke through the ice without her belt on; that one of the children was recovered, but died the following day; and that in spite of her fear, she acted bravely.

In discerning a client's assimilated Stuck Points, it is important to consider how the event is incongruent or congruent with the client's previously held beliefs and schemas. Prior beliefs can be relatively positive, as in the case of the police officer described above, and the trauma may be incongruent or discordant with these beliefs. The police officer had been an exceptionally hardy individual—someone who had overcome significant adversity in childhood and adulthood to become a police officer. Prior to the drowning, she believed that she was capable of good problem solving, especially under pressure, and that she was the person in her relatively chaotic family who took care of others financially, socially, and emotionally. She also held the common belief that children should not die, as well as the *ex consequentia* (i.e., after-the-fact) thinking that good efforts should lead to good outcomes. It was hard for her to accept that despite her heroic efforts (which led to a number of accolades and awards), not all bad things are predictable or preventable. In this case, the officer could have come to the traumatic event believing that she was incapable, became overly emotional under pressure, and served as a "magnet" for bad outcomes. Had she had those premorbid beliefs, the trauma would have confirmed this negative way of thinking.

The pretreatment trauma assessment will give the clinician substantial information about a client's history of traumatization and how the client has made sense of it. For example, a client with traumatic events in his or her childhood, who is subsequently traumatized in adulthood, may use the adulthood trauma as faulty evidence to support previously held negative beliefs stemming from childhood. Even if a client did not suffer a DSM-5 Criterion A traumatic event in childhood, the client may have experienced a generally negative upbringing—one leading to negative beliefs that were self-reinforced in the interpretation of subsequent traumatic experiences. It is our experience that clients with negative preexisting schemas are relatively more difficult to treat, because of their longer-standing, more automatic ways of interpreting the world and its events. With such a client, the therapist will likely need to weave into therapy sessions reminders of where a negative interpretation bias came from and challenges to its origins.

The terms "schemas" and "core beliefs" both refer to deeply entrenched, long-standing, and widely applied beliefs that a person accepts fundamentally as givens. All types of new information (new experiences, etc.) are either fitted into these core beliefs without alteration, are distorted to fit the schemas, or are ignored. Core beliefs are most likely to be dealt with during the latter part of therapy, with the overaccommodated Stuck Points, but can also show up in therapy immediately with a familiar pattern of self- or other-blame. Clients who believe that they "deserved" the traumatic event because they are "bad" or "worthless" have a core belief that was established prior to the index event or has been reinforced through subsequent traumas. Because of the automatic nature of core beliefs, it may take several sessions for a therapist to notice a pattern, and it may take many worksheets on specific events to counteract the core belief with factual information that eventually wears down the automatic assumption. The just-world myth may be a core belief that is accepted without question because it was taught from earliest childhood.

The Impact Statement assigned after Session 1 also provides the therapist with integral case conceptualization information about Stuck Points and possible obstacles to recovery. Specifically, the part of the assignment related to *why* the index traumatic event occurred will help elucidate assimilated beliefs. Sometimes clients do not have an answer to this question, because they have not thought about the traumatic event enough to form a narrative about why it happened. Conversely, a client's narrative may be particularly blaming of self or others, because of the desire for someone to predict the event and prevent it from happening. In the former type of case, the principle is for the therapist to help the client to develop a healthy and balanced appraisal of the event. In the latter, the principle is for the therapist to correct the client's unhealthy appraisal—considering what realistically could have been done at the time in that particular context, and helping the client accept that the event was not preventable (especially after the fact).

As a therapist involved in case conceptualization, it is helpful to ask a client the question, "How would you need to think about this event in order to recover?" In the police officer's case, she might think the following:

"I did the best I could in an extremely unforeseeable case. In fact, I was the most junior officer, and I was offering up suggestions about what we might do when others training me did not know what to do. Others investigating our procedures gave me accolades. And I don't know if reaching the boy I was trying to reach would have necessarily saved him, because the other boy died the next day. While I might use the best procedures and knowledge I have at the time, it still might not work. I am not superhuman; I'm just a person trying to protect our society, and I have to sit with the uncertainty that might be thrown to me in future calls."

These are the types of accommodated beliefs a clinician is looking forward to seeing in the Impact Statement at the end of treatment.

As a clinician, it is key to look for assimilated Stuck Points to work on first, because correcting these beliefs will have downstream effects on overaccommodated beliefs. By definition, a traumatic event is a sentinel event that has consequential effects on a client's beliefs. If the client changes his or her beliefs about a key event, this will have effects on cognitions that result from those appraisals. Thus it is important for the clinician and client to prioritize these emotion-laden beliefs to have effects on other beliefs that can form as a consequence—beliefs related to safety, trust, power/control, esteem, and intimacy. For example, if a client comes to believe that "I did the best I could in an impossible, unpredictable, and helpless situation," then this new belief will have some effect on how much power/control the client has in any given situation. If the client comes to accept that he or she and others did as much as they possibly could do in the situation, the client needs to adjust esteem-related views of self and others to accommodate the new belief that all people, including the client, are human and capable of only so much.

Because of the timing of the topics of overaccommodated Stuck Points in CPT, clients are also more responsible for challenging their thinking in these areas with more cognitive skills. Nevertheless, clinicians should target assimilated Stuck Points until there is increasing resolution before focusing on overaccommodated Stuck Points, in the spirit of efficiency.

PTSD Checklist-5 (PCL-5): Scale and Scoring

Date: _____   Client: _____

The PTSD Checklist (PCL) was recently revised for the DSM-5 (this version is known as the PCL-5).

While this instrument alone is not sufficient to diagnose PTSD, it gives you a sense of whether an individual is experiencing PTSD symptoms and how severe his or her symptoms are.

For your purposes, add up your client's scores on the 20 items. If the total score is 38 or above, refer him or her for a PTSD assessment/evaluation, if needed, for confirmation of the diagnosis. You can track your client's scores by plotting them on the PCL graph at the end of this handout.

There are two versions of the PCL-5:

1. The PCL-5 Monthly is administered before the start of Session 1 of CPT. It uses the past *month* as the time frame reference. There is an alternative format of the PCL-5 Monthly, which may be used before the start of Session 1 in order to assess the Criterion A trauma in more depth (PCL-5 with a brief Criterion A assessment).

2. The PCL-5 Weekly is used during CPT for Session 2 and for all other sessions. Remind the client to use only the preceding *week* as the time frame for each item. Score it immediately upon receipt, and ask the client for any clarifications needed.

If the client's scores have not dropped significantly by Session 6, the therapist should explore whether the client is still avoiding affect, has been engaging in self-harm or other therapy-interfering behavior, or has not changed his or her assimilated beliefs about the traumatic event. Processing the lack of improvement with the client will be important at that point.

Please note: Several important revisions were made to the PCL in updating it for DSM-5. Changes involve the rating scale (now a 0–4 range for each symptom) and an increase from 17 to 20 items. This means that PCL-5 scores are *not* compatible with scores on versions of the PCL for DSM-IV (e.g., the PCL-S, which is in previous editions of the CPT manual), and that the PCL-5 cannot be used interchangeably with these earlier versions.

(continued)

PCL-5 WITH BRIEF CRITERION A ASSESSMENT: MONTHLY

Instructions: This questionnaire asks about problems you may have had after a very stressful experience involving *actual or threatened death, serious injury, or sexual violence.* It could be something that happened to you directly, something you witnessed, or something you learned happened to a close family member or close friend. Some examples are a *serious accident; fire; disaster such as a hurricane, tornado, or earthquake; physical or sexual attack or abuse; war; homicide; or suicide.*

First, please answer a few questions about your *worst event,* which for this questionnaire means the event that currently bothers you the most. This could be one of the examples above or some other very stressful experience. Also, it could be a single event (for example, a car crash) or multiple similar events (for example, multiple stressful events in a war zone or repeated sexual abuse).

Briefly identify the worst event (if you feel comfortable doing so):

How long ago did it happen?

Did it involve actual or threatened death, serious injury, or sexual violence?

☐ Yes

☐ No

How did you experience it?

☐ It happened to me directly

☐ I witnessed it

☐ I learned about it happening to a close family member or close friend

☐ I was repeatedly exposed to details about it as part of my job (for example, paramedic, police, military, or other first responder)

☐ Other (please describe) _____

If the event involved the death of a close family member or close friend, was it due to some kind of accident or violence, or was it due to natural causes?

☐ Accident or violence

☐ Natural causes

☐ Not applicable (the event did not involve the death of a close family member or close friend)

Second, keeping this worst event in mind, read each of the problems on the next page and then circle one of the numbers to the right to indicate how much you have been bothered by that problem *in the past month.*

(continued)

PCL-5: MONTHLY

Instructions: Below is a list of problems that people sometimes have in response to a very stressful experience. Please read each problem carefully, and then circle one of the numbers to the right to indicate how much you have been bothered by that problem *in the past month.*

In the past month, how much were you bothered by:	Not at all	A little bit	Moder-ately	Quite a bit	Extremely
1. Repeated, disturbing, and unwanted memories of the stressful experience?	0	1	2	3	4
2. Repeated, disturbing dreams of the stressful experience?	0	1	2	3	4
3. Suddenly feeling or acting as if the stressful experience were actually happening again *(as if you were actually back there reliving it)*?	0	1	2	3	4
4. Feeling very upset when something reminded you of the stressful experience?	0	1	2	3	4
5. Having strong physical reactions when something reminded you of the stressful experience *(for example, heart pounding, trouble breathing, sweating)*?	0	1	2	3	4
6. Avoiding memories, thoughts, or feelings related to the stressful experience?	0	1	2	3	4
7. Avoiding external reminders of the stressful experience *(for example, people, places, conversations, activities, objects, or situations)*?	0	1	2	3	4
8. Trouble remembering important parts of the stressful experience?	0	1	2	3	4

(continued)

In the past month, how much were you bothered by:	Not at all	A little bit	Moder-ately	Quite a bit	Extremely
9. Having strong negative beliefs about yourself, other people, or the world *(for example, having thoughts such as: I am bad, there is something seriously wrong with me, no one can be trusted, the world is completely dangerous)*?	0	1	2	3	4
10. Blaming yourself or someone else for the stressful experience or what happened after it?	0	1	2	3	4
11. Having strong negative feelings such as fear, horror, anger, guilt, or shame?	0	1	2	3	4
12. Loss of interest in activities that you used to enjoy?	0	1	2	3	4
13. Feeling distant or cut off from other people?	0	1	2	3	4
14. Trouble experiencing positive feelings *(for example, being unable to feel happiness or have loving feelings for people close to you)*?	0	1	2	3	4
15. Irritable behavior, angry outbursts, or acting aggressively?	0	1	2	3	4
16. Taking too many risks or doing things that could cause you harm?	0	1	2	3	4
17. Being "superalert" or watchful or on guard?	0	1	2	3	4
18. Feeling jumpy or easily startled?	0	1	2	3	4
19. Having difficulty concentrating?	0	1	2	3	4
20. Trouble falling or staying asleep?	0	1	2	3	4

(continued)

PCL-5: WEEKLY

Instructions: Below is a list of problems that people sometimes have in response to a very stressful experience. Please read each problem carefully, and then circle one of the numbers to the right to indicate how much you have been bothered by that problem *in the past week.*

In the past week, how much were you bothered by:	Not at all	A little bit	Moderately	Quite a bit	Extremely
1. Repeated, disturbing, and unwanted memories of the stressful experience?	0	1	2	3	4
2. Repeated, disturbing dreams of the stressful experience?	0	1	2	3	4
3. Suddenly feeling or acting as if the stressful experience were actually happening again *(as if you were actually back there reliving it)?*	0	1	2	3	4
4. Feeling very upset when something reminded you of the stressful experience?	0	1	2	3	4
5. Having strong physical reactions when something reminded you of the stressful experience *(for example, heart pounding, trouble breathing, sweating)?*	0	1	2	3	4
6. Avoiding memories, thoughts, or feelings related to the stressful experience?	0	1	2	3	4
7. Avoiding external reminders of the stressful experience *(for example, people, places, conversations, activities, objects, or situations)?*	0	1	2	3	4
8. Trouble remembering important parts of the stressful experience?	0	1	2	3	4

(continued)

In the past week, how much were you bothered by:	Not at all	A little bit	Moder-ately	Quite a bit	Extremely
9. Having strong negative beliefs about yourself, other people, or the world *(for example, having thoughts such as: I am bad, there is something seriously wrong with me, no one can be trusted, the world is completely dangerous)*?	0	1	2	3	4
10. Blaming yourself or someone else for the stressful experience or what happened after it?	0	1	2	3	4
11. Having strong negative feelings such as fear, horror, anger, guilt, or shame?	0	1	2	3	4
12. Loss of interest in activities that you used to enjoy?	0	1	2	3	4
13. Feeling distant or cut off from other people?	0	1	2	3	4
14. Trouble experiencing positive feelings *(for example, being unable to feel happiness or have loving feelings for people close to you)*?	0	1	2	3	4
15. Irritable behavior, angry outbursts, or acting aggressively?	0	1	2	3	4
16. Taking too many risks or doing things that could cause you harm?	0	1	2	3	4
17. Being "superalert" or watchful or on guard?	0	1	2	3	4
18. Feeling jumpy or easily startled?	0	1	2	3	4
19. Having difficulty concentrating?	0	1	2	3	4
20. Trouble falling or staying asleep?	0	1	2	3	4

(continued)

PCL-5 SCORE SHEET

PCL-5 Score

Session #

Patient Health Questionnaire–9 (PHQ-9): Scale and Scoring

Date: _____   Client: _____

Depressive symptom monitoring is optional in the CPT protocol, but it is encouraged when clients endorse depressive symptomatology. In that case, the PHQ-9 may be given every 2 weeks during the course of CPT to monitor depressive symptoms.

While this instrument alone is not sufficient to diagnose depressive disorders, it gives you a sense of whether an individual is experiencing depressive symptoms and how severe his or her symptoms are.

For your purposes, add up your client's scores on the 9 items provided below. The total score guidelines are as follows:

TOTAL SCORE DEPRESSION SEVERITY

Score	Depression severity
1–4	Minimal depression
5–9	Mild depression
10–14	Moderate depression
15–19	Moderately severe depression
20–27	Severe depression

There is one additional item at the end of the measure that assesses the impact of these symptoms on functioning.

Initial of Client's Last Name: _____

Therapist's Initials: _____   Date: _____   Session: ____

Format of CPT: ☐ Individual   ☐ Group   ☐ CPT-C   ☐ CPT

(continued)

PHQ-9

Over the last 2 weeks, how often have you been bothered by any of the following problems? Read each item carefully, and circle your response.

	Not at all	Several days	More than half the days	Nearly every day
1. Little interest or pleasure in doing things	0	1	2	3
2. Feeling down, depressed, or hopeless	0	1	2	3
3. Trouble falling asleep, staying asleep, or sleeping too much	0	1	2	3
4. Feeling tired or having little energy	0	1	2	3
5. Poor appetite or overeating	0	1	2	3
6. Feeling bad about yourself—or that you are a failure or have let yourself or your family down	0	1	2	3
7. Trouble concentrating on things, such as reading the newspaper or watching television	0	1	2	3
8. Moving or speaking so slowly that other people could have noticed— or the opposite: being so fidgety or restless that you have been moving around a lot more than usual	0	1	2	3
9. Thoughts that you would be better off dead or thoughts of hurting yourself in some way	0	1	2	3

If you checked off *any* problems, how *difficult* have these problems made it for you to do your work, take care of things at home, or get along with other people?

Not difficult at all	Somewhat difficult	Very difficult	Extremely difficult
☐	☐	☐	☐

4

Preparing to Deliver CPT

This chapter covers several different topics to consider in anticipation of implementing CPT. First, the introduction of CPT to clients to enhance their engagement in the therapy is discussed. Next, principles of Socratic dialogue—a cornerstone practice of CPT—are presented, along with types of Socratic questions a therapist might pose. The final section of the chapter discusses therapist readiness for CPT, as well as common errors and Stuck Points that may prevent therapists from using CPT, or doing so effectively.

Introducing CPT

The therapist should introduce and describe various treatments that have been found to be effective in the treatment of PTSD. If the therapist is not trained to implement a therapy that the client might be interested in pursuing, then a referral to a therapist trained in that type of treatment is in order. If clients choose CPT, they still need to decide whether they want to participate in CPT or CPT+A. At this writing, the only indicator for CPT+A is a client's also meeting criteria for the dissociative subtype of PTSD (Resick et al., 2013). As described earlier, writing the trauma accounts may help such a client put the fragmented trauma narrative into its proper historical context; may permit better examination of the facts, as well as of the assumptions that the client may have made; and may help ground the client in the trauma memories. Also, some people like to write and want to write their trauma accounts. Some of our clients have stated that having trauma accounts down on paper helped them look at their events more objectively and helped them accept that the events really happened. Others have flatly stated that if they had been asked to write their accounts, they would not have done the therapy.

Having a client choose which version of CPT to pursue is likely to result in better compliance than a therapist's making the decision. There are a few considerations to keep in mind, however. First, a client who decides to do CPT+A and write accounts of the index trauma should *not* be encouraged to change to CPT if the client avoids writing the accounts when the time comes. Reinforcing avoidance is always contraindicated. The client should give an oral account of the index trauma after the therapist discusses the problem of avoidance in maintaining PTSD symptoms. Once the client sees that he or she can give a verbal account of the event without falling apart, it then becomes easier to write an account for the next session.

If a client may only have time for a few sessions, then CPT may be the better choice, because self-reported PTSD symptoms have been shown to improve more immediately with CPT (by Session 4), whereas PTSD scores may not clinically improve in CPT+A until after the two trauma accounts are written and processed (by Session 6; Resick et al., 2008). If fewer sessions are available for treatment, the therapist should focus on the index trauma, assign the Impact Statement, and then use Socratic dialogue, along with the ABC Worksheets, to resolve the most problematic Stuck Points. The goal is to resolve the most pressing Stuck Points, most probably about erroneous self- or other-blame, and not to focus on overaccommodated Stuck Points.

The therapy that is chosen should be described, and any questions the client asks should be answered. Even if clients are not veterans, it may be helpful for them to view the introductory video that is available on the website of the National Center for PTSD (*www.va.ptsd.gov*). The video describes the symptoms of PTSD, and people with PTSD of different ages, genders, and ethnicities describe what it was like for them to have PTSD and how it affected their lives. The video also describes people's experiences in receiving CPT and how participating in CPT changed their lives for the better. Although couple therapy is beyond the scope of this book, there is a couple treatment for PTSD that includes elements of CPT and has been found to be effective (Monson & Fredman, 2012). Even within CPT, it might be helpful to have a session with a significant other and the client together, to explain the symptoms of PTSD, the course of treatment, and ways in which the significant other might help with rather than enable avoidance.

Although the standard course of CPT is established as a 12-session treatment, it is important not to assume that clients will need 12 sessions to ameliorate their PTSD and comorbid symptoms. In line with research discussed in Chapter 2 (Galovski et al., 2012), the therapist should state that the protocol was originally developed to be 12 sessions long, but that some people are able to recover more quickly, and others need a few more than 12 sessions. We do not yet know all the predictors of who might respond more quickly or take longer, but clients should be encouraged to attend all the sessions and to complete practice assignments to the best of their ability.

Once a client agrees to participate in CPT, the therapist and client should sign a therapy contract (see Handout 4.1). Although of course this contract is not legally binding, it can be a helpful agreement regarding the role of the therapist (i.e., to attend sessions on time and be prepared, to keep the session on track, and to monitor the client's progress toward improvement in the symptoms of PTSD and any comorbid disorders) and the role of the client (i.e., to attend sessions on time and be prepared, to participate in trauma-focused sessions, and to complete practice assignments). This contract can be a helpful reminder when the client wants to avoid or change topics.

Socratic Dialogue

A cornerstone practice in most cognitive therapies, including CPT, is Socratic dialogue. This practice involves the clinician's asking a series of questions designed to bring the client into a healthier appraisal of traumatic events and the effects of those traumatic events on here-and-now appraisals of situations. This practice is grounded in the Socratic method of learning, which values the power of individuals' coming to know something new for themselves versus being handed an insight or knowledge from another, as well as the benefits of modeling for clients a method of coming to know something (i.e., curiosity and inquisitiveness) (Anderson & Goolishian, 1992; Padesky, 1993; Thase & Beck, 1993). Like other clinicians and researchers (Rutter, Friedberg, VandeCreek, & Jackson, 1990; Bolten, 2001), we prefer the term "Socratic dialogue" over "Socratic questioning," because "dialogue" connotes that the client and the clinician, in a psychotherapy context, are in a fairly equally balanced exchange with one another. "Questioning," by contrast, suggests a power-imbalanced, teacher–student role in which the "teacher" asks questions of the "student," who needs to learn prescribed knowledge. In Socratic dialogue, the clinician and client are joined as a team: The client brings his or her life experiences, including traumatic experiences and interpretations of those experiences, and the clinician brings his or her expertise to bear on trauma recovery and cognitive interventions.

Various writers have offered different classes of questions that might be posed in Socratic dialogue (e.g., Paul & Elder, 2006; Elder & Paul, 1998; Bishop & Fish, 1999; Wright, Basco, & Thase, 2006). We offer a synthesis of these prior efforts, suggesting a hierarchical approach to the types of questions that a CPT therapist might pose in Socratic dialogue. Monson and Shnaider (2014) also provide an overview and types of Socratic questions that a therapist may pose specific to clients with PTSD.

Clarifying Questions

At the most foundational level, the therapist should be asking as many clarifying questions as possible, to set the stage of what was going on at the time of the index traumatic event and what choices and abilities the client actually had at the time, rather than what the client thought about later. It is extremely important for clinicians doing CPT to be willing to ask sensitive and difficult clarifying questions, and to ask them as nonjudgmentally and matter-of-factly as possible. An example from work with sexual assault/abuse victims is the ability to inquire whether they experienced sexual arousal during their assaults. The clients may have concluded that a sexual response during a traumatic event meant that they wanted to be assaulted or were in some way responsible for the assault. Sometimes differentiating arousal from pleasure can be helpful with rape victims. However, childhood sexual abuse survivors commonly remark that there were pleasurable aspects of their assaults (e.g., feeling "special" or more connected to their perpetrators). For such clients' benefit, it is important to be able to ask these types of questions and discuss the answers as matter-of-factly and supportively as possible to promote recovery. Another example comes from work with veterans, police officers, and other security personnel, who may have experienced positive emotions at the time of committing an act of violence against another. In hindsight, they may have deduced that these positive emotions indicated something negative about their characters (e.g., "What kind of person enjoys killing another person?"), and may not have appreciated the context of the event and the psychophysiological reactions involved in a stressful event.

Challenging Assumptions

At the next level are questions aimed at challenging the assumptions that underlie clients' conclusions about traumatic events. As mentioned in Chapter 3 and discussed in more detail elsewhere, a key assumption held by individuals with PTSD that should be challenged is the "just-world belief" (Lerner, 1980). The just-world belief holds that good things happen to good people, that bad things happen to bad people, and that the world *should* be a fair and just place. This belief emanates from the desire to find an orderly, cause–effect association between an individual's behavior and the consequences of that behavior. In the case of traumatic events, which are construed as bad things, those with PTSD will assume that they did something bad to deserve them and will persist in trying to find the prior bad behavior or bad behavior within the traumatic event that accounts for the bad outcome. It is important to point out that some individuals may not subscribe to the just-world belief (because of their learning history, culture, religiosity, etc.). In these cases, there is no need to push the notion of the desire for a just world. Taking out the notion of justice or fairness, the therapist can describe this desire as a hard-wired, evolutionary need of humans to predict and control events in order to survive. Stressing the universality of this desire, together with the inability to predict and control everything, is most applicable to these cases.

A common overarching assumption that individuals with PTSD make when appraising traumatic events is that they or someone else could have exerted more control over these events or their outcomes. This assumption is evidenced in clients' efforts to exert hindsight bias: "If I had turned left instead of right, I wouldn't have had the accident," "If I'd fought back, I wouldn't have been assaulted," or "I should have jumped into the water after him." Individuals with PTSD fail to appreciate that an alternative action may have had an equally negative or worse consequence. In this way, clients are trying to "undo" negative outcomes through their thinking.

In challenging assumptions, it is important for CPT clinicians not to make their own erroneous assumptions about the contexts surrounding traumatic events. We have observed therapists who assume positive intentions on the part of their clients, leaving their clients reluctant to describe actions, thoughts, or feelings about the traumatic events that they believe might be perceived as running contrary to the therapists' positive assumptions about the event. For example, a service member or police officer might not have followed the rules of engagement that he or she was supposed to follow. If the therapist too quickly assumes that appropriate procedures were followed, the client may be reluctant to disclose the reality of the traumatic event or may feel increasingly worse that he or she did not follow the rules, because the therapist assumes otherwise.

Conversely, we have supervised therapists who made negative assumptions about their clients' behavior, and thus inadvertently blocked the clients' progress in therapy. We understand this tendency, because we all live in a victim-blaming culture, which results from our own desire to predict and control events and to keep others and ourselves safe. However, this type of thinking can be an impediment to processing clients' traumatic events. A common example is that blame should be allocated if a victim consumed substances prior to a traumatic event. Substance use may or may not play a role in traumatic events; it is only with careful consideration of the amount of use, the context, and the client's intentions that the therapist and client can better assess the role of substance use in the event, which ultimately facilitates processing of the traumatic event as a whole. In the case of sexual assault, no amount of substance consumption should result in victim blaming. In fact, the perpetrator may have been that much more predatory in observing a victim who consumed more of a substance. Risky substance-using behavior may need to be addressed in therapy, but later in the CPT protocol (i.e., during the Safety module), when substance misuse should be decreased as an avoidance behavior to increase risk reduction and when the client has effectively dealt with the assimilated belief that "I am responsible [vs. the perpetrator] for the traumatic event because I used substances." If you bring up risk reduction too soon, the client may assume you are blaming him or her.

Evaluating Objective Evidence

Assuming that there are no problematic assumptions underlying clients' conclusions, the next level of Socratic dialogue that we recommend is aimed at helping clients evaluate evidence that may or may not support the conclusions they have drawn. Individuals with PTSD have a cognitive bias toward perceived threat in particular and negative information more generally. Thus clients will have this type of information more readily accessible to them and may overvalue this information relative to data that do not necessarily support their conclusions. A client's overestimation of here-and-now danger is a common example of a PTSD-related thought for which a therapist might use Socratic dialogue focused on evaluating objective evidence for the thought. The overestimation of threat in situations such as being in a crowd, being in open spaces, being in cramped spaces, driving motor vehicles, and being around individuals who resemble perpetrators are examples of situations for which a CPT therapist is likely to encourage clients to evaluate data more objectively.

Challenging Underlying or Core Beliefs

There are times when clients will report that they intellectually understand, but do not emotionally appreciate, that their thinking does not make sense, or will say that emotional changes are not occurring with their new thoughts. Typical statements include "I hear what you are saying, but . . . , " "I know what I am saying doesn't make sense, but it feels that way," or "I do the worksheets on my Stuck Points, but I don't really believe them." On these occasions, we explain to clients first that their emotions may not have caught up with a new way of thinking, so the old way of thinking may seem more "real." We also encourage therapists to consider the possibility that their clients are holding deeper underlying beliefs that may be preventing them from fully embracing alternative ways of thinking. Deeper beliefs often protect clients against the implications involved in changing their thoughts. For example, if a trauma survivor truly embraces the thought that he or she could not have done anything more to prevent the traumatic event from happening, there is the implication that the client could be placed in a traumatic situation in the future in which he or she may or may not be able to change the outcome.

One of us had a client who was a childhood sexual abuse survivor, who was reluctant to change her belief that her father was not at fault for her abuse. The deeper implication of changing this belief was that it would have a negative effect on the relationship she had maintained with her father over the years. In essence, changes in appraisals about traumatic events have cascading implications for both here-and-now and future-oriented beliefs. In this case, the new appraisal was incongruent with the desire to retain the belief that the future is predictable and controllable.

Deeper cognitive intervention may also be necessary when individuals with PTSD have preexisting core negative beliefs or schemas. These preexisting beliefs may serve as risk factors for the occurrence of PTSD upon exposure to a traumatic event. In these cases, the cognitive therapist will likely need to probe more deeply to determine how the client came to these beliefs prior to the trauma (e.g., aversive childhood experiences, invalidating environments), and to work collaboratively with the client to challenge these deeper or core beliefs in order to prevent the client from making trauma appraisals that seem to confirm the negative belief. For instance, if clients have a preexisting schema that they cannot trust their judgment, they are likely to view the traumatic event as confirmative of that schema and to engage in self-blaming appraisals. Changing self-blame appraisals about the trauma runs contrary to the deeper negative belief, often necessitating more cognitive intervention with this core schema to engender emotional and behavioral change. However, a core belief often needs to be changed through having a client complete worksheets every time the belief emerges, because it is difficult to challenge a large belief in the abstract. If there are many examples that disconfirm the underlying belief (e.g., "I am a failure"), then the core belief finally falls under the weight of the opposing evidence on specific examples.

Therapist Readiness

A therapist who is uncertain about using a manualized treatment, cognitive therapy, or structured sessions may intentionally or unintentionally send messages to the client that the client is not ready for CPT, even when the evidence suggests otherwise. We have met many therapists who have told clients they should not do CPT or were not ready for CPT, even when the clients were asking to start the therapy. This can send a message to clients that their therapists do not have faith in them and do not trust the clients' judgment. If the clients must then wait through months of another form of therapy, they may begin to believe that they are too fragile to handle even thinking about their trauma, and that they will "fall apart" if they even minimally talk about the thoughts associated with their traumatic events. We describe this as "fragilizing" clients, which is just as problematic as pushing clients when they are not ready to do trauma-focused therapy. Adding sessions of some other type of therapy can actually do more harm than good for the clients and can lead them to feel disempowered.

Another reason why many therapists do not start clients in CPT may be their own confusion about the role of emotions in CPT. Some therapists were taught, and believe, that clients must fully express all their emotions in session in order to process the trauma. Thus they believe that if the clients are not prepared to cry and grieve outwardly in sessions, they cannot handle CPT. One problem with this belief is the assumption that reliving the emotions tied to an event is necessary to get better. We now know that for many people the emotions related to the trauma have become confused because of their inappropriate self-blaming for the event, which has led to great guilt and shame. In these cases, the clients probably need to spend more time thinking about the messages they are giving themselves about the event that are leading to these painful emotions. An additional problem with this belief is that it assumes that all people process their emotions in the same way, and that outward displays of emotion are required to help clients resolve their feelings about trauma. In fact, many people do not cry when experiencing sadness, but this does not mean that they are not feeling their emotions.

Some therapists are also concerned that if clients show strong emotions in response to their traumatic material, then the therapists are "retraumatizing" the clients. It is important to distinguish between the healthy processing of natural emotions that occurs in CPT and the triggering of PTSD symptoms that can happen daily in clients' lives. In fact, helping the clients understand that they relive the trauma almost every day through the reexperiencing of symptoms, and that addressing the traumatic memories on the clients' own terms (instead of in response to triggers) will actually allow the clients to process their emotions in a safe and healthy manner that allows them to gain control over the triggers. This discussion is one way a therapist can actually encourage a client to participate in CPT if the client is avoidant or skeptical.

Another concern for some therapists is their own reluctance to hear trauma stories in sessions. For example, when a client shows any emotion, a therapist will interrupt the story. This can send a variety of messages to the client: (1) The client should not talk about the trauma; (2) the therapist cannot handle hearing about the client's trauma; (3) the therapist believes that the client is too fragile to talk about the traumatic event; and/ or (4) nightmares and flashbacks should be feared and pushed away. Although perhaps such messages are unintentional, they can all significantly delay the client's recovery. We instead recommend letting clients decide whether they are ready to talk about their trauma, and to let them choose when they start CPT and which version of CPT they engage in (CPT or CPT+A). This empowers the clients and helps them realize they have can have control over both the course of therapy and the trauma memories. If clients are not ready to do trauma work, we do not do "filler" therapy, but ask them to come back when they are ready to work on their PTSD and approach their memories. In addition, we encourage clients to fully experience their nightmares, flashbacks, and intrusive memories, because postponing them only ensures that they will come back again.

We have identified several "therapist Stuck Points" that we recommend reviewing prior to starting CPT (see the discussion below). If therapists find themselves endorsing any of these, we encourage them to use a Challenging Beliefs Worksheet to challenge their own Stuck Points. This will not only help therapists challenge these thoughts, but also help them practice using this worksheet before seeing their first CPT clients.

Therapist Issues: Therapist Errors and Stuck Points

Common Therapist Errors

One of the biggest therapist errors is being poorly prepared to do CPT. Aside from reading this book (in the order in which it is written), we recommend attending a workshop with a qualified CPT trainer, followed by 6 months of case consultation with a qualified consultant. Our website (*www.guilford.com/cpt-ptsd*) includes an email for which we can be contacted about trainers if you or an agency want to sponsor a workshop. There is also a section on the website that lists open workshops. In addition, a free training website, CPT*web* (*https://cpt.musc.edu*), not only reviews the protocol (CPT+A), but also has video examples of each session. This website is designed to be a refresher training and not a stand-alone training.

The CPT protocol should be conducted in the order outlined in the manual (Chapters 5–10 of this book), without adding other skills during treatment. Some common errors therapists make are picking out some components of the therapy and using just those; thinking that they must change the protocol in order to show their creativity; or assuming that CPT must be changed for their clinical populations without trying it as presented in the manual first. CPT was first developed almost three decades ago and has been tested across trauma types and populations, from North America to Third

World countries. Trained and skilled CPT therapists have modified it in collaboration with us over the past decade for particular circumstances, such as brain injury, low literacy, or cross-cultural and language issues; some of these circumstances are discussed in Chapters 13 and 14. We believe there is no reason for therapists new to CPT to modify it without having mastered the existing protocol. CPT has a great deal of flexibility already built into it to adapt it to particular cognitions and different types of traumatic events. If it is modified without testing, then it is not CPT and not an evidence-based therapy.

Probably the most common therapist error in conducting the CPT protocol is trying to convince clients to change their minds about their Stuck Points, rather than using Socratic dialogue to draw out the information and allow them to realize that they keep coming back to their trauma because their assumptions are in conflict with other information that they have within them. Thinking of things they could (should) have done months or years after an event does not change the fact that they didn't have that knowledge or perhaps the necessary skills at the time. The clients may be ignoring facts that don't fit their assumptions, but they do have those facts, and the therapists need to draw them from the clients (e.g., "How big were you? How big was your uncle? Could you really have fought him off? If he threatened your family if you told anyone, did you have another option?"). If a therapist takes one side of the conflict and tries to convince a client that the traumatic event was not his or her fault, the client is likely to become even more rigid in arguing for the other side and tell the therapist, "You just don't understand," "You weren't there," or the like. If the client says, "You don't understand," it is the therapist's responsibility to say, "You are right. I don't. Please tell me what I am missing." It is a good reminder to return to asking questions in a gentle, clarifying manner. The style of the therapist should be curious and even puzzled, but not argumentative or challenging. (A therapist is not a cross-examining attorney!)

Yet another common therapist error is for a therapist to jump to challenging questions (i.e., challenging the evidence; see above) before asking enough clarifying questions. Even if the client writes trauma accounts (see Chapter 11), there may be important information about the context of the situation that is missing and that the therapist needs to know in order to guide the dialogue. When doing CPT, a therapist needs to ask many clarifying questions to understand the context and the actual options the client had. For example, if a man could not save a loved one in a fire, the therapist could ask him where he was and how far away he was when he realized that the house was on fire. How many seconds/minutes did it take for him to realize what was going on and that someone was trapped? What did he do (e.g., did he call the fire department or try to go upstairs)? And what couldn't he do (e.g., was he driven back by the flames and smoke)? The therapist could ask what kind of firefighting equipment he had (e.g., mask, fire-retardant suit) to help him see that he couldn't have done more in that situation. How long did it take for the firefighters to arrive? If they came quickly, then the therapist can ask why the firefighters could not save the person either (or the doctors). If the client has been using the term "blame" or "fault," the therapist can ask him about his intent in the situation. In fact, this man may have been very brave in his attempts to save the other person, which is the opposite of the intention for the person to die.

Because Socratic dialogue early in therapy is entirely verbal and takes place within sessions, with some use of the ABC Worksheets, the therapist should be modeling the questions that will soon be introduced in the Challenging Questions Worksheet. However, while the client is processing the trauma, the therapist will be using more clarifying questions to understand the context of the trauma better and to help the client see how important the context was (e.g., how young the client was, how quickly the event happened, how the client was too surprised to orient quickly to the situation, what options the client actually had and could consider during the event, how the client could not do the impossible). A good expectation is for about 80–90% of the questions in Socratic dialogue to be clarifying questions.

Another common error is for a therapist to stop short and not continue to track through a client's reasoning. Beginning CPT therapists may ask a question about a Stuck Point, get an answer, and then stop or change the subject. They do not know where to go next. Therapists who have been taught not to ask questions in therapy sometimes feel uncomfortable about probing into the facts and their clients' reasoning. The answer to one question should lead naturally to the next, to establish the context of the trauma, what options a client actually had at the time, and (if the client had options at all) why he or she chose a particular one. It has been our experience that, given the brief time that they had to choose, most clients had no good choice, chose the option they perceived to be the least damaging, or had to follow orders or procedures.

If clarifying questions are asked in the spirit of constructive curiosity—that is, trying to understand what happened and how the client came to make the assumptions that have led to ongoing PTSD—there is no question that is off limits. For example, if a male victim of child sexual abuse has a Stuck Point that there must have been something about him that made the perpetrator choose him, there are many questions that could be asked. The following example includes clarifying questions, some education, and summary statements.

THERAPIST: Did [the perpetrator] have access to you when no one else was around?

CLIENT: Yes, but why did he do that to me? Did he think I was a pervert?

THERAPIST: Did he say you were a pervert?

CLIENT: No, he didn't say much.

THERAPIST: Where did the idea come from that he must have thought you were a pervert?

CLIENT: Can I tell you something?

THERAPIST: Of course. You can tell me anything.

CLIENT: I was aroused when he fondled me, so that must mean I am a pervert. I can't believe I was aroused.

THERAPIST: So it was your thought that you were a pervert? Let me explain something to you that may be helpful. When your genitals are stimulated, they have nerve endings that respond whether you want them to or not. It is like being tickled. You react automatically, and if the person doesn't stop or you don't want him to do it, it isn't always pleasant. There is a difference between arousal and enjoyment. Did you always enjoy what he was doing to you?

CLIENT: *No!* I hated it. I felt dirty, but I was just a kid. Sometimes it felt OK, but other times he made me do things that made me feel out of control.

THERAPIST: Do you happen to know the age of consent for sex? How old does someone have to be before they can choose to have sex with an adult and it isn't a crime?

CLIENT: When you are an adult?

THERAPIST: Right. So even if he was making you feel good, which might have happened sometimes, he was committing a crime against you because you were too young to consent. In light of that, who would you say is the pervert?

CLIENT: He was. Not me.

THERAPIST: And I think you said it clearly—he *made* you do things.

CLIENT: But why did he choose me? Was there something about me?

THERAPIST: How about convenience? And do you know whether you were the only one he chose?

A note at this point: Some Stuck Points are so entrenched in some clients' thinking that the clients may not answer questions or will appear to be particularly stubborn about insisting that it must be their fault or erroneously blaming others. First, therapists should remember that Socratic dialogue begins early in the therapy, and that all Stuck Points do not have to be resolved the first time they are broached. If a Stuck Point seems particularly rigid, it is possible that a client may not want to accept that the event happened and is clinging to the Stuck Point in the attempt to deny it after the fact. This is a type of avoidance. It is also possible that the client is protecting a tougher Stuck Point or a core belief that is accepted as fact, as discussed above. If the client appears to be particularly resistant to a particular Stuck Point, the therapist can say something like this: "This idea seems very important to you. I think we will be spending more time on it in therapy."

A further therapist error is jumping from one Stuck Point to another. It is common for clients to use other Stuck Points as evidence for the Stuck Point being worked on, but it is an error for a therapist to start chasing after different Stuck Points without finishing the processing of the first one. The correct response would be to say, "That sounds like another thought, not a fact. Let's get that down on your Stuck Point Log and get back to that one later." Using the worksheets consistently also helps, because the therapist can redirect the client to the thought in column B of the ABC Worksheet, or have the client write a new ABC Worksheet so that the Stuck Point is right in front of him or her (see Chapter 6).

It is also possible that in CPT, therapists may not give enough time for clients to feel their natural emotions because of their emphasis on cognition-based emotions. When a client experiences a natural emotion such as sadness, or relives the genuine fear the client had at the time of the traumatic event, or reexperiences helplessness with the realization that there was nothing the client could have done to stop the event, the therapist should just sit quietly at first and allow the client to experience that emotion. The therapist should then use strategies to amplify the natural emotion by asking the client to name the emotion, asking what physical sensations the client is feeling, or validating the natural emotion (e.g., "It is understandable that you feel sad at the loss of your friends"). Natural emotions can be experienced more subtly than the manufactured emotions that are fueled by cognitions; therapists may forget to look for the natural emotions in pursuit of cognitive change.

Most emotions can be either natural or manufactured. Anger can be a natural emotion if a client is angry at someone who intended to harm him or her. However, if the client is angry at someone who had no control over the situation or did not even know that it occurred, then this is a cognition-based anger, and hence manufactured. Anger can also be used as an avoidance strategy to push people, including the therapist, away. Anger may also be the "go-to" emotion for avoiding more painful and vulnerable emotions (e.g., sadness, fear). A client may experience disgust at what he or she was forced to do during a sexual assault, and that disgust would be a natural emotion. However, if the client says afterward, "I am disgusting because of what happened to me," this is a self-evaluation of the client as a person and is based on his or her conclusions, not on the event itself.

If the therapist does not know whether an emotion is natural or manufactured by thoughts, it is perfectly acceptable to ask about it. In the case of the client just above, for instance, the therapist can ask, "Why do you feel disgust?" If the client says, "Because what [the perpetrator] did to me was disgusting," the therapist should agree with that statement. However, if the client says, "Because now I am permanently damaged and soiled," the therapist can ask a series of questions about who committed the act, the permanence of the effect (e.g., "Do you know how many times your skin has been completely replaced since it happened? Did you know there is not a single spot on your body at this point, inside or out, that [the perpetrator] has touched?"), or whether feeling dirty is a form of emotional reasoning (e.g., "I feel dirty; therefore I am dirty"). It is also helpful to capture this statement in the moment and add it to the Stuck Point Log for further challenging later.

A final common error is not selecting the appropriate index traumatic event to begin the therapy. As discussed in Chapter 3, a therapist should not ask which event is worst, most upsetting, or most disturbing, because doing so could lead to an event that is not even one that would be included in the PTSD diagnosis (e.g., a job loss, a divorce). A better approach is to ask which of the identified traumatic events haunts the client's dreams the most, which one keeps coming back in intrusions, or which one the client tries hardest to avoid thinking about. Some clients may say that a series of events are all similarly distressing, such as combat, sexual abuse, or domestic violence experiences. A therapist error in this case would be to ask the client to consider them all as a group or to write an Impact Statement (see Chapter 5) about the whole series of events. The problem with this approach is that the discussion and Socratic dialogue can quickly become too vague. The client may jump from event to event. It is worthwhile to spend a few minutes to determine whether one event stands out more than the others in memory or intrusions (e.g., first penetration, best buddy being killed in combat, realizing that one's children knew about the abuse or were abused themselves). If the client continues to say that all of the events are equally distressing, or that there are too many to choose from, then the therapist should start with the client's earliest PTSD Criterion A experience. It is likely that the assumptions the client made about the event or the conclusions he or she drew about the self and the world were repeated and reinforced with further traumatic events. For example, a male combat veteran might announce that people can't be trusted, even though the traumatic event he has selected was being shot in combat. Unless someone he trusted betrayed him, there should not be an effect on trust. The person who shot him was a stranger and did not pick him personally. There may have been an earlier traumatic event (perhaps in childhood) that resulted in a betrayal of trust, and the later shooting may have activated the schema.

Therapist Stuck Points

It is not only clients who have Stuck Points; we can all have Stuck Points in our lives, and therapists can certainly encounter them in treating those with PTSD. Therapists can have Stuck Points about themselves as therapists, the approaches they have been taught and have adhered to, or their own fear about trying a new approach (e.g., "Does this mean you are saying I have been doing the wrong thing all this time?"). Therapist Stuck Points may prevent a therapist from trying CPT at all or may affect the course of a client's treatment.

Pretreatment Therapist Stuck Points

Therapist Stuck Points prior to delivering CPT are common, and probably indicate that a therapist is unaware of the research on CPT. In particular, the therapist may not realize that the participants in CPT research have been very similar to those who are treated in general clinical practice (indeed, many cases may have been even more complex). Examples of these Stuck Points and evidence challenging them are presented here.

• *"My client is not ready for trauma-focused therapy."* There is actually an accumulating body of research indicating that clients do not need to be prepared to cope with trauma-focused treatment (e.g., Resick, Bovin, et al., 2012; Resick et al., 2014). Most of the research on CPT for PTSD has started with trauma-focused treatment immediately and has not prepared the clients with coping skills or other preparatory work. In fact, delaying treatment for "stabilization" sends the message that the clients cannot handle the work or that it is too dangerous (i.e., "fragilization," as described earlier). It is important to remember that clients with PTSD have been living with their memories of the traumatic events for years, and doing trauma-focused therapy allows them to take control of when and how they think about the trauma.

- *"My clients' cases are more complex than those of participants in research projects."* As reviewed in earlier chapters, CPT studies, unlike some PTSD treatment studies, have not excluded potential participants because they have comorbid depression, anxiety disorders, personality disorders, or even dissociative disorders. The inclusion of individuals with substance use disorders has been modified over time. Studies of CPT have never excluded people who abuse substances, but earlier studies might have made them wait if they had physiological dependence. Some recent studies have not excluded clients with any kind of substance use disorder. CPT research projects also include clients with suicidal ideation and only exclude them if they are threatening imminent harm to self or others and need hospitalization.

- *"My client is too fragile for trauma-focused treatment."* Akin to the Stuck Point above about a client's not being ready for CPT, this therapist Stuck Point indicates that the therapist is nervous about the possibility that the client may get worse. A recent study (Bryan et al., 2016) examined whether CPT increased suicidal ideation among active-duty military personnel. The researchers found that in fact suicidal ideation decreased over time, and that there were no suicide attempts during or following CPT. This question has also been investigated in regard to PE (see Chapter 2), another trauma-focused therapy that requires clients to reexperience their index trauma over and over with the aim of habituation. Across a number of studies, PE researchers found that clients did not worsen as a result of trauma-focused treatment (Jayawickreme et al., 2014).

- *"If I use a manual, it will stifle my creativity and interfere with rapport,"* or *"Manuals are too restrictive."* It is unrealistic to expect that a new therapy be created for every client. Of course, CPT looks different across different clients, based on individual case conceptualizations and different client–therapist relationships. It is our experience, however, that rapport comes immediately and naturally with the therapist's rapt attention and interest in what the client thinks about the index traumatic event. Many clients have had the experience of prior therapy in which the therapist avoided talking about PTSD or traumatic events, so the fact that the therapist is interested in how the client uniquely thinks and feels about the trauma is an immediate rapport builder.

- *"CPT won't work with comorbidities (depression, substance abuse, personality disorders)."* Please see Chapter 2 for evidence contrary to this Stuck Point.

- *"Clients won't do this amount of homework."* Whether a client completes worksheets during CPT (and, if so, how many) depends on how well the therapist sets the stage for the out-of-session work. This issue is addressed in more detail in Chapter 5.

Some clients do not do as much practice as others, but this should be discussed in the context of avoidance, as well as the importance of practice in learning a new skill—a new way to think.

Therapist Stuck Points Regarding Assessment and Treatment in General

• *"It will take too long to assess the client regularly."* The PCL-5 and the PHQ-9 take about 5 minutes each to administer. It is possible to ask the client to come to the therapy session 10 minutes early, so that he or she can complete the assessment scale(s) before starting the session. If the therapist has a receptionist, that person can give the client the measure(s) on a clipboard, much like the forms one completes at a physician's office. An envelope can be left in the waiting room for the client with the measures if there is no receptionist. At the beginning of the session, the therapist can quickly score the instruments and note whether the scores indicate stability, worsening, or improvement in symptoms. If the scores are worsening, the therapist needs to determine whether the client was rating a different event, whether the client is using the scale as a general distress measure for current events, whether the client is using the wrong time frame (i.e., not just the past week), or whether the scores are truly worsening. It is possible that as the client stops avoiding thinking about the traumatic event, he or she may have a temporary increase in scores because of greater intrusive memories, nightmares, and negative emotions, as well as the emergence of Stuck Points. If this is the case, the client should be reassured: "This is actually a good sign that you are not avoiding thinking about the event, as you have done ever since the trauma, and that your brain is getting you to face the event."

• *"If the client's PTSD scores are not decreasing, this means . . . [e.g., I am doing CPT wrong, I am a bad therapist, etc.]."* It is important that the therapist not take it personally if the client's scores are not decreasing. Some therapists avoid doing assessment during treatment for this exact reason: They are focusing on themselves and their own insecurities, rather than on the progress of their clients. As the CPT manual (Chapters 5–10) indicates, there are many reasons why a client's scores may not be decreasing, especially early in therapy. The client may not be doing the practice assignments, may be canceling sessions frequently, or may be working on the wrong traumatic event first. Or the client may not have told the therapist what the real index event is, due to avoidance or shame. A lack of reduction in symptoms should indicate to the therapist that it is time to stop and ask the client what is going on or to recalibrate the assessment.

• *"If the client's scores are not decreasing, I need to change the therapy."* As reviewed in Chapters 3 and 11, clients who do not complete their recovery in 12 sessions are likely to do so by continuing to use CPT with the Stuck Point Log and Challenging Beliefs Worksheets. Changing to a different type of therapy may be quite confusing to a client, especially if the underpinnings of the new therapy are quite different from those of CPT. The therapist may want to seek consultation, but should probably stay the course and go back to check the content of the client's flashbacks, intrusive recollections, and nightmares, as well as to see what the client is still avoiding. The thoughts about the avoided memories or reminders of the trauma may be Stuck Points that have not yet been dealt with thoroughly.

- *"If I interrupt, I will offend my client," "If I don't listen to everything my clients say, I will invalidate them,"* or *"If I address avoidance, I will damage our relationship."* These Stuck Points are variations on a theme: A therapist is concerned about what a client thinks of the therapist and worries that the therapist will somehow offend the client. Some therapists have been taught to reflect or provide interpretations, never to interrupt clients, or to allow clients to talk about whatever they want in therapy. In CPT, a therapist allowing this to happen would be considered to be colluding with avoidance, and so these beliefs are antithetical to the principles of CPT. It is typical for clients to come to therapy sessions and announce they want to talk about something else that session, take the floor, and begin storytelling that lasts much of the session. They may try other ways to get the topic away from the assignments for that session or away from the index trauma. All of this is avoidance, and it is important for the therapist not to contribute to such avoidance.

The therapist may need to set some ground rules about digressions and avoidance early in treatment. For instance, because there is a lot to cover in each session, the therapist may either interrupt verbally or give some nonverbal sign (e.g., a hand up like a stop sign, or a "T" for "time out") to get the session back on track. The therapist can set these ground rules gently but firmly, so that sessions do not become 2 hours long. It is quite possible to achieve all the goals for each session within 50–60 minutes, but not if the therapist has one of these Stuck Points. A review of the treatment rationale with the client will demonstrate why bringing the client back to the content of the session is neither rude nor invalidating, but is in the best interests of the client's treatment.

CPT-Specific Therapist Stuck Points

- *"I can't get through the material for the session."* Experienced CPT therapists are able to get through the material prescribed in each session, so this is likely to be a Stuck Point held by a therapist who is new to CPT. It is not necessary to go through every worksheet the client has completed in detail during the session. The therapist and client can look at the worksheets generally, and the therapist can see whether the client has had problems completing them or understands the concepts. They may pick out one or two important ones to focus on, particularly those regarding the most important assimilated Stuck Points, worksheets the client struggled with, or those on one of the themes being covered during the second half of treatment.

- *"We can't move on if the client has not mastered the material,"* or *"Everything [handouts, sessions, etc.] has to be perfect."* We have sometimes consulted with therapists who kept assigning ABC Worksheets over and over as assignments and did not move on to the Challenging Questions Worksheet because they were not sure that their clients could label their emotions accurately or the clients had trouble getting their thoughts into good Stuck Point form. The purpose of these sequential assignments is to get to the Challenging Belief Worksheet as soon as possible, because it includes alternative, more balanced, and more fact-based statements to counter the Stuck Points. The Challenging Belief Worksheet includes the ABC Worksheet, so the client will have many opportunities to learn how to differentiate facts from thoughts and how thoughts lead to specific emotions. Perfection is not a goal for therapists any more than it is for clients. As we have emphasized throughout this chapter, we encourage therapists to stay consistent with the CPT manual.

- *"If I have the manual out, I look incompetent."* We advise therapists to keep their manuals on their laps or on the edge of the desk in front of them, just as the clients have their binders for therapy materials out. We have never heard of a client's complaining if a therapist says, "I am going to leave the manual open to refer to it, so that I don't miss anything we need to cover in this session. I want to give you the best possible therapy."

- *"I can't make the client choose one trauma."* It is important to validate that all of a client's traumatic events are important, but to make it clear that it is best to start treatment with the one that currently causes the most PTSD symptoms. After the initial sessions, the client can weave any other traumas into the therapy with extra worksheets. Trying to process all the traumatic events at once is going to end up being too vague for challenging Stuck Points, and it is likely that many of the traumatic events resulted in similar Stuck Points.

- *"I won't know where to go with the client's Stuck Points."* This is a common concern by therapists who are new to CPT and have not yet mastered Socratic dialogue. Instead of worrying about what to ask next, a therapist should listen to what the client is saying, notice what does not make sense (e.g., "How could the client have been in two places at once?" or "How could a 6-year-old understand what was unacceptable adult behavior?"). An obvious place to start is to wonder about the client's intention in that situation and the client's expectations based on his or her prior experience. The therapist can then focus on finding out more about the actual context of the situation and what options the client realistically had under those circumstances. This therapist Stuck Point reflects anxiety and self-focus, and the solution is to focus on what the client was thinking, feeling, and doing during the index trauma.

- *"If we don't do the written account/exposure, the client can't get better."* This last Stuck Point stems from a common belief underlying the proliferation of exposure research that began the field of PTSD—namely, that it is necessary to have clients reexperience their traumatic events as a necessary component of treatment. The Resick et al. (2008) dismantling study of CPT reviewed in Chapter 2 demonstrated that CPT+A did not improve the outcomes of therapy, and, in fact, slowed the progress of achieving a clinically significant improvement. Schumm et al. (2015) have also demonstrated that changes in cognitions predict changes in PTSD symptoms.

Cognitive Processing Therapy
for Posttraumatic Stress Disorder: Contract

Date: _____   Client: _____

What is cognitive processing therapy?

Cognitive processing therapy (CPT) is a cognitive-behavioral treatment for posttraumatic stress disorder (PTSD) and related problems.

What are the goals of CPT?

The overall goals of CPT are to improve your PTSD symptoms, and any associated symptoms you may have (such as depression, anxiety, guilt, or shame). It also aims to improve your day-to-day living.

What will CPT in this clinic consist of?

CPT in this clinic consists of 6–24 individual (one-on-one) therapy sessions; the average is 12. Each session lasts 50–60 minutes. In these sessions, you will learn about the symptoms of PTSD and the reasons why some people develop it.

You and your therapist will also identify and explore how your trauma or traumas have changed your thoughts and beliefs, and how some of these ways of thinking may keep you "stuck" in your symptoms. CPT does not involve repeatedly reviewing the details of your trauma(s). However, you will be asked to examine your experiences in order to understand how they have affected your thoughts, feelings, and behaviors.

What is expected of me in CPT?

Perhaps the most important expectation of CPT is for you to make a commitment to come to sessions.

In addition, after each session you will be given practice assignments to complete outside the sessions. These assignments are designed to improve your PTSD symptoms more rapidly outside the treatment sessions. You are also encouraged to ask any questions that you might have at any point in doing CPT.

(continued)

What can I expect from my CPT therapist?

At each session, your therapist will help you figure out how your trauma has affected your thoughts and emotions, and help you make changes to feel better and function better.

In order to do this, your therapist will review your practice assignments and share what he or she notices about your trauma-related thoughts, feelings, and behaviors. Your therapist will ask questions to examine what you have been thinking about your trauma(s) and their effects on your life, and will help you to challenge thoughts that might be inaccurate. Your therapist will also teach you skills to change the way you think about events and about yourself and others. Another part of your therapist's job is to notice and point out when you are avoiding working on the trauma, even when you may not notice that you are doing it. Avoidance is a key PTSD symptom that keeps you stuck in nonrecovery.

Can I choose to stop this therapy?

Your decision to do CPT is voluntary. Therefore, you may choose to stop the treatment at any time. If this should happen, you will be asked to come in for one final session to discuss your concerns before terminating.

With my signature, I am indicating that I have reviewed these materials and received information about CPT for PTSD. I commit optimistically to myself, to this treatment, and to the goals listed above. I will receive a copy of this agreement.

_____   _____

Client signature   Date

_____   _____

Clinician signature   Date

Part III

CPT Manual

5

Overview of PTSD and CPT
Session 1

Goals for Session 1

The overall goals for the first session of CPT are for clients to understand what PTSD is, how they got stuck in their recovery, and what CPT will do to put the clients on the path to recovery. However, the most important immediate goal is to engage them in treatment so that they don't avoid it by quitting before or after the first session, which is not uncommon in PTSD treatments. First, therapists describe the symptoms of PTSD and engage clients in describing examples of their symptoms. Next, therapists explain what happens to the body and thinking during traumatic events. Therapists then move into the cognitive theory of PTSD; they explain how people attempt to maintain their prior beliefs about prediction and control, and their faith in the just-world myth. Finally, therapists explain how CPT teaches clients to become their own therapists by giving them tools to examine their thoughts and label their emotions in ways they were not taught previously, with the goals of feeling the natural emotions arising from the trauma and changing thoughts that are keeping them stuck.

Procedures for Session 1

1. Set the agenda.
2. Describe the symptoms of PTSD and the theory of why some people get stuck in recovery.
3. Describe cognitive theory.
4. Discuss the role of emotions in trauma recovery.

5. Briefly review the index trauma.
6. Describe the overall course of therapy.
7. Give the first practice assignment.
8. Check the client's reactions to the session.

Setting the Agenda

Therapists should explain to clients that the first session of CPT is somewhat different from the rest of the sessions, because the therapists will be educating the clients about the symptoms of PTSD, explaining how PTSD is a problem of nonrecovery, discussing the role of avoidance in maintaining PTSD symptoms, and describing how CPT works. The session ends with the first assignment. Therapists tell clients that they (the therapists) will do most of the talking in the first session, but that this will change over time, with clients doing more of the talking while the therapists serve as consultants regarding any problems with practice assignments. The therapists will ask questions to guide the clients to think about their trauma differently.

Discussing the Symptoms of and a Functional Model of PTSD

PTSD for Therapists: Diagnostic Criteria

Rather than just listing the symptoms and clusters of PTSD, a therapist needs to help a client understand why some people are later diagnosed with PTSD. Therefore, it is important for the therapist not just to know the list of DSM-5 or ICD-10 symptoms, but to understand how they interact to prevent some people from recovering. Several major changes have been made to the diagnosis and classification of PTSD in DSM-5 (American Psychiatric Association, 2013). One of the most important is that PTSD is no longer considered an anxiety disorder, as it was from DSM-III to DSM-IV-TR (American Psychiatric Association, 1980, 2000). The various negative emotions that clients with PTSD experience, such as guilt, anger, shame, disgust, and sadness, have been demonstrated sufficiently well that PTSD is now considered much more than an anxiety disorder. PTSD has been included in a new DSM-5 category called "trauma- and stressor-related disorders."

Criterion A for PTSD (the definition of traumatic experiences) has been tightened up to exclude media-related exposures as traumas (unless such an exposure occurred as part of one's job), and learning about a traumatic event is considered a traumatic experience only if the event occurred to a close friend or relative. In addition, there are now four rather than three symptom clusters. According to DSM-5, the Criterion B cluster should be described not as thinking about the event repeatedly, but as unexpected, intrusive memories that are either cued by something in the environment or emerge when individuals are not keeping their minds preoccupied with other matters (e.g., chronic working). When they are tired, sick, or not busy, clients may have memories of their traumatic events that emerge in the form of images, sounds, or flashbacks—or, during sleep, in the form of nightmares about the traumatic events. More severe flashbacks may include dissociative responses, in which an individual becomes lost in an event and loses the sense of present time. Even without full recall of the traumatic event, it is possible to have emotional or physiological reactions upon reminders of the event. The Criterion B symptoms are thus largely sensory and brief, but highly distressing.

Criterion C, the avoidance criterion, is now composed of just two avoidance items: avoiding internal memories of the event, and avoiding external reminders. However, these two types of avoidance can be manifested in myriad ways. For example, the most common types of avoidance related to therapy are for clients not to come to sessions, to come late, or not to do their out-of-session practice. They may also attempt to change a distressing topic to something more mundane in a session. The use of substances or other self-harm behaviors to numb memories and emotions or to sleep without nightmares are other forms of avoidance. All these types are effective in the short run, but prevent processing of the traumatic event. There are probably as many forms of avoidance as there are clients; therapists must always be vigilant for avoidance, label it as a symptom, and emphasize that it is not an effective form of coping in the long term. Criterion C does not appear in the graphic at the top of Handout 5.1 because this figure illustrates the process of natural recovery. The graphic at the bottom of Handout 5.1 includes the avoidance criterion in PTSD, and should be discussed last rather than in the order in which it appears in DSM-5.

Criterion D is new to DSM-5, but includes a range of cognitive and emotional responses that have been found repeatedly in the literature. Although the cognitive symptoms are described as part of the cognitive theory of PTSD later in the session, it is good to elicit clients' responses at this point for reference. Cognitive symptoms include persistent negative expectations about oneself, others, or the world; persistent distorted blame of self or others for a traumatic event; and even dissociative amnesia for parts or all of the event. Although it is usually quite easy for clients to blame themselves for causing or failing to prevent traumatic events, they may not recognize that blaming other people who did not cause or intend the events might not be accurate. For instance, clients who were abused as children may blame their mothers for not protecting them from perpetrators, without understanding that (1) their mothers might not have known about the abuse, or (2) the mothers might have been abused themselves and unable to extricate themselves and their children from the situation. Military service members may have been taught implicitly or explicitly that if all personnel do their jobs correctly, all will come home unharmed. If service members or veterans cannot find any way in which they made a mistake—for example, if their units were ambushed—they may look to blame other service members, superior officers, or the military itself, rather than recognizing that the nature of an ambush is a surprise and that perhaps no one could have foreseen the event except the person(s) who planned the attack.

Emotional reactions in DSM-5 no longer focus only on fear and anxiety, because PTSD is no longer classified as an anxiety disorder. Disrupted emotions can include any kind of pervasive negative emotional states (e.g., fear, horror, anger, guilt, disgust, shame); markedly diminished interest or participation in significant activities; or feelings of detachment or estrangement from others. In DSM-IV/DSM-IV-TR, there was an emphasis on emotional numbing. However, it has since become clear that despite their attempts to numb their emotions, people with PTSD have breakthroughs of negative emotions when reminded of their traumatic events. The only emotions that they are truly successful at numbing are positive emotions, such as joy, happiness, and love. The lack of positive emotions and the presence of negative emotions also contribute to diminished interest in previously enjoyed activities or estrangement from others.

Criterion E includes the arousal items that were present in DSM-IV/DSM-IV-TR, and some behavioral reactions have been added. So, in addition to hypervigilance, pronounced startle responses, problems with concentration, sleep difficulties, and irritability/anger, DSM-5 now also includes aggression as the typical expression of irritability/anger, as well as reckless or self-destructive behavior. The latter can include self-harm behaviors, driving erratically or too fast, driving a motorcycle without a helmet, indiscriminate sexual behavior, or other risk-taking behavior suggesting that clients may not care whether they live or die.

Therapists who are using the ICD-10 (World Health Organization, 1992) classification system should note that ICD-10 also includes five criteria, but that the focus is slightly different from that of DSM-5. These differences should be taken into account in discussing how a client's PTSD symptoms are affecting the client today. Criterion A in ICD-10 still refers to experiencing a stressful event, but clarifies that the event must have been "exceptionally threatening or catastrophic" and would be likely to cause ongoing distress in almost everyone. Like its counterpart in DSM-5, Criterion B focuses on experiencing intrusive flashbacks or dreams and/or feeling distressed when exposed to trauma triggers. Criterion C is also similar to that in DSM-5, it its focus on avoidance of stimuli that are either related to or resemble the stressor event(s). ICD-10 Criterion D offers a departure from DSM-5, in that an individual needs to have either (1) the inability to remember important aspects of the event, or (2) persistent arousal that is shown by any two of the following symptoms: sleep difficulties, irritability/anger, difficulty concentrating, hypervigilance, or exaggerated startle response. Finally, Criterion E in ICD-10 requires that the onset of symptoms must occur within 6 months of the stressor, unlike DSM-5, which specifies only that the symptoms must have a duration of greater than 1 month (although the label "with delayed expression" is used if full diagnostic criteria are not met within 6 months of the event).

The preparation of ICD-11 is well underway, with a projected release date of 2018. Initial comparisons of ICD-11 drafts with DSM-5 indicate that ICD-11 is moving to a narrower definition of PTSD that focuses on it as a fear-based, stress-induced anxiety disorder. The ICD-11 system also includes complex PTSD as a separate diagnosis, whereas DSM-5 does not. Studies of the two systems (O'Donnell et al., 2014; Stein et al., 2013) suggest that ICD-11 PTSD prevalence, comorbidity with depression, and disability rates are all lower than those obtained in research using the DSM-5 classification system. Practitioners who will be using ICD-11 may find that fewer individuals in their practice will meet full criteria for PTSD than when they were using either the DSM-5 or the ICD-10 system.

PTSD for Clients: A Functional Model

In reviewing Handout 5.1 with a client, a therapist should refer to the top portion of the handout as a description of normal recovery, noting that if a trauma is severe enough or if a person has experienced repeated traumas, PTSD symptoms are normal rather than abnormal, at least for a period of time. Once the trauma has ended, it becomes a memory that people have to integrate in a balanced way into their understanding of experiences and why they happen, as well as into their view of themselves, others, and the world. A review of the PTSD symptom clusters, and a discussion of which symptoms a client is experiencing and when they occur, is a good starting place. As an example of such a review, the therapist could say something like the following (in his or her own words, not in a verbatim reading):

"One set of PTSD symptoms has to do with intrusive memories, or memories that 'intrude' on you in an unwanted way. They come at you when you don't expect or want them to—maybe when you are falling asleep or aren't feeling well. They can come as images, sounds of the event, or physical or emotional reactions when you encounter something that reminds you of [the index event]. Can you give me any examples of the types of intrusive symptoms you have? When you have these experiences intrude on you, it is natural to experience strong feelings as well. These emotions need to run their course. When you think about the trauma, what emotions do you experience?

"You also have thoughts about why the event happened, and, in an attempt to prevent future events, you may blame yourself or look for mistakes you think you made. Those kinds of thoughts are also associated with emotions, but different emotions from those that come from the event naturally. Your natural emotions about the event might be fear, anger, or sadness. If you blame yourself, however, you may feel guilt or shame, which is not a natural emotion but one based on your thoughts. Have you had any of these kinds of thoughts or feelings?

"If your intrusive symptoms, emotions, or thoughts are unbearable to you, you may attempt to escape or avoid them. There are many ways that people avoid thinking about or feeling their emotions about a traumatic event. Keeping very busy, drinking or using drugs, not coming to therapy sessions, coming late, or not doing your practice assignments are all examples of avoidance. Although it is understandable that you would want to avoid dealing with the traumatic event, and you may have been doing that for a long time, the avoidance prevents you from recovering."

When describing natural recovery from a traumatic event, the therapist should point out that when intrusive memories, strong emotions, arousal, and so forth are triggered, individuals are more likely to hear corrective feedback about the actual causes of the events and receive support for their natural emotional reactions if they allow themselves to feel their emotions, think about the trauma, and talk to supportive people about their thoughts. Natural emotions that emerge directly from the flight–fight–freeze response (e.g., fear, anger) are likely to decrease rather quickly, along with other emotions that are not based on thoughts (except grief, which is an ongoing process). As emotions decrease, individuals become more receptive to other points of view and acceptance of the traumatic event. The top portion of Handout 5.1 shows how thoughts, emotions, and arousal interact in natural recovery, and how they decrease and disconnect from one another over time. After a while, the survivor may be able to say, "I remember how awful that event was and how bad I felt at the time," rather than continuing to feel strong emotions and needing to push away the memories. It becomes part of his or her life history.

The lower portion of Handout 5.1 shows how people can get stuck in these symptoms and be diagnosed with PTSD. Instead of feeling natural emotions, talking about their traumatic events with other people and taking in others' perspectives, and approaching rather than avoiding their symptoms in order to integrate their experiences appropriately into memory (the process of accommodation; see Chapter 1), persons with PTSD stop the natural recovery process by avoiding any or all emotions, thoughts, and other reactions to the traumatic event, at all costs. Unfortunately, although avoidance is not an initial part of posttraumatic reactions, it ultimately prevents recovery. Also unfortunately, most forms of avoidance (such as aggression, substance abuse, and withdrawal from others) work in the short term—but because they do not work in the longer term, the persons increase their use, often to such an extent that these behaviors can become comorbid disorders in their own right. In fact, if clients had a tendency to engage in any of these dysfunctional behaviors before the trauma, they may worsen after the trauma. As depicted in the lower portion of Handout 5.1, the symptoms of PTSD may appear smaller because the avoidance is larger. However, if a person with PTSD stops engaging in the avoidance behavior, the symptoms of PTSD reemerge. For example, it is well known that people with PTSD and substance abuse are more likely to relapse than people with substance abuse alone. As soon as these clients stop drinking or using drugs, they may experience more flashbacks or nightmares, and then are more likely to relapse into using substances to diminish these PTSD symptoms.

It is important for clients receiving PTSD treatment to understand the role of avoidance in maintaining PTSD symptoms, and to accept that in order to recover, they need to cease the forms of avoidance in which they are engaging. Furthermore, one of therapists' major roles is to help clients identify avoidance behaviors when these occur so that they can stop the behaviors. Therefore, the importance of attending sessions on time, completing practice assignments, and not relying on other forms of avoidance is emphasized and included in a therapy contract (see Handout 4.1 in Chapter 4).

Therapists will also assist clients in examining their thoughts about the causes and consequences of their traumatic events, help them differentiate thoughts from facts, facilitate their learning how specific thoughts lead to different emotions, and help them learn the skills involved in examining their experiences in a balanced way. After reviewing the symptoms of PTSD, therapists then give clients an explanation of cognitive theory, with an emphasis on the role of thoughts in PTSD and on how changing thoughts can change PTSD symptoms.

Describing Cognitive Theory

Part of engaging clients in CPT is helping them to understand the cognitive model of emotional and psychological disorders. Clients may have heard nothing about cognitive theory or the cognitive model, or they may have misconceptions of the model—for example, that it is superficial, or cold, or a form of mind control. Therapists will provide a good start to treatment if they give their clients a clear working model of the conceptual underpinnings of CPT and the rationale for the approach.

Below is a typical explanation of cognitive theory as presented by a therapist. (Again, this is *not* meant as a script to be followed word for word, but simply as an example of how to introduce these concepts to clients.)

"From the time we are born until the time we die, we are bombarded with information. Information comes in through our senses, through our experiences, and through what people teach us. All this information would be completely overwhelming if we didn't find a way to organize it, and to figure out what to pay attention to and what we can ignore. As human beings, we have a strong desire to predict and control our lives, and we often believe we have more control over other people and events than we really have. Without organizing all the incoming information, we would have difficulty determining what is dangerous or safe, what we like and what we don't like, or how we want to spend our time and with whom.

"As small children, we begin to learn language as a way to organize information. In the beginning, our environment and experiences are very limited, and we have only a few words to describe them. A child may call an animal with four legs, a tail, and a nose a 'dog,' because that is the only word the child knows—even if the animal is a cat, a pig, a horse, or a lion. As we grow older, we develop more categories that are more fine-tuned, so that we can communicate with others and so that we have a greater sense of control over our world.

"The 'just-world myth' is taught to children by parents, teachers, religions, or society in general, because as small children we are too young to understand probabilities or more subtle outcomes to behaving or misbehaving. The just-world myth goes something like this: 'People get what they deserve. If something bad happens to someone, then that person must have committed some wrong previously and is being punished. If something good happens, then the person must have done something courageous or smart or kind before, or must have followed the rules. In other words, good things happen to good people, and bad things happen to bad people.'

"Parents don't usually announce to their children that if they behave, they may or may not be rewarded. They don't say, 'If you misbehave, you may or may not be punished.' It is only through the course of time and greater learning that people realize that good things can happen to criminals (for instance, they may get away with crimes), or that bad things can still happen to people who follow the rules and are kind to others. Unfortunately, early learning is not erased, and people often revert to the 'Why me?' question when they experience a negative event. They believe that they are being punished for something they did, and if they can figure out what they did wrong, then they can prevent bad things from happening in the future. This is probably one of the reasons why we hear so much self-blame following traumatic events.

"The flip side of the 'Why me?' question is the 'Why not me?' question. This is the source of survivor guilt. We have often heard service members say something like this: 'It is not fair that my buddy was killed. He was a great guy who was married with two small kids. I'm single and don't have kids. Why was I spared?' Or someone may wonder why the tornado spared his or her house but destroyed every other house on the street. The person may feel guilty about being spared when so many other people were not. Both questions ('Why me? Why not me?') are assuming that all life events are explainable, fair, and potentially controllable.

"When a traumatic event occurs, it is a big event, and there are very natural emotions like being terrified, angry, grief-stricken, or horrified that accompany the event. Your mind also has to find some way to reconcile what happened with your previous beliefs and experiences. If you have never experienced a traumatic event before, your expectation might be that only good things should happen to you. The traumatic event pulls the rug out from under you, and you have to figure out a way to take in this new information that bad things can happen to you. Another thing that people often do is to try to change the event so that it matches previous positive beliefs about the world and the sense of control over future events. They may distort their memory of the event like saying to themselves that they made a mistake, it was a misunderstanding, or they should have prevented the event. If they can just figure out what they did wrong, they think that they can prevent bad things from happening in the future. [Therapist note: This is assimilation.]

"If someone came from an abusive or neglectful home, the event may not be so difficult to accept. That person already has negative beliefs about him- or herself, and this new traumatic event is used as proof of the prior beliefs. The person may think, 'I am a trauma magnet,' or 'Bad things always happen to me.' In fact, if the person already has PTSD, and negative beliefs stemming from prior traumas, these negative beliefs may be activated after a new trauma event even if they don't quite fit the new event. An example would be a rape victim who is assaulted by a stranger and says afterward, 'I don't trust anyone in my life in any way.' Why would a stranger's actions affect one's beliefs about trust? That belief probably arose from earlier events and is now being reactivated.

"One thing that people with PTSD try to do is distract themselves or avoid memories of a traumatic event, as we talked about earlier. But it is pretty difficult to ignore an event so important, and the avoidance is not successful in the long run.

"Recovery from traumatic events consists of changing negative beliefs about the self and the world enough to include this new information. It means learning and accepting that traumatic events can happen. A new thought might go something like this: 'I didn't do anything wrong. Maybe bad things can happen to good people, and the person who harmed me is the one who is at fault.' For some people, this thought is frightening, because if it is not their fault, then perhaps all bad things cannot be prevented. If other people blamed you for your traumatic incident, it would also reinforce the idea that you must have done something wrong for the event to occur to you. In fact, if you were abused a lot as a child, you may come to believe an extreme and unhelpful version of the just-world myth: Bad things will always happen because of something about you as a person. Instead of self-blame regarding a single incident, you may experience shame and a deep belief that you are a bad person or deserve only mistreatment.

"If you were not alone during the event, and had someone else to blame besides the perpetrator and yourself, you might blame someone nearby who didn't actually cause the event or intend harm. This is another way some people think, to try to get a false sense of control that blaming a perpetrator does not give them. In the military, it is often taught that if all personnel do their jobs correctly, then everyone will come home unhurt. But what if there is an explosion and people are killed, and you cannot see anything you did wrong? In order to keep the idea that your side has control, you might blame someone else in your unit or someone higher up the chain of command. Similarly, a child who is abused by one parent may blame the other parent the most, even if the other parent didn't know about it.

"Another way to cope with a traumatic event is to change your beliefs about yourself and the world to extremes. Here are some examples: 'I used to trust my judgment and decision-making ability, but now I can't make decisions,' 'I must control everyone around me,' 'The world is always dangerous, and you must stay on guard at all times,' 'People in authority will hurt you.' Such extreme negative beliefs may come from flipping from one belief to the exact opposite, or from attending only to negative events and people and deciding that avoiding these is the best way to protect and control your future. Instead of saying, 'That person hurt me, so I will stay away from that person in the future,' a trauma victim may blame everyone who falls into a shared class with that person (such as men, women, the military, or people in authority). So the person may conclude that people cannot be trusted in any way, and withdraw from anyone who reminds him or her of the presumed cause of the event. Beliefs can go overboard after a trauma in many ways, but common ones are related to the themes of safety, trust, power and control, esteem, or intimacy. These themes may be related to yourself or to others. [Therapist note: This is overaccommodation.] The more you say something to yourself, the more you may come to believe that it is a fact, and you may stop noticing any evidence that contradicts what you have decided. The problem is that these kinds of beliefs have serious negative effects on your life and continued PTSD symptoms. You have to ignore or distort anything or anybody who doesn't fit the new beliefs, and you end up isolating yourself from others. We call these thoughts that prevent recovery 'Stuck Points.'"

At this point, therapists should give clients Handout 5.2 and review with them what a Stuck Point is and isn't.

Discussing the Role of Emotions

After discussing the role of thoughts in impeding recovery from traumatic events, therapists turn to the role of emotions. A major negative life event should naturally generate intense emotions. These may be generated during the event itself as part of the fight–flight–freeze response. If one has been trained to fight, as in the military or other first-responder positions (e.g., firefighters, police), one might expect an approach response to threat, and fight may be accompanied by anger. The flight response is to run away and is accompanied by fear. The freeze response may be one of two types. At the first perception of danger, the person may freeze briefly to orient to the situation, determine whether there is a threat, and decide what is going on or what to do. Sometimes clients who have done this blame themselves for having frozen for a few seconds, as if that could have changed the outcome of the event. The other type of freezing may be associated with tonic immobility and dissociation. If threat continues and neither fight nor flight is working, the freeze response may be the survival response; this may be accompanied by dissociation, a flattening of affect, or a complete sense of objectivity about the event, as if watching it from outside (i.e., derealization, depersonalization). The emotions that are paired with automatic responses are all perfectly natural emotions generated directly by the event without the need for time-consuming appraisal. Humans are hard-wired to have natural emotions in response to threat, loss, something disgusting, or even something pleasant. From an evolutionary perspective, they provide important information about how to respond in a situation. However, once the danger is over, a person should return to a steady state. In the case of PTSD, people bottle up their emotions and do not allow them to run their natural course. In fact, therapists often use the example of a carbonated beverage bottle that has been shaken. If a person starts to lift off the lid, there may seem to be an enormous eruption that is perceived as never-ending, and the person immediately puts the lid back on. However, if the person left the lid off, the energy would abate after the initial eruption, and the beverage would become flat fairly quickly.

Biologically, what happens in the brain during the fight–flight response is that when danger is detected, the amygdala activates emotions (fear or anger) and sends out neurotransmitters to the brain stem, which start the emergency response to fight or flee (see Chapter 1). In the process, unnecessary functions are turned off. The prefrontal cortex (the reasoning center, abbreviated here as the PFC) is quiet, as well as the immune system, digestion, and other functions that are not relevant to fighting or fleeing. There is a circular relationship between the amygdala and the PFC: When one is responding strongly, the other is relatively weak. A person who is calm can think clearly, and the amygdala is kept in check. If the amygdala is highly active in an emergency, the person does not need to be engaged in higher-order thinking, "What is my philosophy of life?" or "Do I want to change jobs?", so the PFC is less active. However, in a normal fight–flight response, the PFC detects when the danger is over; it sends a message to the amygdala to stop the fight–flight response; and in turn the amygdala lowers the levels of neurotransmitters being sent to the brain stem. The PFC comes back online, and balance is restored. In someone with PTSD, the PFC shuts off too much, and there is no message to the amygdala to stop the high-level response. It takes much longer to calm down. A client may experience "speechless horror" because Broca's area, the brain's speech center (which is part of the PFC), is turned off. Talking may bring the PFC back online. Labeling ones' emotions and keeping the PFC active by talking about the trauma rather than reliving it may be the most effective means of teaching the client affect regulation.

Emotions of the other kind are generated by the client's thoughts following the event. These emotions produced by thoughts are what we call "manufactured emotions" in CPT (and what others might call "secondary emotions"). For instance, instead of being angry with the perpetrator of an assault—which leaves the victim wondering whether such an event could happen again—the victim engages in self-blame and feels either guilt or self-directed anger. With new information, and with help in looking at the event in different ways, the person can learn to change the manufactured emotions quickly. The analogy we often use to make the distinction is that of a fire. We may say something like this:

"A fire in a fireplace has a lot of heat and energy, like emotions, and you may not want to get too close. If you just sit there and watch the fire and do nothing to it, what happens? [A client usually says, "It burns out."] Yes, it can't keep burning forever unless it is given more fuel. That's what natural emotions from the traumatic event do: They burn out if you just feel them until the energy has burned out of them. But what if you throw 'thought logs' on this emotion fire, like 'It's all my fault,' 'I'm so stupid,' or 'I should have known it was going to happen'? You can keep that fire blazing as long as you keep throwing thought logs on that fire. The problem is that these are not the natural emotions from the event. The fire does not burn out, because it is being fueled by different thoughts like self-hatred, blaming people who weren't responsible for that particular event, thinking that all people are bad or untrustworthy, and so on.

"In this therapy, what we want to do is allow the natural emotions to burn down naturally, which does not take very long, and to take away the fuel that has been keeping the other emotions burning hot by changing any extreme or inaccurate thoughts. Does this make sense?"

Reviewing the Index Trauma

After a therapist has answered any questions a client has about the cognitive theory of PTSD and natural versus manufactured emotions, the therapist and client agree on the index event (the traumatic event causing the most distress and impairments to be addressed first in the therapy). In some cases, an assessor has met with the client before the first session, has gone through the trauma history, and has picked what the client considered the most troubling trauma to use as the index event for conducting the clinical interview (preferably the Clinician-Administered PTSD Scale for DSM-5; see Chapter 3) to determine whether the person has PTSD and, if so, how severe it is. Even if this has been done, however, the therapist should review the trauma history and help the client decide on the index event in the first session, because a client may be afraid during a first interaction in assessment to discuss the actual most distressing trauma, may worry about being judged, or may confuse "distress" or "worst life event" with "worst traumatic event and PTSD symptoms" (e.g., "When my father died of cancer, that was the worst event of my life. Everything changed after that"). Grief and PTSD are not the same, and the client may report an event that has not actually produced the symptoms of PTSD. The therapist should review the events reported as traumatic and ask about any that the client has thought about since the assessment. Sometimes it is helpful for the therapist to ask questions such as these: "Is there any other event that you left out or thought of since the assessment?", "Is there an event that you hope I don't ask about or doesn't come up in therapy?", or "Which event do you have the most nightmares about or most often pops into your head when you least expect it?"

The reason for starting CPT with the most distressing traumatic event is that other events are likely to have the same Stuck Points attached to them, and if treatment starts with a lesser event, a client may have to begin again with the most difficult event, prolonging the therapy unnecessarily. Once clients learn that they can tolerate their emotions about the most distressing events, the other traumas can be dealt with during the course of therapy by completing Challenging Questions Worksheets and listing any unique Stuck Points on the Stuck Point Log.

Once the index trauma has been determined, the therapist asks the client to give a brief description (no more than 5 minutes long) of the trauma, if this was not done during the pretreatment assessment. The purpose for this short description is for the therapist to hear a few facts about what happened, in order to start generating a plan for how to guide the therapy. It is important that this description not become a detailed description with lots of emotion. At this point in therapy, clients occasionally have an urge to speak about the trauma, but if they become too emotional, they may well flee from therapy and may assume that their therapists are judging them as they have been judging themselves. At this early point in the therapy, they have no reason to trust that their therapists will be supportive, and no sense that there may be other ways to look at their traumatic event than how they have been viewing the events since they happened. If a client starts to get too detailed, a therapist can help keep the session on course by asking questions, moving the client on to describe the next part of the event, and asking how it ended. However, we have found that most clients do give brief versions of their events, because they have likely developed short, emotionless versions for public consumption.

Describing the Therapy

A therapist should now give a brief overview of the therapy course. If the therapist and client have not agreed before the first session on whether to do CPT+A or CPT, this is the time to decide. Some people like to write, but other people would quit therapy if they had to do so. This issue is discussed at greater length in Chapter 6. If clients can choose the version of therapy they want to do, they will be more empowered and more likely to engage in the treatment. The only instances in which therapists may recommend the addition of written accounts are (1) when clients are highly dissociative, and thus would benefit from writing the accounts to put events back into proper order with a beginning, middle, and end and to stay more engaged with their trauma memories; or (2) when clients are particularly emotionally numb, because sometimes the written accounts can elicit natural emotions that talking about the traumatic events cannot. If clients are extremely emotional, or have severe comorbid mental illness and are at risk of decompensation, it would probably be better to do CPT, which helps with affect regulation through the activation of the PFC and speech areas of the brain, and corresponding inhibition of the amygdala. Writing the accounts, with the associated imagery and emotions, may be unnecessarily distressing for these latter clients and as reviewed in Chapter 2, do not add to the outcomes of therapy.

The brief overview of the therapy can be as simple as saying something like this:

"As with every skill we learn, practice is necessary. And, as with most new things you learn, the more you put into something, the more you will get out of it. These facts may seem in stark contrast to your desire to avoid thinking about or talking about your traumas, and to escape feeling the emotions that emerge when you do. However, what you have been doing—avoiding—has not been working for you, as we have determined. Therefore, this treatment is going to be asking you to take the opposite stance, and approach dealing with the traumas. CPT will do this by teaching you new skills a step at a time, to help you look at your thoughts, tell the difference between a fact and a thought, ask yourself questions about the thought, and decide how you feel when you think it. You will be given handouts that will help you put your thoughts down on paper, and will show you new skills to question the facts surrounding your trauma and to determine how you might think about it differently. Ultimately, you may come up with different, more effective ways to think about the trauma and its effects, and you will notice a change in your emotions.

"We are going to spend the first half of this therapy focusing on the trauma or traumas themselves and determining what you have been saying to yourself. Together, we will ask questions to help you figure out what the facts were in that situation and whether your conclusions about them are accurate. If they are not, then we will work to find more factual statements you can learn to think. People can change their minds, and if you have been thinking the same things ever since the trauma happened without really reconsidering them, these thoughts might have become habits that could use a bit of exploration. We will use a series of informational handouts and worksheets to help you learn some skills for examining your thoughts that you were never taught in school. If you are thinking in certain ways that have become habits, it could take some practice to change your mind and make the new, more factual ways of thinking into new habits. The handouts and worksheets will help you do this. In fact, we are going to keep a list of these kinds of thoughts that have interfered with your recovery on a log, which we call the Stuck Point Log. A Stuck Point is a thought that you probably formed during or shortly after the trauma about why the trauma happened or what it means about yourself, others, and the world. It serves to keep you stuck in place and stops your recovery and growth. These Stuck Points will be examined throughout therapy, and you will learn new ways of dealing with them by using the Stuck Point Log and the other worksheets.

"Because your PTSD is out in your life and not only in this room, it is important that you practice these new skills with the worksheets every day, where they will do the most good. There are 168 hours in a week, and if you practice the new way of thinking only in 1 or 2 hours of therapy each week and the old way the other 166 or 167 hours, you will make little progress.

"Toward the end of the therapy, we will touch base on some specific themes of thoughts that are often affected by traumatic events: safety, trust, power/control, esteem, and intimacy. I mentioned these themes earlier, and each theme may relate to yourself or others. You will be given handouts to help you think about whether you have changed your beliefs too much as a result of the trauma(s) and haven't considered all the exceptions to these negative beliefs in your life."

Giving the First Practice Assignment

In order to start to understand how the index trauma has affected a client's thinking, the therapist asks the client to complete the first practice assignment, called an Impact Statement (see Handout 5.3). The Impact Statement consists of a short (typically one-page) essay describing the *reasons* why clients currently believe the traumatic event happened, and the *consequences* of the trauma in terms of their beliefs about themselves, others, and the world. In determining the effects of the trauma on their thinking, clients are encouraged to consider each of the themes (see above and Chapter 1) with regard to themselves and others.

Therapists should not only describe the assignment and give it to clients in writing; they should also encourage clients to start on it as soon as possible, to add to it over the days until the next session, and not to avoid it. The therapist may need to problem-solve when and where they can do their practice assignments if they don't have much privacy. Clients should be reminded that they are not being asked to write about *what* happened, but what they think about *why* it happened and *how* it has affected their thinking and behavior. This may be the first chance that a therapist has to ask a client some clarifying questions. If the client expresses apprehension about writing at all, or about writing about the meaning of the event (e.g., "I'm afraid you will judge me and throw me out of therapy," or "I might feel too many emotions and become over-whelmed"), the therapist can label these as Stuck Points and ask a few questions. Here are some examples of such questions:

> "So you are wondering if I think just like you? . . . In CPT we call that 'mind reading.' Why don't you ask me under what conditions I would throw you out of therapy?"
>
> "What happens when you feel emotions? . . . And then what happens? . . . And then what happens?"
>
> "What are too many emotions? Have you ever seen anybody whose emotions never stopped?"

"What emotions are you likely to feel if you think about what the event means to you?"

"What could you do so that you don't feel overwhelmed?"

"What could you do if you feel overwhelmed?"

It is important for the therapist to stay calm and reassuring but firm that the client can do the assignment. For example, the therapist can say:

"I wouldn't have suggested this therapy if I didn't think you could handle it. In talking with you and doing the assessment, I can see that you have the ability to benefit from CPT. In fact, once you get over the hump of the first few sessions, you may enjoy it."

A common therapist error is to scare clients by saying that they may get worse before they get better, or by overemphasizing how much work they have to do. Many clients, especially in CPT, have an immediate decrease in symptoms. Those who do have an increase in nightmares or flashbacks at the beginning of treatment may do so because they are not avoiding for the first time. Therapists can actually help such clients notice that this is a good start and that the flashbacks and nightmares will decrease over time. An increase in PCL-5 scores by a few points is not clinically significant.

Therapists can also remind clients that most of the out-of-session therapy assignments do not take a lot of time and are geared to helping them to take over as their own therapists by the end of treatment with a new set of skills. Moreover, therapists can remind clients that they have been having memories of their traumatic events for a long time, and that the goal of CPT is to relieve them of the pain of those intrusive memories and find a satisfactory way to accept what happened without all of the symptoms of PTSD.

Checking the Client's Reactions to the Session

A therapist should end Session 1 by asking about a client's reactions to the session and answering any questions the client may have about the session content or the practice assignment. Normalizing any negative emotions and praising the client for taking this important step toward recovery are both essential. The therapist should remind the client that he or she may have the urge to avoid both doing the practice assignment and coming to the next session, but that both are important for the recovery process.

Recovery or Nonrecovery from PTSD Symptoms Following Traumatic Events

In normal recovery, intrusions and emotions decrease over time and no longer trigger each other.

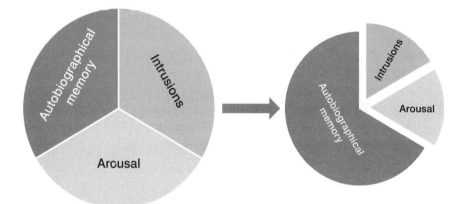

When intrusions occur, natural emotions and arousal run their course and thoughts have a chance to be examined and corrected. It is an active "approach" process of dealing with the event.

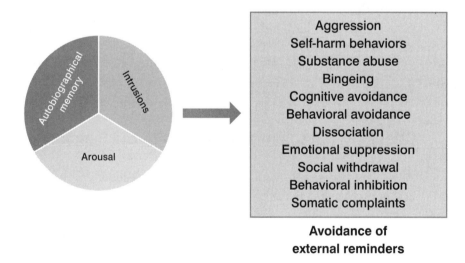

**Avoidance of
external reminders**

However, in those who don't recover, strong negative emotions lead to escape and avoidance. The avoidance prevents the processing of the trauma that is needed for recovery, and it works only temporarily.

What Are Stuck Points?

Stuck Points are:

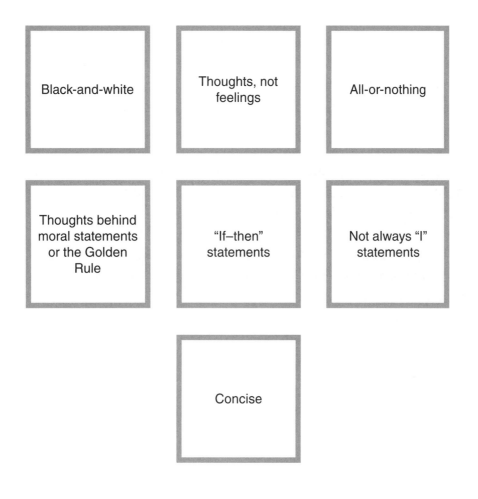

Black-and-white	Thoughts, not feelings	All-or-nothing
Thoughts behind moral statements or the Golden Rule	"If–then" statements	Not always "I" statements
	Concise	

Practice Assignment after Session 1 of CPT

Date: _____   Client: _____

Please write at least a one-page statement on *why* you think your most distressing traumatic event occurred. You are *not* being asked to write specific details about this event. Write about what you have been thinking about the *cause* of this event.

Also, consider the effects this traumatic event has had on your beliefs about yourself, others, and the world in the following areas: safety, trust, power/control, esteem, and intimacy.

Bring this statement with you to the next session. Also, please read over the two handouts I have given you on PTSD symptoms and Stuck Points (Handouts 5.1 and 5.2), so that you understand the ideas we are talking about.

6

Finding Stuck Points

Sessions 2 and 3

Goals for Sessions 2 and 3

The overall goals for Sessions 2 and 3 of the CPT protocol are to review the Impact Statement each client writes as the first practice assignment, with a primary goal of finding Stuck Points that have interfered with the client's recovery after traumatization. These sessions are foundational to the client's developing understanding of the association between thoughts and feelings—an understanding that is fostered through the use of psychoeducational materials and self-monitoring of these associations. The therapist also initiates Socratic dialogue in these sessions, focusing on assimilated Stuck Points (i.e., historical appraisals of the index trauma) in order to facilitate the client's more accurately appreciating the context of the event and the roles of self and others in the event. The therapist should encourage the client to express natural emotions that emanate from this more accurate understanding, both within and outside sessions. Following these sessions, the client engages in daily self-monitoring of events, thoughts, and feelings, including at least one event related to the index trauma, as a practice assignment.

Session 2: Examining the Impact of Trauma

Procedures for Session 2

1. Review the client's scores on the self-report objective measures.
2. Have the client read his or her Impact Statement aloud, and assist the client in identifying Stuck Points in this statement.

3. If the client has not completed the Impact Statement as a practice assignment, address the nonadherence with the assignment. (Do this for all practice assignments in CPT.)

4. Begin helping the client to identify and recognize the connections among events, thoughts, and emotions, and to differentiate facts from thoughts.

5. Introduce the ABC Worksheet.

6. Describe and discuss Stuck Points more fully.

7. Give the new practice assignment.

8. Check the client's reactions to the session and the practice assignment.

Reviewing the Client's Scores on the Self-Report Measures

As a reminder, each client should complete the PCL-5 (Handout 3.1; and perhaps the PHQ-9 [Handout 3.2]) on a weekly basis at the beginning of the therapy session or in the waiting room beforehand. The PCL-5 total scores should be graphed on Handout 3.1 to share with the client. The therapist should record the scores and add them to the client's records, and the client given feedback on symptoms at each assessment.

Having the Client Read the Impact Statement, and Identifying Stuck Points

One objective of the Impact Statement (which the client has been assigned to write as the practice assignment at the end of Session 1) is to elicit the client's appraisals about the cause of the traumatic event and to have the client examine the effects the event has had on his or her life in several different areas (i.e., safety, trust, power/control, esteem, intimacy). When the client reads this statement, it is important for the therapist to determine whether or not these goals have been achieved. While listening to the Impact Statement, the therapist should also be attuned to Stuck Points that are interfering with acceptance of the event (i.e., assimilation) and extreme, overgeneralized beliefs (i.e., overaccommodation).

Here is an example of an assimilated Stuck Point: A client who has been physically assaulted by her husband may write, "The reason that the assault happened was that I burned dinner." After the therapist discusses the event with the client, she may put on her Stuck Point Log (Handout 6.1), "When I am not perfect, I cause my husband to hit me." This switches the focus of the statement from the burned dinner to the husband's reaction to any mistakes the client might make. The therapist can move forward over the sessions to the evidence about whether it is possible to be perfect, and whether an assault is an appropriate response to imperfection.

An example of overaccommodation, along these same lines, might be "I can't do anything right." The client can write it down just as stated, because it will be addressed later in therapy. The therapist can also use the opportunity to practice a little Socratic dialogue to assess the client's cognitive flexibility. For example, the therapist may say, "You can't do anything right? I thought you did a good job on the Impact Statement. Are there some things that you can do right?"

Another objective of the initial Impact Statement is to increase the client's motivation for change. In the process of examining the myriad ways that the traumatic event has affected the client's beliefs about self and others, it is possible for the therapist to help the client see that the cost of avoidance is very high, and that remembering traumas and feeling painful natural emotions are worth the risk. The therapist might notice how many different areas of the client's life have been affected by the client's interpretation of the traumatic event(s): social life, work, self-esteem, confidence, control, intimacy, and attachment to others. Still another reason why the Impact Statement is important is that it is used as a benchmark for changes at the end of therapy, when it is compared with the client's final Impact Statement.

The therapist should begin this session and all subsequent sessions by asking the client about practice assignment completion. Based on social convention or other models of therapy, the therapist may be inclined to begin sessions with open-ended questions such as "How was your week?" or "How are you doing?" Asking such questions allows the client to avoid working on the traumatic material, and much of the session could be lost to irrelevant storytelling. Consistently beginning sessions with an inquiry about practice assignments reinforces the importance of these assignments in the client's recovery and helps shape the client toward the goal-focused and active nature of the treatment. The therapist should praise the client for completing assignments, especially the first Impact Statement, which sets the stage for further adherence. (Addressing nonadherence with practice assignments, particularly this one, is covered in a separate section below.)

The client is asked to read the Impact Statement aloud (i.e., the therapist does not read it either aloud or silently). This is done to support the client's approach behavior over avoidance behavior, and to reinforce the client's active role in therapy. After listening to the Impact Statement, the therapist should normalize the impact of the event, but should also begin to instill the idea that there may be other ways to interpret traumatic events—ways that will allow the client to move beyond them. Next, the therapist should review the Impact Statement in depth, by asking clarifying questions and determining how the content of the statement makes the client feel. The therapist should also help the client to identify Stuck Points that are hindering recovery, which will be objects of focus during treatment. It is possible to put the Stuck Points on the Stuck Point Log without phrasing them in optimal format; this may save time in the session, and the therapist and client will be working with the Stuck Points one at a time as they arise over the course of therapy. However, the therapist may want to spend some time on the most salient assimilated Stuck Point, to get it into a good "If–then" format rather than "I should have" or "I would have" phrasing (e.g., "If I hadn't frozen for a few seconds, I would have stopped the event"), because the most important assimilated Stuck Point is the beginning of therapy.

Any and all Stuck Points should be placed on the Stuck Point Log (Handout 6.1). If the client tries to argue that some statement is not a Stuck Point (a thought) but is a fact, the therapist can suggest writing it down anyway, so that they can decide about this together later. If the client still insists that this thought is a fact, the therapist can write it on his or her copy of the Impact Statement so that it can be revisited later. The therapist may even say, "Given how strongly you are saying that, I expect we may be spending more time on this later."

It is our experience that clients are relatively more capable of identifying over-accommodated thoughts that are consequences of traumatic events than of identifying assimilated thoughts. This is likely to be a result of avoiding retrospection on the trauma itself, or simply of being more attuned to here-and-now thoughts in daily life. Thus the therapist should pay special attention to drawing out assimilated thoughts, or specific thoughts about why the traumatic event occurred, given their importance in the therapist's individual case conceptualization. As a reminder, overaccommodated thoughts are consequences of assimilated thoughts. Accordingly, the therapist can often deduce from overaccommodated thoughts the likely assimilated thoughts that the client holds.

Some clients have avoided thinking about the trauma to such an extent that they actually do not recognize the assimilated thoughts that they hold or have not taken the time to form a trauma narrative. In these cases, the therapist should gently probe for possible problematic interpretations of the traumatic events. For example, in response to a client's statement of a thought about ways he or she could have handled a traumatic situation differently, the therapist might say, "How do you think you should have handled it? What were your options at the time?" Hindsight bias ("I should have known that it would happen"), self-blame ("It is my fault that it happened"), and denial of various sorts (e.g., "I keep thinking that if I had been there, he wouldn't have been killed," or "I always think there must have been something I could have done to stop it") are all examples of assimilation or trying to alter perceptions of the event to fit with prior beliefs. Keep in mind that if the client denies any self-blame, undoing, or just world thoughts, their assimilation of the event may be erroneous blame of someone who did not commit the trauma or have intent for it to occur. Examples of overaccommodation include "We are in grave danger all the time," "I can't trust my own judgment," and "I can never feel close to anyone again." The therapist can mildly point out that those extreme statements, while intended to make the client feel safer and more in control, have a heavy price and ultimately do not work. The therapist might say, "How do these thoughts relate to what you think caused the trauma?"

As discussed in Chapter 3 regarding case conceptualization, the therapist should recognize Stuck Points that reflect assimilation or overaccommodation, in order to prioritize and order the Stuck Points that will be addressed in treatment. Although it is important for the therapist to be able to recognize assimilated versus overaccommodated beliefs, because the therapist needs to begin therapy with trauma-focused assimilated beliefs, it is not necessary to use the actual terms "assimilation" and "overaccommodation" with the client.

The following is an example of an Impact Statement written by a 34-year-old man who was sexually abused as a child and was the victim of several adult assaults. Although he is clearly blaming himself for the events (i.e., assimilation), he is intimidated by other people and has overgeneralized beliefs about danger in the world. His problems with self-esteem are also evident.

> The overall feeling of what it means to have been assaulted is the feeling that I must be bad or a bad person for something like this to have occurred. I feel it will or could happen again at any time. I feel only safe at home. The world scares me, and I think it is unsafe. I feel all people are more powerful than me, and I am scared by most people. I view myself as ugly and stupid. I can't let people get real close to me. I have a hard time communicating with people in authority, so plainly I haven't been able to work. My fiancée and I rarely have sex, and sometimes just a hug revolts me and scares me. I feel if I spend too much time out in the world, an event like my past [events] will take place. I feel hatred and anger toward myself for letting these things happen. I feel guilty that I've caused problems with my family [this man's parents were divorced]. I feel dirty most of the time and believe that's how others view me. I don't trust others when they make promises. I find it hard to accept that these events have happened to me.

After reviewing the Impact Statement, the therapist and client should turn to the Stuck Point Log, adding Stuck Points to the log based on the discussion of the Impact Statement. The therapist should work to distill the Stuck Points so that they are thoughts versus feelings and challengeable (without using up the entire session time). Based on the sample Impact Statement given above, examples of Stuck Points would include the following:

"I must be bad for this to have occurred."
"I will be abused at any time again."
"All people are more powerful than me."
"I am ugly and stupid."
"The world is unsafe."
"Home is the only safe place."
"I can't work."
"If I spend too much time out in the world, an event like my past [events] will take place."
"I am dirty."
"Other people view me as dirty."
"Others can't be trusted when they make promises."

The therapist keeps each client's first Impact Statement in his or her records for this client, so that the client does not use it in writing the final Impact Statement. Also, the therapist should make a copy of the client's Stuck Point Log periodically or keep his or her own Stuck Point Log for each client during therapy, so that if the client forgets the log or loses the therapy binder or workbook, the therapy can proceed anyway.

Addressing Nonadherence with the Impact Statement and Other Practice Assignments

As with any form of cognitive-behavioral therapy, it is imperative that therapists quickly and effectively address practice assignment nonadherence, in order for clients to receive an adequate dose of CPT. Addressing nonadherence is especially important in the treatment of PTSD, because avoidance is an integral factor maintaining this disorder. Moreover, of all the various possible factors in treatment outcomes that have been examined (e.g., type of trauma, length of diagnosis, chronicity of traumatization), the amount of practice done outside sessions is among the most robust predictors of improvement. It may be tempting to allow clients to do no or minimal work on practice assignments, but then the clients may complete the treatment with no or minimal improvements, and may be left believing that they are "treatment failures." They are then less likely to profit from future treatments, and future therapists will have to overcome the clients' socialization that they can do no or minimal work outside sessions. For these reasons, it is incredibly important that therapists quickly address nonadherence to the practice assignments in CPT.

If a client does not write the Impact Statement assigned at the end of Session 1, the therapist should begin by querying what prevented the client from completing the assignment, using Socratic dialogue skills. In some cases, the difficulty may be a knowledge deficit: The client may not have understood the assignment. However, it is our experience that most people with a true knowledge deficit will at least attempt the assignment. In most cases, the problem is pure avoidance, or motivational issues have gotten in the way. For example, clients may feel hopeless that treatment will work, or may be embarrassed about their literacy or comprehension skills. The therapist should identify such issues and assign them as topics for ABC Worksheets to be completed before the next session (see the later discussion of ABC Worksheets), to help sensitize clients to their ways of thinking and the effects of this thinking on adherence.

Because in most cases avoidance of thinking about the trauma gets in the way of clients' completing this assignment, an important second step is to reiterate the role of avoidance in keeping clients stuck in their recovery. We recommend asking clients what they remember about the psychoeducation provided in Session 1 regarding the role of avoidance, in order to assess the clients' understanding of the rationale for facing the trauma-related thoughts. This also creates a situation in which the clients are arguing for approaching versus avoiding. This method decreases any tendency for therapists to sound as if they are "lecturing" clients or heightening the shame the clients may be feeling about not completing the assignment.

The third step in addressing nonadherence with the Impact Statement assignment is to have clients share orally in session what they would have written if they had completed their Impact Statements (or what they wrote, if they say they forgot to bring it in). A therapist should *not* stop the session to have a client write the statement. This is a crucial step, because the therapist should not collude with nonadherence (a/k/a avoidance). Instead, the therapy proceeds. It is advisable to have clients take some notes or use the Stuck Point Log to jot down some of their thoughts about what they would have written, in order to facilitate the completion of this assignment after Session 2. The fourth step in addressing nonadherence is to have each nonadherent client complete the Impact Statement at home, in addition to the next practice assignment (i.e., the use of ABC Worksheets for self-monitoring). This strategy of reassigning uncompleted practice assignments circumvents any possibility of a therapist's reinforcing avoidance of addressing the Stuck Points that are maintaining PTSD and comorbid conditions. If the therapist does not move on with the next assignment, as well as having the client complete the previous assignment, the client will get the message that it is acceptable to do the assignments every other session or only occasionally. The therapist will then be colluding with avoidance.

Finally, we recommend that therapists ask clients during the portion of each session focused on assigning the next practice assignment what the clients will concretely do to ensure completion. Some suggestions therapists can make include beginning each assignment the day it is assigned, scheduling time in the clients' calendars, using reminders in their calendars or on their cell phones, and enlisting trusted others to inquire about how each assignment is going. (Note: There is a CPT application available for free through iTunes called CPT Coach, in which all the assignments are available, as well as methods to record reminders for practice completion and the next appointment.)

Examining Connections among Events, Thoughts, and Feelings

After a therapist and client have discussed the client's Impact Statement, the therapist begins to assist the client in identifying and labeling thoughts and emotions; starts to help the client see the differences and connections among events, thoughts, and feelings; and introduces the client to the idea that changing thoughts can change the level and type of emotions the client experiences. The therapist first gives the client the Identifying Emotions Handout (Handout 6.2), to help provide psychoeducation about the different types of emotions and their range and intensity. The therapist needs to allow at least a third of the session for this new rationale and material. One way of beginning this discussion is to say something like this:

"Today we are going to work on identifying different feelings, and we will also be looking at the connections between your thoughts and feelings. Let's start with some 'basic' or 'natural' emotions: angry, disgusted, sad, scared, and happy. All humans are hard-wired to experience basic emotions, which occur automatically and give us important information about how to behave in the current and future similar situations. Can you give me an example of something that makes you angry? When do you feel sad? How about happy? What frightens you? How do you feel physically when you are feeling angry? How do you feel physically when you are feeling scared? How are angry and scared different for you?

"There are other kinds of emotions that are based on our thoughts, not directly resulting from an event. We call these 'manufactured' emotions, because it is like we have a little factory inside our minds that keep producing negative thoughts about why the event happened or what it means, and we end up with different emotions like feeling guilty or ashamed. We can even blame someone who didn't intend the outcome or harm, because it feels safer to blame that person than the actual person who caused the event. These emotions, natural or manufactured, can be combined to create other emotions like being jealous (angry + scared) or can vary in intensity (for instance, 'angry' can be described as ranging from 'irritated' to 'enraged'). With natural emotions, we encourage you to allow yourself to finally feel them, and they will lessen naturally and fairly quickly. With manufactured emotions, you will have to learn to say something more accurate to yourself, and the emotions will change with the changes in thoughts. Some of the thoughts you have had about why the trauma occurred were assumptions you made after the trauma, and you may have been young or may not have had all of the facts. Because you have been avoiding remembering the trauma, you have not had the opportunity to examine the facts behind your thoughts. We will look at these together."

The therapist can use as an example an acquaintance's walking down the street and not greeting the client, or a friend's promising to call and not calling. The client is next asked, "What would you feel?" and then "What would you say to yourself?" (e.g., "I'm hurt. He must not like me," or "I am angry. She is being rude"). If the client is unable to generate alternative statements, the therapist should present several other possible self-statements (e.g., "He must not have his glasses on," "I wonder if he is ill," or "He didn't see me," "Maybe her cell phone died"). Then the therapist can ask what the client would feel if he or she said any of the other statements. It should then be pointed out how different self-statements elicit different emotional reactions. The client's Impact Statement should be used as material for personalizing the client's event–thought–feeling connections:

"Now let's go back to the Impact Statement you wrote. What kinds of things did you write about when you were thinking about what it means to you that [the index event] happened to you? What feelings did you have as you wrote it?"

When clients are unable to label their emotions accurately, therapists can help them differentiate emotions by focusing on how different emotions feel in the body. As a parenthetical note, some emotions have multiple functions, and it may take some clinical judgment as well as Socratic dialogue to determine the particular function in a particular instance. For example, anger can be a natural emotion that is a response to being attacked—the fight response or righteous anger (cognitively mediated but accurate). Anger can also be cognitively mediated and may be erroneously self- or other-directed ("It is my fault that it happened," "My mother should have prevented her brother from abusing me"). Finally, some clients use anger to cover more painful emotions such as sadness or grief, or to push their therapists and other people away as avoidance.

If clients do not recognize their emotions or the connections of their emotions to their beliefs, therapists can help them tie their thoughts to feelings and behaviors by asking such questions as "How do these thoughts influence your mood? How do they affect your behavior?" Therapists should make sure that clients see the connections among thoughts, feelings, and behaviors. Some clients cannot tell the difference between a thought and a fact; sometimes a simple "why" question can help elicit a client's thinking.

THERAPIST: Why were you angry?

CLIENT: Because I should have known better.

THERAPIST: So your thought was "I should have known that this was going to happen"?

CLIENT: Yes.

THERAPIST: And your anger was directed toward yourself? [Note: It is always important to ask about the direction of anger.]

This exchange also allows the therapist to begin some gentle Socratic dialogue to further assess the flexibility of the client's thinking, and to determine whether the client has made some simple "blind" assumptions (e.g., "I just should have known") or has developed complex and convoluted thought patterns.

THERAPIST: I don't understand; how could you have known that this was going to happen?

CLIENT: I had a strange feeling that morning, like something was going to happen.

THERAPIST: Have you ever had those kinds of feelings when nothing happened?

CLIENT: Yes, but it was very strong. I should have done something.

THERAPIST: Did your feeling tell you what was going to happen or when it was going to happen?

CLIENT: No.

THERAPIST: Then what could you have done?

CLIENT: I don't know. I just should have done something.

THERAPIST: Were you certain about your feeling? You said that sometimes you have had feelings and then nothing happened.

CLIENT: No, I wasn't positive.

THERAPIST: So you didn't quite trust those feelings and wouldn't have known what to do, even if you were sure?

CLIENT: No, but I still feel guilty that I should have done something.

THERAPIST: Let's pretend for a second that you had a clear vision of exactly *what* was going to happen and exactly *when* it was going to happen, and knew exactly *who* to call to warn. What do you think their reaction would have been?

CLIENT: They wouldn't have believed me. They would have thought I was crazy.

THERAPIST: And then how would you feel?

CLIENT: Well, I wouldn't feel guilty or angry at myself; I would be angry at them and frustrated at not being able to do anything.

THERAPIST: Yes, it's frustrating not being able to do anything to stop an event that is out of your control, isn't it?

CLIENT: Yes, I hate it.

THERAPIST: It is very difficult to accept that some events can be out of our control. But is it your fault that it happened?

CLIENT: No, I suppose not.

If the client begins to argue with the therapist or becomes defensive about his or her beliefs, the therapist should back off immediately and say something like this: "This seems like an important topic that we will return to," or "I hear what you're thinking. Would you be open to discussing it more later?"

Although some clients have very convoluted thinking that justifies their Stuck Points, often a therapist will obtain few answers in response to questions in Socratic dialogue, especially early in therapy. Consider this example:

CLIENT: I let it happen.

THERAPIST: How did you *let* it happen?

CLIENT: I don't know; I didn't prevent it.

THERAPIST: How could you have prevented it?

CLIENT: I don't know. I just should have.

In cases such as this one, clients are making an unconsidered assumption: They drew a conclusion after the traumatic event that they *could* have prevented it, believed it without question, and never examined it further. This is particularly common when traumatic events happened in childhood, because the clients' level of thinking at the time would have been rather simplistic. Once they determine an unexamined belief, the clients then respond as if the statement were true, just because they thought so.

If clients become uncomfortable because they do not have answers to the questions, therapists should back off and gently reassure them that this is exactly what they will be working on in therapy. In other words, therapists and clients will be working together to help the clients think about the reality of the situation and experience the natural feelings associated with that reality.

Introducing the ABC Worksheet

The ABC Worksheet (Handout 6.3; we provide completed samples of this worksheet in Handouts 6.3a, 6.3b, and 6.3c) is the first of several worksheets that build on each other and are used across CPT; the ultimate aim of these worksheets is to have clients become their own cognitive therapists. The ABC Worksheet is designed to heighten clients' awareness of how their interpretations of day-to-day events, as well as trauma appraisals, influence how they feel.

Therapists should first orient clients to the ABC Worksheet by pointing out the different columns and demonstrating how to complete them. We initially encourage that only one event be put on a worksheet at a time, to simplify the process of monitoring; ultimately, more than one event can be written on each worksheet, with a line between one event and the next as clients gain a better grasp of the task. In addition, multiple thoughts can be activated in reaction to the same event. Therapists should help clients see the links between different thoughts and different emotions.

The client and therapist should complete one worksheet together during the session. An event that the client has already brought into therapy, or an event that has occurred within the past few days, should be used. We recommend that the client write on the worksheet that is used as an example, to ensure that the assignment is understood. One or more of the completed sample ABC Worksheets (Handouts 6.3a, 6.3b, and/or 6.3c) that have some relevance to the client's presentation should also be given to the client. Enough copies of the ABC Worksheet for daily self-monitoring before the next session should be given to the client. In addition, the client should be prompted to do at least one worksheet related to the index event.

"These practice worksheets will help you to see the connections between your thoughts and feelings following events. Anything that happens to you, or anything you think about, can be the event to look at. You may be more aware of your feelings than your thoughts at first. If that is the case, go ahead and fill out column C first. Then go back and decide what the event was (column A). Then try to recognize what you were saying to yourself (column B). Ask yourself why you feel that way, and the answer is likely to be your thought. Try to fill out these worksheets as soon after the events as possible. If you wait until the end of the day (or the end of the week), you are less likely to remember what you were saying to yourself. Also, the events you record don't have to be negative events. You may also have thoughts and feelings about pleasant and neutral events. However, I want you to do at least one ABC Worksheet about the traumatic event that we decided to start with."

At the bottom of the ABC Worksheet are two questions that introduce the notion of alternative interpretations of events. At this point in CPT, the client's primary focus in completing ABC Worksheets should be on identifying the links between thoughts and feelings before moving on to challenging cognitions. Thus the therapist should use his or her judgment about introducing these questions in this session to the client, depending on the client's grasp of the basic thought-monitoring process. Typically, the therapist doesn't assign the bottom two questions at this point, because the client is likely to say that the thought is realistic and that there is nothing else to say. If, during the Socratic dialogue about the ABC Worksheet, the client insists that the extreme thought is realistic, then the therapist has obtained important information about the client's cognitive rigidity.

However, if the client answers the question spontaneously with an appraisal that the thought is unrealistic, this may be an indicator that the client is already beginning to challenge his or her own thoughts. The two questions at the bottom can be assigned in such a case, but do not have to be. The two questions at the bottom can also be used in addition to the rest of the form as an alternative to the progressively more sophisticated worksheets (i.e., the Challenging Questions Worksheet, Patterns of Problematic Thinking Worksheet, and Challenging Beliefs Worksheet) if these later forms prove to be too difficult for the client because of low intelligence, comprehension problems, head injury, literacy issues, or the like.

Describing and Discussing Stuck Points More Fully

The concept of Stuck Points, of course, has already been introduced in connection with the client's reading of the Impact Statement and the client and therapist's review of this statement. However, because therapists themselves are not always clear about what a Stuck Point is or isn't, we have included a guide for therapists to help clients identify Stuck Points (see Figure 6.1). An informational handout for clients (Handout 6.4) is also provided as part of the session materials for the same purpose. As noted above, a therapist may choose to give the client one of the completed sample ABC Worksheets, to help the client learn how to fill out this form. Clients usually don't need all three of these samples, and it is helpful to pick one that is closer to each individual client's index trauma. Therapists who are working with particular types of trauma clients (e.g., refugees, survivors of motor vehicle crashes) may want to make up their own completed sample ABC Worksheets for these populations.

Here are some additional suggestions for describing and discussing Stuck Points:

1. Stuck Points are often more easily understood when they are first described in *nontraumatic* terms.
2. Because reminders of the trauma often bring up anxiety, people may have difficulty "hearing" the description of Stuck Points, so describing them by using

Therapist Stuck Point Guide

Stuck Points are concise statements that reflect thoughts—not feelings, behaviors, or events. They are usually phrased in "If–then" format. When clients provide what they think are Stuck Points, but are not in Stuck Point format, Socratic dialogue can be used to clarify the underlying Stuck Points.

A. Examples of statements commonly misidentified as Stuck Points:

1. Not a Stuck Point: "Trust."

Why not? This is a concept, not a thought. It is not specific, and you need to identify what the person thinks about trust. In this example, you might ask the client what about "trust" is a problem.

Possible related Stuck Points: "I can't trust anyone in any way," "If I let anyone get close to me, I will get hurt," "I can never trust my judgment."

2. Not a Stuck Point: "I am nervous whenever I go on a date."

Why not? This statement is describing a feeling and a fact, not a thought. In this example, you might ask what the client is telling him- or herself about the date, to help the client identify potential Stuck Points.

Possible related Stuck Points: "If I go on a date, I will get hurt," "People always take advantage of me."

3. Not a Stuck Point: "I fight with my daughter all the time."

Why not? This is describing a behavior, a fact, not a thought. In this example, you might ask more about the client's thinking before, during, and after a recent fight with her daughter to identify possible Stuck Points.

Possible related Stuck Points: "I don't mean anything to her," "I must be in control to keep her safe."

4. Not a Stuck Point: "I witnessed people die."

Why not? This statement is describing a fact, not a thought. In this example, you might ask for the client to describe the impact of witnessing others die. What thoughts did the client have at the time? What thoughts does the client have now? Or after that statement, you can ask, "And therefore . . . ?"

Possible related Stuck Points: "It was my fault that people died," "I should have done something to prevent it."

5. Not a Stuck Point: "I don't know what will happen to me," or "What will happen to me?"

Why not? This is a question about the future. In order to find the Stuck Point in this example, you might ask the client, "When you ask yourself that question, what is the answer you come up with? What is the meaning of that answer?"

Possible related Stuck Points: "I will not have a future," "I am not deserving of good things in my future."

(continued)

FIGURE 6.1. Guide to Stuck Points for CPT therapists.

6. Not a Stuck Point: "Parents should love their children."

Why not? This is a moral statement/rule, and you want to identify the thought behind it. In this example, to find the Stuck Point, you might ask what the moral statement means to the client with respect to his or her own life.

Possible related Stuck Points: "My parents failed me," "I can't trust people even if they are family members."

B. A few reminders about good Stuck Point structure:

1. Make sure that each Stuck Point is one concise thought. If a client provides multiple Stuck Points as one, make sure to break them apart and challenge them separately. For example, "It is my fault Joe died, I am a terrible person, and I deserve to be punished" can be broken down into three different Stuck Points: "It is my fault Joe died," "I am a terrible person," and "I deserve to be punished," which all should be challenged separately, starting with the assimilated thought "It is my fault Joe died."

2. If you are struggling, put a statement into the "If–then" format if possible, and have the client fill in the blank. For example, "If I had seen the land mine, then Joe would not have died." On the client's Impact Statement, you can underline Stuck Points and put them into "If–then" format on the Stuck Point Log.

3. Stuck points are typically black-and-white statements couched in extreme language. Extreme language can sometimes be hidden. For example, often when a client says, "It was my fault," the client usually means "It was *all* my fault." The second statement can be easier to get some movement on.

4. Stuck Points are harder to challenge when they are too vague. Make it more specific by asking, "How did you come to this conclusion?" For example, "I trust no one" can be refined to "If I trust others, then I'll get hurt."

5. Keep your eye out for words that can have multiple interpretations. Stuck Points are easier to challenge when they are specific and do not make assumptions about the meaning of words. For example, you can make the statement "If I was normal, then I wouldn't have fallen apart" more specific by asking, "What do you mean by 'normal'?" and "What do you mean by 'fallen apart'?"

C. Examples of Stuck Points:

1. If I had done my job better, then other people would have survived. (assimilated)

2. Other people were killed because I messed up. (assimilated)

3. Because I did not tell anyone, I am to blame for the abuse. (assimilated)

4. Because I did not fight against my attacker, the abuse is my fault. (assimilated)

5. I should have known he would hurt me. (assimilated)

FIGURE 6.1 *(continued)*

6. It is my fault the accident happened. (assimilated)

7. If I had been paying attention, no one would have died. (assimilated)

8. If I hadn't been drinking, it would not have happened. (assimilated)

9. I don't deserve to live when other people lost their lives. (overaccommodated)

10. If I let other people get close to me, I'll get hurt again. (overaccommodated)

11. Expressing any emotion means I will lose control of myself. (overaccommodated)

12. I must be on guard at all times. (overaccommodated)

13. I should be able to protect others. (overaccommodated)

14. I must control everything that happens to me. (overaccommodated)

15. Mistakes are intolerable and cause serious harm or death. (overaccommodated)

16. No one can understand me. (overaccommodated)

17. If I let myself think about what has happened, I will never get it out of my mind. (overaccommodated)

18. I must respond to all threats with force. (overaccommodated)

19. I will go to hell because of the things that I have done. (overaccommodated)

20. I am unlovable. (overaccommodated)

21. Other people should not be trusted. (overaccommodated)

22. My hypervigilance is what keeps me safe. (overaccommodated)

23. If I have a happy life, I will be dishonoring my friends. (overaccommodated)

24. I have no control over my future. (overaccommodated)

25. Men cannot be trusted. (overaccommodated)

26. People in authority always abuse their power. (overaccommodated)

27. I am damaged forever because of the rape. (overaccommodated)

28. I am unlovable because of [the trauma]. (overaccommodated)

29. I am worthless because I couldn't control what happened. (overaccommodated)

30. I deserve to have bad things happen to me. (overaccommodated)

more routine examples can be more helpful. Such a description can be given as follows:

"In this therapy, we focus on how your thinking or your thoughts can get in the way of your recovery from your trauma. We call these kinds of thoughts 'Stuck Points,' because they are thoughts that keep you 'stuck' in your symptoms. They create barriers to your recovery. Examples of some Stuck Point thoughts are 'It's my fault,' 'I should have done something differently,' or 'We should have gone left instead of right.' Remember, these are thoughts, not feelings.

"Let me give you an example of how thoughts can keep us stuck and be barriers: When you were getting ready to come to the session today, you probably had some thoughts about coming. What were your thoughts? [The therapist should write down these thoughts on a whiteboard or a piece of paper. Typical thoughts are "I don't know if I can do this," "I don't know if this will help," "This isn't for me," "You'll think I'm stupid."]

"If this is what you were telling yourself, how did that make you feel? [The therapist should write down the corresponding feelings on the whiteboard or paper.] Wow, you can see how these thoughts made you feel and how they could have gotten in the way of your coming here today and working toward recovery. But somehow you got yourself here. You told yourself something that got you here. What were those thoughts? [There is no need to write these thoughts down; the therapist should simply have the client answer. Examples may include 'I need to do this,' 'I am tired of living this way,' or 'I want to do this for my family and myself.']

"See how the thoughts that got you here are different from the first ones that we wrote down? The thoughts that got you here moved you forward, while the other thoughts can hold you back and keep you stuck, and so we call those types of thoughts Stuck Points. In this therapy, we want to look at your Stuck Points and see how they are keeping you stuck in your recovery from your traumas."

Giving the New Practice Assignment

The practice assignment after Session 2 (see Handout 6.5) is for the client to do daily self-monitoring on the relationships among events, thoughts, and feelings, using the ABC Worksheets. At least one of the worksheets needs to give the index traumatic event as the event. If the client did not write an Impact Statement, writing this statement will be reassigned, in addition to daily completion of ABC Worksheets.

Checking the Client's Reactions to the Session and the Practice Assignment

The therapist should conclude Session 2 by eliciting the client's reactions to the session and asking whether the client has any questions about the content or the new practice assignment. The therapist should reinforce any important ideas or discoveries made in the session, and should note the important take-home messages that the client offers.

Session 3: Working with Events, Thoughts, and Feelings

Goals for Session 3

The main goals for Session 3 are for clients to identify events, thoughts, and feelings; to determine how they are connected; and to begin discovering how feelings can change when thoughts change. An important goal of this session is to make sure that clients can identify different emotions and can label them accurately, and are beginning to understand which ones came directly from a traumatic event (i.e., natural emotions like fear or sadness) and which ones were based on their appraisals or conclusions about the event (e.g., guilt, shame, erroneous other-blame). Although it is ideal for clients to start to change what they are saying (e.g., "You know, I have been thinking that I should have done something different, but everything I come up with wasn't possible at the time"), this is not usually the case at this stage. Clients who have been making assumptions for a long time come to believe that these assumptions are true, merely because they think they are. They come to assume that their thoughts are facts through repetition. It is important for therapists to be patient with the process and allow clients to come to the new knowledge themselves, rather than to try to convince them. By the end of this session, if clients can recognize their thoughts and matching emotions, and put them into the correct columns, the session has been successful.

Procedures for Session 3

1. Review the client's scores on the self-report objective measures.
2. Review the client's completion of the practice assignments given to this point. If the client did not bring a completed Impact Statement to Session 2, but has brought one to Session 3, the therapist should have the client read it first and add any new Stuck Points to the Stuck Point Log. If the client has not completed any of the assignments, the therapist needs to address the nonadherence before doing anything else.
3. If the client has completed some ABC Worksheets, assist the client in labeling thoughts and emotions in response to events, and introduce the notion that changing thoughts can change the intensity or type of emotions experienced.
4. If the client has completed one or more trauma-related ABC Worksheets, use these to begin challenging assimilated thoughts about the index traumatic event.

5. Give the new practice assignment.
6. Check the client's reactions to the session and the practice assignment.

Reviewing the Client's Scores
on the Self-Report Measures

As in Session 2, and in each subsequent session, each client should complete the PCL-5 (Handout 3.1; and perhaps the PHQ-9 [Handout 3.2], if the client has depression in addition to PTSD) on a weekly basis at the beginning of the therapy session or in the waiting room before the session. The therapist should look over the scores on the self-report measure(s) and notice whether there has been a decrease in overall scores or if avoidance has decreased, resulting in an increase in intrusions. If the client says that he or she feels worse, the therapist should check the PCL-5 scores to see whether they have increased overall, or whether there is just an increase in the intrusive or hyperarousal symptoms. (The therapist can say, "Good job. You are not getting worse; you are avoiding less and beginning to process the traumatic event. What is your brain trying to get you to think about?")

Reviewing the Client's Completion
of Practice Assignments

Addressing Continued Nonadherence with Practice Assignments

If a client did not write the initial Impact Statement after Session 1 for review in Session 2, and fails to bring the completed Impact Statement and ABC Worksheets to this session, the therapist and client should have a serious discussion about the client's motivation to continue in treatment at this time. As discussed earlier in this chapter, therapists should be careful not to proceed with an evidence-based treatment if there is poor or no adherence with assignments, because of the potential for creating greater recalcitrance to treatment. An analogy we recommend using to help clients understand the importance of doing the practice assignments as prescribed is that of antibiotic treatment. Taken as prescribed, antibiotics are effective for many bacterial infections; if these drugs are not taken at their recommended dosage for the prescribed length of time, bacteria can become treatment-resistant. Unless a client can clearly commit to CPT with a plan for changing the nonadherent behavior, we recommend terminating the protocol until the point at which the client can fully commit. The therapist might consider whether any therapy at the current time makes sense in light of the client's motivational deficits, or whether some other form of treatment may be recommended (e.g., dialectical behavior therapy, anger management, substance use treatment, panic disorder treatment) before a commitment to trauma-focused PTSD treatment can be made. We also recommend that the client be referred to someone other than the CPT therapist when switching to another therapy, thus reinforcing the avoidance.

Reviewing the Impact Statement and Dealing with ABC Worksheet Nonadherence

If the client did not bring an Impact Statement to Session 2, but has brought one to this session, the therapist should strongly reinforce the client's improved adherence and then have him or her read the Impact Statement aloud, with attention to fleshing out Stuck Points and putting those Stuck Points on the Stuck Point Log. It is important to note that the therapist will need to pace this session more carefully because of the additional time needed to read and discuss the Impact Statement, while also delivering the prescribed interventions for this session. If the Impact Statement was thoroughly discussed in Session 2, the therapist could ask about and log new Stuck Points that emerged without having the client read the statement. The therapist would then take the Impact Statement to keep for the final session.

If the client completed the Impact Statement and shared it in Session 2, but has not brought completed ABC Worksheets to this session, the therapist should follow the steps to addressing overall nonadherence outlined above. Given that the client is still nonadherent with treatment, it may be helpful to look for Stuck Points regarding doing practice assignments or getting better, and do ABC Worksheets on these Stuck Points. In our experience, clients will generally continue to do their practice assignments if they complete the first Impact Statement assignment. However, sometimes there are knowledge deficits or waxing and waning motivational issues that need to be addressed over the course of treatment. Clients should be consistently reminded of the tried and true adage that they will get out of the therapy what they put into it. Every new assignment should be preceded with a compelling rationale.

This raises the important question of "How much is enough?" when it comes to adherence. There are risks in continuing the treatment protocol when a client is doing only minimal amounts of practice. We recommend consistently urging and supporting such a client in doing more practice, but we ultimately recommend using the results of ongoing objective assessment of PTSD and comorbid symptoms as the litmus test of whether the client is getting a sufficient dose. More specifically, if the client's scores are not improving or only minimally improving across sessions, and the client is not doing the recommended amount of practice, then the therapist should address the level of effort more directly to improve the client's ultimate outcomes.

Reviewing ABC Worksheets and Using These to Examine Events, Thoughts, and Emotions

If the client has completed and shared the Impact Statement in Session 2, and has brought completed ABC Worksheets to this session (i.e., the client has completed all practice assignments in a timely manner), the therapist should begin this session by reviewing the ABC Worksheets. In looking over the completed worksheets, the therapist should consider several things. First, it is very common for clients to label thoughts as feelings. For example, one client brought in an ABC Worksheet with the activating event (in column A) of "Get yelled at before I even have my coffee." Her belief (in column B) was "I try so hard but never get rewarded," and her consequent feeling (in column C) was "I feel like I'm fighting an unsuccessful battle." The therapist reminded the client of the emotions to be identified in column C of the ABC Worksheet by referencing the Identifying Emotions Handout (Handout 6.2). The therapist then asked her which of the feelings fit the statement best. She replied, "Sad and angry." The therapist pointed out that what she had listed in column C was actually another thought that could be listed in column B, and then drew an arrow from the statement over to column B. The client was then better able to understand the distinction between thoughts and feelings. The therapist also pointed out that using the words "I feel . . . " in front of a thought does not make that thought a feeling. Clients are encouraged to use the words "I think . . . " or "I believe . . . " for thoughts, and to reserve "I feel . . . " for emotions. This is an equally important reminder to clinicians, because the misuse of the word "feel" is so common that therapists may also catch themselves misusing the term. It is quite acceptable, and in fact better, for therapists to correct themselves during the session if this occurs; doing so illustrates for clients how our spoken language can be misapplied.

Another common problem in ABC Worksheet completion is that the thoughts may not flow logically to the reported feelings. If there is not a logical connection, there are probably other intervening thoughts that are being experienced but not recognized or recorded. For example, an identified thought might be "I can't do anything right," with the identified feeling of guilt. The intervening thought in this case might be "I let my team down when I didn't protect them." The therapist should also consider whether there is a match between the thoughts and the magnitude of the emotions (i.e., small event, disproportionately large feelings). In this case, the client may not be recording his or her actual thoughts; that is, the client's self-talk may be more inflammatory than what was written down to be shared with the therapist or may have been a sequence of thoughts leading to greater emotion. The therapist should encourage the client to record exactly what he or she is thinking, as opposed to a more socially desirable version. The therapist should also consider whether a particular dominant emotion repeatedly occurs (e.g., anger at self, guilt). And related to the possibility of recurring emotions is a particular theme of thoughts emerging across situations, which might indicate greater schema/core belief distortion (e.g., "I can't do anything right"—low self-esteem)?

In helping a client to become more proficient at completing the ABC Worksheets, it is important for the therapist to praise the client's efforts and provide corrections in a low-key manner, particularly if the client has issues with negative self-evaluation (e.g., "OK, let's move this thought over to column B. Now what feeling goes with that thought? Just one word"). Also, any new Stuck Points should be recorded on the Stuck Point Log. Occasionally, when clients use the worksheets as evidence that they are stupid or cannot do anything right, it is helpful to ask the clients whether they were ever taught about emotions and thoughts in school; if not, they can be reminded that they should not be expected to know something they were never taught.

Using Trauma-Related ABC Worksheet(s) to Begin Challenging Assimilated Cognitions

When reviewing the worksheet(s) about the index traumatic event, the therapist has an opportunity to use the content to begin challenging assimilated cognitions via Socratic dialogue. If the client does not complete an assimilated thought about the index trauma, a reminder here is that the therapist can often determine underlying assimilated thoughts from the client's overaccommodated thoughts. For example, if the client records the thought "Parking lots are dangerous," the therapist can deduce that there is likely to be an assimilated thought about the trauma itself, such as "If I had avoided the parking lot that day, I wouldn't have been assaulted." The therapist can simply ask the client a question like "How did you come to the conclusion that parking lots are dangerous?" to get to assimilated thoughts about the index event. As noted previously, it is important to focus on assimilated thoughts at this point in the therapy.

Below is an example of Socratic dialogue that followed the review of a client's ABC Worksheet related to traumatic bereavement:

CLIENT: In the A column, I wrote, "I sent my men into an ambush, and half of them were killed." My thoughts were "It is my fault," and "I am worthless." In the C column. I wrote, "Shame, anger, and I canceled my plans for the evening."

THERAPIST: Let's start with the emotions. Who were you angry at?

CLIENT: Myself.

THERAPIST: OK. Can you help me understand how it is your fault that you were ambushed?

CLIENT: I don't know—it just is.

THERAPIST: (*Waits silently*)

CLIENT: Well, I am responsible for my men, and some were killed, so it is my fault.

THERAPIST: Can you control everything in a war zone?

CLIENT: No, but I should have anticipated the attack on that road.

THERAPIST: (*Pause*) Let me understand something. What is an ambush?

CLIENT: It is a surprise attack.

THERAPIST: So, if it was a surprise, how could you have anticipated it? Had you been given information that they were waiting for you?

CLIENT: Well, no, but that just means our intel [intelligence] wasn't good. It has to be someone's fault.

THERAPIST: What about the people who intended the harm? What amount of blame do they get?

CLIENT: They get a lot of blame. They attacked us.

THERAPIST: If blame and fault go with intention, who had the intention to kill your men?

CLIENT: They did.

THERAPIST: So if the intel wasn't there and you didn't have any way to know this was going to happen, how much blame do you and your command get? Did they intend this outcome?

CLIENT: No, of course not. If they had known, they wouldn't have sent us out there with so few men. And I certainly wouldn't have sent my men there.

THERAPIST: You are saying now that the enemy gets a lot of blame. Who else gets blame? Who intended the harm and ambushed your men?

CLIENT: They did. I guess they get all the blame. I just wish I had known.

THERAPIST: I agree. I wish you had known as well, and that they hadn't died. It is a hard thing to accept that you might not have been able to predict the situation and that your men died. Does that feel different from the blame you have been heaping on yourself?

CLIENT: Yes, I have really been beating myself up—but when you make me look back at it, it was an ambush, and there was no way to know that we would be facing such big forces against us that day.

THERAPIST: So how do you feel then when you look at it this other way?

CLIENT: Still sad, very sad.

THERAPIST: That makes sense. You need to let yourself grieve for their loss. You have been focused on your guilt and anger at yourself, because you couldn't see the unforeseeable. Sadness is the natural emotion, and it is important to let yourself feel it in order to recover.

Giving the Practice Assignment

The practice assignment after Session 3 (see Handout 6.6) is for the client to continue daily self-monitoring with the ABC Worksheets, but this time the client should complete one of these worksheets each day on the index event or other traumas. The client can do other ABC Worksheets on day-to-day events, in addition to several trauma-related ABC Worksheets.

Checking the Client's Reactions to the Session and the Practice Assignment

As with Session 2, the therapist should conclude Session 3 by soliciting the client's reactions to the session and asking whether the client has any questions about the session content or the new practice assignment. The therapist should reinforce any important ideas or discoveries made in the session, and should note the important take-home messages that the client offers.

Stuck Point Log

Date: _____   Client: _____

We will be using this Stuck Point Log throughout therapy, and you will always leave it in the front of your therapy binder or workbook. You will add to this log as you recognize Stuck Points after writing your Impact Statement. Throughout therapy, we will add to it or cross off thoughts that you no longer believe.

_____

_____

_____

_____

_____

_____

_____

_____

_____

_____

_____

_____

_____

_____

_____

_____

_____

_____

_____

Identifying Emotions Handout

Date: _____ Client: _____

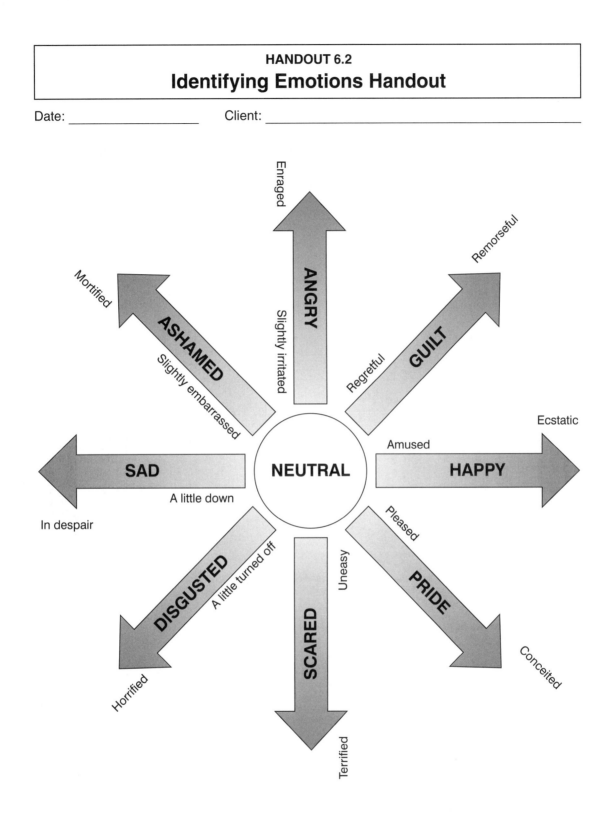

ABC Worksheet

Date: _____   Client: _____

Activating Event A *"Something happens"*	Belief/Stuck Point B *"I tell myself something"*	Consequence C *"I feel something"*

Are my thoughts above in column B realistic or helpful? _____

_____

_____

What can I tell myself on such occasions in the future? _____

_____

_____

Sample ABC Worksheet

Activating Event A *"Something happens"*	Belief/Stuck Point B *"I tell myself something"*	Consequence C *"I feel something"*
Shooting a Vietnamese woman while in combat	*"I am a bad person because I killed a helpless civilian."*	Guilt and anger at myself

Are my thoughts above in column B realistic or helpful? No. One mistake does not make me a bad person. People make mistakes, and high-stress situations, like combat zones, increase the probability of such mistakes.

What can I tell myself on such occasions in the future? *"I may have made mistakes in my life, but that does not make me a bad person. I may have done things that I regret, but I have also done good things in my life."*

Sample ABC Worksheet

Date: _____   Client: _____

Activating Event **A** *"Something happens"*	**Belief/Stuck Point** **B** *"I tell myself something"*	**Consequence** **C** *"I feel something"*
My uncle raped me	*"I let it happen and didn't tell anyone."*	*Guilt and shame*

Are my thoughts above in column B realistic or helpful? _____

_____

_____

What can I tell myself on such occasions in the future? _____

_____

_____

Sample ABC Worksheet

Date: _____ Client: _____

Activating Event A "Something happens"	Belief/Stuck Point B "I tell myself something"	Consequence C "I feel something"
I build a porch and the railing comes loose.	"I can never do anything right."	Anger at myself and sadness

Are my thoughts above in column B realistic or helpful?   No. It wouldn't hold up in a court of law, because I do some things right.

_____

_____

What can I tell myself on such occasions in the future?   "There are some things that I do all right. It is not true that I 'never do anything right.'"

_____

_____

Stuck Point Help Sheet

Date: _____   Client: _____

What is a Stuck Point?

Stuck Points are thoughts that you have that keep you stuck from recovering.

- These thoughts may not be 100% accurate.

- Stuck Points may be:

  - Thoughts about your understanding of why the traumatic event happened.

  - Thoughts about yourself, others, and the world that have changed dramatically as a result of the traumatic event.

- Stuck Points are concise statements (but they must be longer than one word—for example, "trust" is not a Stuck Point).

- Stuck Points can often be formatted in an "If–then" structure. Here is an example: "If I let others get close, then I will get hurt."

- Stuck Points often use extreme language, such as "never," "always," or "everyone."

What is *not* a Stuck Point?

- **Behaviors.** For example, "I fight with my daughter all the time" is not a Stuck Point, because it is describing a behavior. Instead, consider what thoughts you have when you are fighting with your daughter.

- **Feelings.** For example, "I am nervous whenever I go on a date" is not a Stuck Point, because it is describing an emotion and a fact. Instead, consider what you are telling yourself that is making you feel nervous.

- **Facts.** For example, "I witnessed people die" is not a Stuck Point, because this is something that actually happened. Instead, consider what thoughts you had as this happened and what you think about it now.

- **Questions.** For example, "What will happen to me?" is not a Stuck Point, because it is a question. Instead, consider what answer to your question is at the back of your mind, such as "I will not have a future."

- **Moral statements.** For example, "The criminal justice system should always work" is not a Stuck Point, because it reflects an ideal standard of behavior. Instead, consider how this statement pertains to you specifically, such as "The justice system failed me," or "I can't trust the government."

Examples of Stuck Points

1. If I had done my job better, then other people would have survived.

2. Because I did not tell anyone, I am to blame for the abuse.

(continued)

3. Because I did not fight against my attacker, the abuse is my fault.

4. I should have known he would hurt me.

5. It is my fault the accident happened.

6. If I had been paying attention, no one would have died.

7. If I hadn't been drinking, it would not have happened.

8. I don't deserve to live when other people lost their lives.

9. If I let other people get close to me, I'll get hurt again.

10. Expressing any emotion means I will lose control of myself.

11. I must be on guard at all times.

12. I should be able to protect others.

13. I must control everything that happens to me.

14. Mistakes are intolerable and cause serious harm or death.

15. No civilians can understand me.

16. If I let myself think about what has happened, I will never get it out of my mind.

17. I must respond to all threats with force.

18. I can never really be a good, moral person again because of the things that I have done.

19. Other people should not be trusted.

20. Other people should not trust me.

21. If I have a happy life, I will be dishonoring my friends.

22. I have no control over my future.

23. The government cannot be trusted.

24. People in authority always abuse their power.

25. I am damaged forever because of the rape.

26. I am unlovable because of [the trauma].

27. I am worthless because I couldn't control what happened.

28. I deserve to have bad things happen to me.

29. I am dirty.

30. I deserved to have been abused.

31. Only people who were there can understand.

Practice Assignment after Session 2 of CPT

Please complete the ABC Worksheets (Handout 6.3) to become aware of the connections between events, your thoughts, and your feelings. Complete at least one worksheet each day. Remember to fill out the worksheet as soon after an event as possible, and if you identify any new Stuck Points, add them to the Stuck Point Log (Handout 6.1). Complete at least one worksheet about the traumatic event that is causing you the most PTSD symptoms. Also, please use the Identifying Emotions Handout (Handout 6.2) to help you determine the emotions you are feeling.

Practice Assignment after Session 3 of CPT

Please continue to self-monitor events, thoughts, and feelings with the ABC Worksheets (Handout 6.3) on a daily basis, to increase your mastery of this skill. You should complete one worksheet each day on the trauma causing you the most distress, or other traumas, but you can do additional worksheet items on day-to-day events. Please put any newly noticed Stuck Points on your Stuck Point Log (Handout 6.1) as you use the ABC Worksheets.

7

Processing the Index Event

Sessions 4 and 5

Goals for Sessions 4 and 5

The goals for Sessions 4 and 5 are to make sure clients can label events, thoughts, and emotions and can see the connections among them, as well as to introduce two new worksheets (i.e., the Challenging Questions Worksheet and the Patterns of Problematic Thinking Worksheet) that are designed to help clients begin to become their own cognitive therapists by challenging their individual thoughts and considering their characteristic ways of thinking. Socratic dialogue is used throughout these sessions to help the clients challenge their Stuck Points. Assimilated Stuck Points about each client's index trauma (and, potentially, other traumas) should be prioritized in these sessions. In Session 4, a therapist will probably be doing more Socratic dialogue—especially asking clarifying questions—than in any other session.

Session 4: Examining the Index Event

Procedures for Session 4

1. Review the client's scores on the self-report objective measures. (See the discussions of this review for Sessions 2 and 3 in Chapter 6.)
2. Review the client's ABC Worksheets.
3. Address the client's assimilated Stuck Points, using Socratic dialogue to clarify and

examine these. Identify the context in which the index trauma occurred, and help the client differentiate among blame/intent, responsibility, and the unforeseeable.

4. Introduce the Challenging Questions Worksheet.
5. Give the new practice assignment.
6. Check the client's reactions to the session and the practice assignment.

Reviewing the Client's ABC Worksheets

At the end of Session 3, the therapist has assigned the client to complete at least one copy of the ABC Worksheet each day on the index trauma, and additional copies as needed on other traumas or life events that may occur between sessions. Any new Stuck Points that emerged during the previous session should be added to the Stuck Point Log and put into good Stuck Point format. Clients are likely to say in column B that an event was their fault or that they should have done something different. Occasionally, they will say that they do not blame themselves (e.g., "I was only a child"), but they may doubt that the event happened, perhaps because other people (e.g., their parents) deny it. This is also assimilation (i.e., "It didn't happen"), and it may include underlying sentiments of unfairness about the trauma (i.e., just-world thinking). Sometimes, as noted in earlier chapters, clients also erroneously blame others; they may blame persons in their proximity who did not intend the harm or outcome, rather than the persons who did.

The elucidation of assimilated thoughts should lead directly into Socratic dialogue. Those who have internalizing presentations are likely to be focused on their role in the trauma, to be engaging in self-blame, and perhaps to have comorbid depression. Some clients have more angry presentations and tend to have related externalizing thoughts. This may be particularly true if there were other people with them or in their proximity whom they can blame (not the perpetrators), or if they do not construe that they made any mistakes. Erroneous other-blame is also a form of just-world thinking that focuses on how the event could have been averted by someone else. Examples include military personnel who blame their commanders or unit leaders, while ignoring the people who set up an ambush or buried a land mine; blaming nonoffending parents who actually did not know that their children were being abused; or blaming bystanders rather than perpetrators. Once these emotions have been labeled, a therapist should begin asking questions focused on a client's distorted (i.e., assimilated) thinking about the trauma.

Cognitive Processing: Addressing Assimilated Stuck Points

A large portion of Session 4 is spent on Socratic dialogue focused on the trauma itself. The therapist needs to start with clarifying questions to understand what the facts were, so that he or she can determine whether each statement the client is making is factually correct or is a Stuck Point. As a rule of thumb, an 80–20% split between clarifying questions and examining the actual evidence or alternative thoughts is desirable. Below is an example—a therapist's exchange with a client who was raped and believed that it was her fault that it happened. The therapist starts by asking clarifying questions and making summarizing statements.

THERAPIST: Can you tell me what options you had at the time of the rape?

CLIENT: I should have said "No" more times. He might not have heard me or misunderstood.

THERAPIST: How many times did you say "No"?

CLIENT: Four or five. Then he told me to shut up.

THERAPIST: If he told you to shut up, might that mean that he did hear you?

CLIENT: I guess, but maybe he didn't believe me. He said, "You know you want this."

THERAPIST: And did you want this?

CLIENT: No.

THERAPIST: And you told him so?

CLIENT: Yes, and I was trying to push him off of me, but he was too big.

THERAPIST: Given those circumstances, at what point do you think it stops being your fault and becomes his fault? Is there something in the law about how many times you have to say "No" before it becomes a crime?

CLIENT: I think just once.

THERAPIST: Let me make sure I understand you correctly. You said you did not want to have sex with him, and you told him "No" a number of times, and you tried to push him off but couldn't. Is that correct?

CLIENT: Yes.

THERAPIST: In light of that, what other options do you think you had at the time?

CLIENT: I should have fought harder.

THERAPIST: (*Puzzled tone*) Can you explain how you could have fought harder? You said you couldn't get him off you. Did he have you pinned down?

CLIENT: Yes. I couldn't move my legs, so I couldn't kick him, and he had one of my arms pinned under my back. When he told me to shut up, he hit me across the face.

THERAPIST: Oh, I didn't hear that part before. That's important. You were saying "No" repeatedly and pushing him with one arm, while the other arm was under you and your legs were pinned down. Then he hit you. As I say it back with you, does this sound like a misunderstanding to you?

CLIENT: (*Quietly crying*) No, he raped me.

In such a case, after allowing the client to feel her natural emotions and then helping her label them, the therapist should go on to find out what would normally happen during a consensual sexual interaction or on a "normal day," to help the client further realize that she did not want the rape nor is it her fault. The therapist may also ask what the typical "protocol" would be if the client perceived a dangerous situation. Below is a therapist–client exchange involving a combat-related Stuck Point.

> THERAPIST: The Stuck Point that seems the strongest for you is "If I had been able to cover my buddy, he wouldn't have been killed."
>
> CLIENT: That's right. He would be alive today if I had been there to cover him.
>
> THERAPIST: And when you say that, what do you feel?
>
> CLIENT: I feel angry.
>
> THERAPIST: Who are you angry at?
>
> CLIENT: At the unit commander. It is his fault. But I am also angry at myself for not just going with my friend.
>
> THERAPIST: Regarding yourself, are there other emotions that you feel about your belief that you should have gone with your friend?
>
> CLIENT: Guilt, too.
>
> THERAPIST: It sounds like there are two Stuck Points you are grappling with. One is about being able to cover your buddy, and the other is that if you could have done that, he wouldn't have been killed. Let's take them one at a time. What stopped you from providing him cover fire?
>
> CLIENT: I was sent by my commander to a different location. We were given word that there was an insurgent at a particular house who we were supposed to apprehend, and my friend was with the group that was going in the front door. I was sent around back to cover the back door and windows with a couple of other guys.
>
> THERAPIST: And was this a usual way to enter a house like this?
>
> CLIENT: For us to cover the front and the back? Yes. We were heading in our usual positions, but something didn't feel right that night.
>
> THERAPIST: How so?
>
> CLIENT: There were fewer people on the street than usual. It was really quiet. I should have known what was going to happen.
>
> THERAPIST: I think that this is another Stuck Point we should write down on your Stuck Point Log. This sounds like you are saying you should have had the ability to predict the future. I wonder if that is where some of the guilt comes from. Let's get back to the first Stuck Point now, though. It was quieter than usual. Did that mean, according to the usual protocol, that you should have changed your position and moved to the front of the house?
>
> CLIENT: No. I started feeling more nervous, because this should have been a

simple extraction and it didn't feel that way—but I was not sent to the front of the house, so I kept my position. The insurgents could have tried to leave out a back window or door.

THERAPIST: What happened then?

CLIENT: All hell broke loose. It was a set-up. Insurgents came pouring out the front door and killed three of the men in my unit. Two others were wounded. We came running around from the back, and I shot one guy; two others were also shot; and two got away. We didn't have a medic with us, so we did what we could for our guys until we could get help.

THERAPIST: Given that your thought has been, "If I had been able to cover my buddy, he wouldn't have been killed," what evidence do you have that if you had been in the front of the house instead of someone else, you would have been able to protect him? Given that everyone in the front was shot, why do you think you wouldn't have been shot also?

CLIENT: I don't know. I just imagine that if I were there, I could have shot the guy first who killed Mark. I shot him too late.

THERAPIST: (*Quiet for a moment*) Can I ask you a question?

CLIENT: Yes.

THERAPIST: Did you see the guy who shot Mark? I ask, because I thought you didn't come around the house until after you heard the shots.

CLIENT: Huh. Let me think a minute. You know, I don't know if that was the guy who shot Mark. By the time we got to the front of the house and started shooting, our guys were down. The guy I suspect was closest to Mark, so I assume it was him.

THERAPIST: But you said you shot him "too late." Before you heard the shots, was there any reason to leave your position?

CLIENT: No, not really. I just wish I could have saved Mark.

THERAPIST: I wish that Mark hadn't been killed, also. (*Pause*) However, what you are saying is a bit different from what you said before. What do you feel when you say you wish he hadn't been killed?

CLIENT: Sad. I wish I could "rewind it all" and make it come out different.

THERAPIST: That is a human tendency. It is sad when we lose someone we care about, and it is sometimes hard to accept that you can't change it, no matter how much you wish you could. Sadness is a natural emotion that we need to feel. (*Pause*) I'm wondering if that is different from saying it was the commander's fault or being angry at yourself?

CLIENT: Yeah, it just feels better to think that we should have known it was an ambush. I know he wouldn't have sent us into the usual positions if he had known there was going to be an ambush. I just want to blame somebody.

THERAPIST: That is also a human tendency. Is it possible to blame the insurgents who intended the harm and set up the ambush?

CLIENT: Yeah, but it is hard to let go of the idea that there was something we could have done.

THERAPIST: We will continue to work on that. While we do, I want you to let yourself feel sad about losing your friend. That is a very natural emotion when we lose someone we care about. Do you think it is possible that you are feeling anger at yourself or your command to avoid feeling a more difficult emotion—sadness? You've told me that you take it out on people who had nothing to do with your friend's death, like your wife and kids.

CLIENT: I do. It is hard for me to just be sad.

The examples above illustrate how a therapist can elicit information with questions about the trauma that are associated with a client's assimilated beliefs and related emotions. The questions are designed to help both the therapist and the client understand the context of the situation; determine whether it was actually possible for the client to change the outcome; and, if so, consider whether the outcome could have been even worse. Putting traumatic events into their proper context is integral to cognitive processing. The goal is to recognize that clients may well have had little forewarning of impending danger, and very little time to make decisions or take action. Indeed, the events may have been unforeseeable and unpreventable.

Notice in the examples above that the therapists did not ask about the graphic details of the woman's rape or the ambush in which the soldier was involved. Although the clients may have had flashbacks or nightmares about these incidents, such reactions have been shown to decrease with cognitive interventions, and without the need to focus on repeating those details or eliciting strong emotions. The same principle applies to any type of trauma (child abuse, a car accident, a fire, etc.). The gory or painful images may not be the reasons why the persons have PTSD, and research shows that they do not need to be recounted in depth. Also note that when the soldier brought up a second Stuck Point, the therapist did not chase after it but redirected the client to working on the first Stuck Point, in order to bring more resolution to one Stuck Point before moving to another.

If there is time in the session, the therapist may focus on another Stuck Point, but it should again pertain to the causes of the trauma. In the combat case above, the therapist might focus on the second Stuck Point. In this example, if the client had been at the front of the house, would the results have been different? Could they have been even worse? Or the therapist might focus on the Stuck Point that lead to anger at the commander, even though the client was already showing some cognitive flexibility regarding this other-blame. In the first example, because the rape victim showed more cognitive flexibility, the therapist might ask her, "Does it feel different when you describe what happened to you as a rape versus a misunderstanding?"

Typical common assimilated Stuck Points involve (1) hindsight bias; (2)

outcome-based reasoning; and (3) failure to differentiate among intention for the act, responsibility (playing a role), and the unforeseeable. "Hindsight bias" means that after the trauma, clients think of all the things that they could or should have done to prevent or stop the event. They even may come to believe that they had such knowledge at the time and made a mistake or failed to act on their foreknowledge. It is not accurate to assume this reasoning to be correct, because their thinking may in fact be quite distorted about what they should or could have known or done at the time. At times, clients have very unrealistic beliefs about what they should have done and whether it would have worked (e.g., a 5-year-old's stopping paternal abuse, a motorist's being able to see around a blind corner to avoid a drunk driver). The bottom line is that hindsight bias is an assumption that there should have been some way to stop the event—that perhaps the clients had foreknowledge that something was going to happen, and that they failed in some way by not preventing it.

"Outcome-based reasoning" is closely related to the just-world myth and the desire to be omniscient and omnipotent. It stems from the belief that because an event had a bad outcome, a client *must* have done something wrong; otherwise, the outcome would have been better. It is common for clients to hear and think that "everything happens for a reason," and that if they just knew what the reason was, they could have changed the outcome or could prevent future negative events from happening. A client typically makes some version of this statement: "I must have made a bad decision, because it had a bad outcome." Younger people in particular (or those who were traumatized at a younger age and have never examined their thoughts about the trauma) are particularly prone to believing that there are only right or wrong decisions, and that if there was a bad outcome, they must have made the wrong choice. Clients who believe this often give up making choices and let others make decisions for them, or become immobilized when they have to make decisions themselves. They do not recognize that not making a choice is, in fact, making a decision.

Because differentiating among intention, responsibility, and the unforeseeable is somewhat more complex, we discuss it separately below.

Differentiating among Intention, Responsibility, and the Unforeseeable

In most societies, there are distinctions among intention for an act, responsibility, and an accident or the unforeseeable. Legal consequences based on these distinctions can help in clarifying these constructs. For example, if someone was driving very slowly and carefully through a neighborhood, and a child suddenly bolted out from between parked cars chasing a ball and was hit by the car, this would be considered an accident. Although the driver might be quite traumatized by the event, he or she would not be prosecuted and punished by the law if the police determined that the event was an unavoidable accident. However, if the driver was going too fast, was drunk, and killed the child, he or she might well be prosecuted for vehicular homicide or manslaughter. In this case, the punishment would be somewhat mitigated by the fact that the driver did not intend to kill the child; he or she had responsibility for the crash, but did not have intention to kill. If someone, in a fit of anger, swerved and hit someone, this driver might be charged with second-degree murder. Or, finally, if someone waited to run over and kill a person with premeditation, this driver might be charged with first-degree murder. In the latter two cases, the behavior was fueled by intentionality, either in the heat of passion or with premeditation, and blame/fault/guilt would be assigned. Most criminal justice systems make these distinctions, and the related punishments increase accordingly. If a victim of a crime says, "It is my fault for not stopping the crime," this is an inappropriate use of the term "fault." The victim did not intend the outcome and probably did not foresee it. The Levels of Responsibility Handout (Handout 7.1) should be used to help explain these concepts to clients.

It is important for therapists to help clients to change their language and stop using the phrases "It is my fault," or "I blame myself," as if they are being punished for something they did or failed to do. For instance, when a client says, "It is my fault that I was raped, because I was in a bar with friends, had been drinking, and was wearing a short skirt," the therapist might respond by looking puzzled and asking, "So you were intending someone to commit a crime against you?" Then, when the client answers in the negative, the therapist might ask, "What were your intentions that evening?" (to have a good time with friends, presumably) or "How were all of the other women in the bar dressed?" There are many other questions a therapist could ask, such as "Have you ever been in that bar—or any bar, for that matter—and not been raped?", "Have you ever heard of anyone who was sober or not wearing a skirt who was raped?", "Are all rape victims to blame for what happens to them?", or "What about the rapist? What level of intent and fault does he have?"

Ultimately, clients should come to realize that they may have somehow provided the occasion for their traumatic events, but that they were not the causes of these events. In other words, they need to understand that they happened to be in the wrong place at the wrong time, and that this may have had major effects on them, but that the events say nothing about them as people. When clients have been singled out for crimes, this can be a hard concept for them to grasp.

There are some cases in which clients used poor judgment, had some level of responsibility, committed some intentional act, or did not act when they could have. PTSD can result, even when someone actually intended harm at the time of the traumatic event. Prisons are full of people with PTSD from a lifetime of victimization who then committed criminal acts. Sometimes in gang territory, the rule is "Join the gang and commit crimes and kill, or be killed." Or military personnel may commit acts or not prevent something from happening that they later regret when they come home and have time to reflect on their actions or inactions. It is important to remember and convey to such clients that if they had no consciences, they would not have guilt or shame over these acts, and therefore would not be haunted by their traumatic events. The fact that someone comes for treatment for PTSD and has committed some act against another person (or did not act when he or she could have) is a good sign that the person does have a conscience.

We are often asked what to do if someone comes to therapy who insists that he or she did play a role in the traumatic event or actually had intent to commit a crime. First, it is important to determine through Socratic dialogue whether the person's perception represents false blame, a Stuck Point, or an accurate belief. The therapist also has to consider whether the client really has remorse and is not currently committing the same or similar acts. If someone indeed held some responsibility or intended harm against someone else, then regret or guilt is the appropriate response, and the therapist should not try to take that away. The client may have to accept what he or she did and consider whether any type of restitution is possible, for the victim(s) or for the community in general. Could the person volunteer at a shelter for homeless people or otherwise give back to the community in some way?

Typically, in these cases of PTSD, we are talking about events that occurred in the past for which clients feel guilt and remorse. They sentence themselves more harshly than a jury would. If this is the case, then the task is to "right-size" the Stuck Points (e.g., "I am nothing but an evil monster"), put the event into the context in which it occurred and then into the larger context of the clients' lives. Therapists can ask clarifying questions to determine the context in which the clients' acts occurred. They can also ask questions about whether the clients are still committing similar acts or whether they have changed their lives. We have yet to have a client who sought PTSD treatment while still committing the same crime they are feeling guilty over. Typically, a therapist can draw a circle to create a pie chart and can then ask a client, "What proportion of your life was spent committing crimes, and what proportions have you spent in different roles?" (See the example below.) Next, the therapist can ask the client who he or she currently is and to imagine how it would feel to say, "Even good people can do bad things in certain contexts," instead of "I must be evil." The therapist should also help the client to consider the learning environment in which he or she was raised, and to consider how that might have played a role in the client's understanding of the behavior at the time.

Generally, if someone kills another person or persons during war, this is typically not considered murder and is not prosecuted as a crime, especially if the person was following the rules of military engagement at that time. However, if the client says, "People shouldn't kill; I have killed; therefore I am a monster," the thought does not match the event. The therapist can ask, "What emotion do you feel when you say, 'I am a monster'?" Then the therapist can ask a series of questions about context, such as whether the client had killed people before the war, has done so since the war, or has the urge to kill people now. The answers to these questions will guide the therapist to understand whether this is a pattern of behavior or whether it only occurred in the context of war. Below is an example of a therapist–client Socratic dialogue regarding this issue.

THERAPIST: What do you mean by "monster"?

CLIENT: Not human, not fit for the company of others.

THERAPIST: Is that why you have isolated yourself, even from your family at times?

CLIENT: Yes, I suppose so. Who would want to be around me when I am so dangerous?

THERAPIST: Dangerous? Why do you think you are dangerous?

CLIENT: I have killed before. I could do it again.

THERAPIST: Under certain circumstances, couldn't most people kill? What if someone were attacking a child? Might not the mother kill in the defense of her child?

CLIENT: Well, yes, but that's different. She would be doing it to save someone else.

THERAPIST: And what was your mission when you killed? What was going on?

CLIENT: Well, we were on patrol in the jungle, and the Viet Cong attacked our platoon.

THERAPIST: And were you just killing someone, or were you trying to save yourself and others?

CLIENT: We didn't have a choice.

THERAPIST: So how is that different from the mother protecting her child? Are you both monsters?

CLIENT: I hadn't really thought about it that way before. No, she wouldn't be a monster. And I was shooting to protect myself and my men. However, there is something that I haven't told you. When I killed the guy, I felt a physical rush, and I was happy. That can't be right.

THERAPIST: When your life is in danger, your body produces all sorts of chemical reactions to help you fight or flee. When the adrenaline rush happened, you were probably also relieved to have survived and happy to have saved others. Sometimes people experience dissociation and even may have endorphins flood their system, which shuts off pain, kind of like a runner's high. What is wrong with that?

CLIENT: I don't know, but I saw it happen to other guys too, and some of them didn't stop killing. They were just shooting everyone they saw.

THERAPIST: Remember when I told you about different parts of the brain that get turned on or off when there is danger? The survival part of your brain turned on. That goes along with the fight–flight–freeze response. That survival part includes emotions, too, like anger and fear. At the same time, the front part of your brain—the thinking part—turns off, at least temporarily. For you, after the danger and that rush of emotions was over, your frontal lobes—the thinking part—came back, and then you calmed down and didn't keep killing. Some of the other guys you were with may not have had your level of control. They were young, 19 or 20, and their brains hadn't even finished developing yet. It sounds like the thinking parts of their brains didn't put on the brakes, and their emotional parts kept them in fight mode. However, I expect that they are probably not still killing either, and they may have great regrets over things that they did in the heat of the war. (*Pause*) But let's go back to the word "monster." Words are powerful to how we feel about ourselves. Is that accurate?

CLIENT: No, I suppose not. But I am a "killer."

THERAPIST: Yes, you have killed. Is that different from being a "killer"?

CLIENT: I guess being a killer implies that you do it all the time.

THERAPIST: So are you a killer versus someone who has killed?

CLIENT: Hmmm . . . I guess someone who has killed.

THERAPIST: And when you say it that way, how do you feel?

CLIENT: Less despicable.

THERAPIST: OK. We're getting somewhere. I'm also curious: What else are you besides someone who has killed?

CLIENT: What do you mean?

THERAPIST: Are you a son?

CLIENT: Yes.

THERAPIST: Are you a monster or a killer as a son?

CLIENT: (*Laughs*) Well, I might have been a little monster when I was a kid from time to time. But, no, I am a good son and take care of my mother.

THERAPIST: Are you a husband and father?

CLIENT: Yes, I get your point. I am more things than just a killer.

THERAPIST: Right. If we were to take a pie and slice it up into all the things you are—a son, a father, an uncle, a worker, a boss, a caretaker, a gardener, a door-knob fixer, a dishwasher, a friend, a deacon in your church—how big a slice of the pie would "killer" realistically take up?

CLIENT: A small slice, but an important one.

THERAPIST: I agree that some slices are more important than others, but it seems important not to ignore all the other slices that make you up. Don't they also make part of who you are and what your whole life is?

CLIENT: Yeah, you have talked before about thinking about everything and not just some parts. I guess I was losing that with this Stuck Point.

THERAPIST: When you say, "I killed during the war to protect myself and my men," how do you feel?

CLIENT: Well, not so bad. Better.

THERAPIST: Better in what emotional way?

CLIENT: I don't feel so ashamed. I'm not there yet, but I guess I might be proud if I remembered that I protected my men.

THERAPIST: It's good that you're imagining how you could feel if you held onto that new thought. Now comes the practice to embrace that thought. Let's use this as an example for the next worksheet that we are going to start using.

At this point, the therapist introduces the Challenging Questions Worksheet (Handout 7.2).

Introducing the Challenging Questions Worksheet

It is important to leave enough time in the session to introduce new worksheets and help a client practice with them prior to the end of the session. Up to a third of the session may be needed, depending on the complexity of each worksheet. Every time a new worksheet is introduced, the rationale for using it needs to be explained, and the therapist should walk the client through it with one of the Stuck Points the client and therapist have just been working on during the session, or one from the Stuck Point Log. The purpose of the Challenging Questions Worksheet is for clients to begin to challenge their own thoughts about their trauma, and later their ongoing beliefs about themselves, others, and the world, with a series of questions.

Giving the New Practice Assignment

The practice assignment after Session 4 is to have a client complete one Challenging Questions Worksheet (Handout 7.2) each day on a Stuck Point from the Stuck Point Log (Handout 6.1). In addition to presenting copies of this blank worksheet for practice, the therapist can use the completed examples of Challenging Questions Worksheets (Handouts 7.2a and 7.2b) to demonstrate how some Stuck Points can be challenged, and the Guide for the Challenging Questions Worksheet (Handout 7.3) to help explain exactly what each question is asking. It is important to use this discussion to make sure that the client has a clear idea of how to proceed before attempting to complete a Challenging Questions Worksheet each day before the next session. The client should also be reminded that the Challenging Questions Worksheet includes a variety of questions, because not every question applies to every Stuck Point.

Checking the Client's Reactions to the Session
and the Practice Assignment

The therapist should conclude Session 4 by eliciting the client's reactions to the session and asking whether the client has any questions about the session content or the new practice assignment (see Handout 7.4). The therapist may even mark on the Stuck Point Log or at the top of the blank Challenging Questions Worksheets which assimilated

Stuck Points the therapist wants the client to focus on. The therapist should reinforce any important ideas or discoveries made in the session, and should note the important take-home messages that the client offers.

Session 5: Using the Challenging Questions Worksheet

Procedures for Session 5

Review the client's scores on the self-report objective measures. (See the discussions of this review for Sessions 2 and 3 in Chapter 6.)

1. Review the client's Challenging Questions Worksheets.
2. Introduce the Patterns of Problematic Thinking Worksheet.
3. Give the practice assignment.
4. Check the client's reactions to the session and the practice assignment.

Reviewing the Client's Challenging Questions Worksheets

At the end of Session 4, the client has been asked to complete a Challenging Questions Worksheet each day prior to Session 5. The first thing the therapist should do is check to see how many worksheets the client has completed, and discuss the role of avoidance if no or very few worksheets have been done. If the therapist has written in the relevant Stuck Points at the tops of the blank worksheets, he or she can check to see which (if any) of these Stuck Points have been dealt with and which have been avoided. This may be a clue as to which Stuck Points are particularly entrenched or threatening. Although the majority of the therapy time will be focused on assimilated Stuck Points about the index trauma, the therapist and client should spend some time with the questions in general if the client has trouble understanding any of them.

If the client has resolved all assimilated Stuck Points about the index traumatic event (or has moved on to other traumatic events), this resolution should still be the focus of the therapy session. Even if clients say that they do not believe a particular Stuck Point any more (e.g., "I don't believe it is my fault now"), it is still good practice to have them complete a copy of the worksheet on this Stuck Point, to have it available for reference in their therapy binders or workbooks and to reinforce new learning. When learning to use the Challenging Questions Worksheet, clients should attempt to answer every question—and not just with a "Yes" or "No," but with an explanation of the reason(s) for this answer.

The most common error clients make in completing the Challenging Questions

Worksheet is that they try to use another Stuck Point as evidence for the Stuck Point they are working on. For example, if a client's Stuck Point is "The rape was my fault," and evidence for it is given as "I must have done something that made him think I wanted sex," the therapist should devote some time to explaining the difference between a thought and a fact. Opinions cannot be used as evidence to support a Stuck Point. Common examples of evidence that can be used include evidence that would be accepted in a court of law or that would be published in reputable news media. Here is an example of a therapist–client dialogue regarding this:

> THERAPIST: When we talk about "evidence" in CPT, we are talking about evidence that would stand up in a court of law or would be published by a reputable newspaper or news website. For instance, do you think a jury would say, "You must have done something to make him think you wanted sex"? Remind me what you said to him that night.
>
> CLIENT: I said I liked his shirt.
>
> THERAPIST: Can you explain to me how saying you liked his shirt was sending him a message that you wanted to be raped?
>
> CLIENT: But isn't that flirting?
>
> THERAPIST: Maybe. But even if your intention was to flirt at that time, is that a message to say that you want to be attacked?
>
> CLIENT: No.
>
> THERAPIST: And even if you wanted to have sex with him, does that give him the right to rape you?
>
> CLIENT: No.
>
> THERAPIST: So, going back to the worksheet, what is the evidence for the Stuck Point that the rape was your fault? Did you intend to be raped? Who had the intention to rape?
>
> CLIENT: He did. But then there is no evidence for the rape being my fault.
>
> THERAPIST: OK, let's get that down on the worksheet: "There is no evidence that the rape was my fault." What is the evidence against the idea that it was your fault?
>
> CLIENT: He told me that he would drive me home, and he took me out into the countryside and attacked me.
>
> THERAPIST: OK, he took you out in the countryside and raped you. And did you say "No"?
>
> CLIENT: Yes, and I fought him as hard as I could, and I tried to run away, but he caught up with me and knocked me down.
>
> THERAPIST: So it sounds like to me that there is lots of evidence against the rape being your fault. Let's write that down in the space about evidence against the Stuck Point.

Some clients have trouble with question 3 on the Challenging Questions Worksheet: "In what ways is your Stuck Point not including all of the information?" This is a question aimed at contextualizing the situation and considering elements that a client has been ignoring. In the example above, the client didn't include her saying "No," her fighting back, and the perpetrator's saying he would drive her home but then driving her into the countryside as part of the context of the rape. Or soldiers may blame themselves or others in their units, but ignore what it means to be ambushed by the enemy. By definition, an ambush is unanticipated—a surprise attack. This is part of the context in which the trauma occurred. Similarly, could a child who weighs 50 pounds have fought off a 200-pound adult? Could a client have known in advance that someone she knew and had no reason not to trust would suddenly commit an attack? Can a family member go into a house engulfed in flames and rescue someone upstairs? When clients say, "I should have known," or "I should have stopped [the traumatic event] from occurring," it is important for the therapist to ask what they knew at the time that it happened and what they could have realistically done, given who they were, what the context was, and what choices they really had.

Questions 4 and 5 on the Challenging Questions Worksheet are similar, but the first of the two asks whether the person is using all-or-none terms, as if there are only two categories (as opposed to various intermediate categories). Question 5 asks whether the client is using phrases that are extreme or exaggerated. In the latter case, "should" may be an extreme word (e.g., "I should have prevented the shooting") but is not absolutely black-and-white, as is "I would have prevented the event if I had been able to change positions." The therapist can ask the questions both ways, to capture the client's various thoughts regarding assimilation.

The therapist should also look for hidden words in a thought. If a mother says, "It is my fault that my daughter was abused," is she really saying that it is *all* her fault? What about the perpetrator? Did the mother even know that it was happening, or did she have some responsibility in entrusting her daughter to someone she suspected might hurt her daughter? Even in the latter case, the mother would have a level of responsibility, but she did not intend harm to her daughter and did not commit the act(s). The perpetrator had intent, and therefore was at fault. The mother might share the blame if she offered up her daughter to the perpetrator, but she could not force him to violate the daughter. The perpetrator would still be blameworthy.

Question 6 on the Challenging Questions Worksheet is concerned with overfocusing on one aspect of the situation and disregarding other aspects. For example, a woman who had been drinking prior to an assault may assume that alcohol was the cause of the event: "If I hadn't been drinking, I wouldn't have been assaulted." This client may be ignoring the fact that everyone else in the environment had been drinking that night, or the possibility that she might have been assaulted whether she imbibed alcohol or not. Although alcohol may be a risk factor for victimization or problems in following procedures, it may or may not be a factor in the outcome of an event. For example, alcohol cannot cause someone else to perpetrate a crime. It is important to avoid victim blaming in these situations.

Question 7 asks where the Stuck Point originated. Sometimes the source of the information is the client. However, if the client decided that the traumatic event was his or her fault when the client was a child, the source thus might not be a reliable, mature person. The Stuck Point may even represent magical thinking in a post hoc effort to exert control over an uncontrollable situation (e.g., "I should have beaten him up"). Or the Stuck Point might have come from someone else. If a rapist says, "You know you want this," is he an accurate or reliable source of information? If an abusive parent says, "You made me hit you," is that possible? It is important for the client to identify the source of the information that resulted in the Stuck Point, and to recognize that this source may not have been reliable. A question that therapists sometimes ask is "What do the people you respect the most say?"

Question 8 is "How is your Stuck Point confusing something that is possible with something that is likely?" In other words, is the client confusing a rare or low-probability event (e.g., a terrorist attack in North America) with a high-probability event (e.g., the sun's coming up in the morning)? People with PTSD often assume that because something happened once or twice, it *will* happen again if they are not hypervigilant. Much of the avoidance behavior seen in PTSD is an attempt to prevent bad events from happening. Soldiers or veterans with PTSD will avoid going into large stores or restaurants because of their assumption that crowds are dangerous and something bad will happen. A rape victim may leave all the lights on at night because the rape happened when it was dark. After a car accident, some clients refuse to drive on busy highways or other types of roads reminiscent of the accident. So question 8 often pertains to safety-related Stuck Points.

Question 9 pertains to emotional reasoning. Emotional reasoning occurs when clients use their emotions as "proof" of their Stuck Points. In other words, instead of looking at the facts and then noticing how they feel, clients notice their feelings and assume them to have legitimate causes or to confirm that their Stuck Points are correct. Clients may feel fear and presume that there is danger, or anger and presume that someone wronged them, or guilt and assume that they did something wrong. To take an example from the preceding paragraph, a traumatized soldier or veteran may walk into a large, crowded store and begin to feel anxious. He then assumes that he is in danger and leaves. He does not stay long enough to discover that nothing bad would have happened, and his rapid departure thus simply reaffirms his belief that stores are dangerous. Many triggers are conditioned at the time of traumatization and then generalize. Clients with PTSD use those conditioned emotional responses as proof of their thought in a form of backward reasoning.

The final question on the Challenging Questions Worksheet asks clients whether they have been focusing on irrelevant factors as to why the event happened. In the example of the rape victim earlier in this section, she assumed that she was raped because she complimented the rapist about his shirt. She thought that she must have been flirting (and might have been), but she was focusing on that factor instead of all the other events surrounding the forcible rape. Flirting does not force someone to attack and should not be confused with an invitation to have consensual sex. For someone who has PTSD after a car accident, focusing on the driver's alcohol consumption might well be a relevant factor, but the fact that it happened in a certain city would not be. Yet therapists often hear clients with PTSD say things about moving away so that more bad things won't happen. If someone lives in a very high-crime neighborhood, this might be a risk factor—but living in a safe neighborhood and blaming the neighborhood, city, or state would probably be an inaccurate appraisal of a crime or a car accident, because it would represent a focus on an unrelated part of the event.

Introducing the Patterns of Problematic Thinking Worksheet

After spending about two-thirds of the session reviewing the client's completed Challenging Questions Worksheets, the therapist introduces the next worksheet, the Patterns of Problematic Thinking Worksheet (Handout 7.5). Instead of focusing on just one Stuck Point, this worksheet helps the client look for tendencies in his or her ways of thinking that can be problematic. The therapist should go over the worksheet with the client and have the client think about Stuck Points or even reactions to daily events that fit into one of the patterns. These patterns may have existed before the traumatic event occurred and may even be core beliefs. Some clients will find examples under each of the categories, and others will be "specialists" (e.g., they tend to jump to conclusions, but may not engage in emotional reasoning). A therapist should describe how these patterns become automatic, creating negative feelings and causing a client to engage in self-defeating behaviors (e.g., avoiding relationships because of the conclusion that no one can be trusted).

The one item that is newly introduced in this worksheet is mind reading (specifically, the tendency to assume that people are thinking badly of a client when there is no actual evidence for this). The therapist may have the opportunity to discuss this item within the context of the therapy, if the client assumed at the start of treatment that the therapist was going to behave in a certain way or react to the trauma story with revulsion or rejection. The therapist can point out that the client was incorrect in this mind reading, and that it may have been a better indicator of what the client was thinking than of what another person (the therapist) was thinking. The therapist should give the client several copies of the blank Patterns of Problematic Thinking Worksheet, so that the client can work on them every day between sessions. An example of a completed worksheet (see Handout 7.5a) should also be provided, to help the client in understanding and completing the assignment.

Giving the New Practice Assignment

The therapist should assign the client to complete a copy of the Patterns of Problematic Thinking Worksheet every day (see Handout 7.6). The patterns can be taken from everyday events, as well as from items on the Stuck Point Log. The purpose is to discover whether the client has these tendencies in one specific area (e.g., mind reading), or is more of a "generalist" and uses most or all of these patterns. Noticing everyday thoughts as well as traumatic event Stuck Points will enable the client to examine his or her habits of thinking.

Checking the Client's Reactions to the Session and the Practice Assignment

The therapist should conclude Session 5 by eliciting the client's reactions to the session and asking whether the client has any questions about the session content or the new practice assignment. The client should be encouraged to examine everyday patterns of problematic thinking as well as those on the Stuck Point Log, in order to identify any particularly strong tendencies that the client will need to watch out for. The therapist should reinforce any important ideas or discoveries made in the session, and should note the important take-home messages that the client offers.

Levels of Responsibility Handout

Date: _____   Client: _____

Your role in the traumatic event: What are the facts?

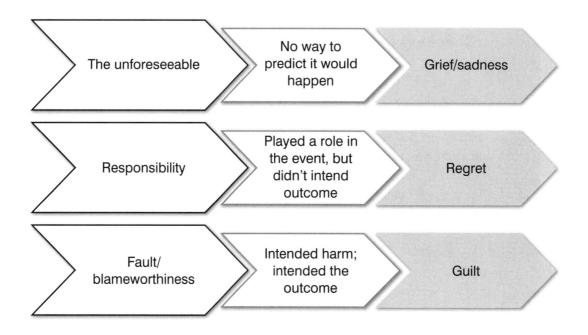

Challenging Questions Worksheet

Date: _____   Client: _____

Below is a list of questions to be used in helping you challenge your Stuck Points or problematic beliefs. Not all questions will be appropriate for the belief you choose to challenge. Answer as many questions as you can for the belief you have chosen to challenge below.

Belief:

1. What is the evidence for and against this Stuck Point?

   For:

   Against:

2. Is your Stuck Point a habit or based on facts?

3. In what ways is your Stuck Point not including all of the information?

(continued)

4. Does your Stuck Point include all-or-none terms?

5. Does the Stuck Point include words or phrases that are extreme or exaggerated (such as "always," "forever," "never," "need," "should," "must," "can't," and "every time")?

6. In what way is your Stuck Point focused on just one piece of the story?

7. Where did this Stuck Point come from? Is this a dependable source of information on this Stuck Point?

8. How is your Stuck Point confusing something that is possible with something that is likely?

9. In what ways is your Stuck Point based on feelings rather than facts?

10. In what ways is this Stuck Point focused on unrelated parts of the story?

Sample Challenging Questions Worksheet

Date: _____   Client: _____

Below is a list of questions to be used in helping you challenge your Stuck Points or problematic beliefs. Not all questions will be appropriate for the belief you choose to challenge. Answer as many questions as you can for the belief you have chosen to challenge below.

Belief:

It is my fault that my uncle had sex with me. [Therapist asked whether the Stuck Point had a hidden word, "all."]

1. What is the evidence for and against this Stuck Point?

    For:

    ~~*I must have done something that made him think it was OK.*~~ [After more questions by therapist about fault and intent:] *There is no evidence for its being my fault.*

    Against:

    I didn't want to do it, and I told him so. He threatened to hurt my little sister. He said no one would believe me. He was an adult, and I was a child. He was bigger and stronger than me.

2. Is your Stuck Point a habit or based on facts?

    Habit. I have been saying this to myself for 25 years.

3. In what ways is your Stuck Point not including all of the information?

    How could it be my fault? I didn't even know what sex was when he started. You don't do that to kids. Just because he read me stories and babysat me didn't give him the right to do that.

4. Does your Stuck Point include all-or-none terms?

    Well, we talked about the hidden word "all." I thought it was all my fault and didn't even think about really blaming him. I was too scared of him, and my mother loved him.

5. Does the Stuck Point include words or phrases that are extreme or exaggerated (such as "always," "forever," "never," "need," "should," "must," "can't," and "every time")?

    "All my fault."

6. In what way is your Stuck Point focused on just one piece of the story?

    Because he did it to me, I assumed it was about me. I didn't think about the fact that I was a child or that what he did was a crime. I told him "No," and he threatened my family.

(continued)

---

7. Where did this Stuck Point come from? Is this a dependable source of information on this Stuck Point?

   Mostly from me, but I think he said things that made it seem like it was my fault. I was so pretty, that he couldn't keep his hands off of me, I was special, etc.

8. How is your Stuck Point confusing something that is possible with something that is likely?

   N/A.

9. In what ways is your Stuck Point based on feelings rather than facts?

   Because I felt guilty and shameful, I thought it must be my fault.

10. In what ways is this Stuck Point focused on unrelated parts of the story?

    I must have thought that I had more control over the situation than I did.

Sample Challenging Questions Worksheet

Date: _____ Client: _____

Below is a list of questions to be used in helping you challenge your Stuck Points or problematic beliefs. Not all questions will be appropriate for the belief you choose to challenge. Answer as many questions as you can for the belief you have chosen to challenge below.

Belief:

It is my fault that my brother was killed in the car accident, because I should have done things differently.

1. What is the evidence for and against this Stuck Point?

   For:

   I should have made him wear his seat belt. He refused, and I thought it was only a few blocks so it didn't really matter. We were laughing and talking.

   Against:

   I didn't cause the crash. The other person was texting and ran the red light. The officer said that even with a seat belt, being hit from the side like that, my brother would have been killed anyway.

2. Is your Stuck Point a habit or based on facts?

   Habit. I have been blaming myself for 2 years. I guess it was wishful thinking.

3. In what ways is your Stuck Point not including all of the information?

   When the light turned green, I did look both ways before I entered the intersection. He was coming so fast that there was nowhere for me to go.

4. Does your Stuck Point include all-or-none terms?

   I thought it was all my fault because my brother died, and I didn't even think about the driver of the other car. I kept saying I should have done something different to avoid the crash.

5. Does the Stuck Point include words or phrases that are extreme or exaggerated (such as "always," "forever," "never," "need," "should," "must," "can't," and "every time")?

   "All my fault." "Should have done things differently."

6. In what way is your Stuck Point focused on just one piece of the story?

   I was focused on the fact that my brother refused to put on his seat belt, and I didn't really listen when the officer said that with that kind of side crash, it wouldn't have made a difference. I was also focused on the fact that we were talking and laughing, but I overlooked the fact that I did look both ways.

(continued)

7. Where did this Stuck Point come from? Is this a dependable source of information on this Stuck Point?

The Stuck Point came from me, but when it first happened my parents' first reaction was that it was my fault, and that I shouldn't have started the car until he put his seat belt on. Later they were more supportive, but I think they were so upset at the time that they took it out on me.

8. How is your Stuck Point confusing something that is possible with something that is likely?

I kept thinking that I could have done something different to avoid the crash. Maybe there was something I could have done, but it isn't likely.

9. In what ways is your Stuck Point based on feelings rather than facts?

Because I felt guilty, I thought it must be my fault.

10. In what ways is this Stuck Point focused on unrelated parts of the story?

I was focused completely on the seat belt. I didn't kill my brother. The other driver did. He shouldn't have been texting and driving too fast. Focusing on the fact that we were laughing was irrelevant. I was paying attention and following the rules.

Guide for the Challenging Questions Worksheet

Date: _____   Client: _____

Below is a list of questions to be used in helping you challenge your Stuck Points or problematic beliefs. Not all questions will be appropriate for the belief you choose to challenge. Answer as many questions as you can for the belief you have chosen to challenge below.

Belief: *Put a Stuck Point here. You can use your Stuck Point Log to find one.*

*The belief should **not** be a feeling or behavior, and should **not** be too vague. Use "If–then" statements if possible.*

1. What is the evidence for and against this Stuck Point?

   *Evidence consists of the type of facts that will hold up in court. We are not challenging that the event happened. We are looking for evidence that **supports** and does **not support** the Stuck Point you have given above.*

   For: *Do **not** use another Stuck Point! Make sure you are identifying facts.*

   Against: *Only **one** exception is needed to make a belief **not** a fact. A fact is 100% and absolute. If you can identify one exception to your Stuck Point, then it is not a fact, and therefore would not hold up in court.*

2. Is your Stuck Point a habit or based on facts?

   *Have you been telling yourself this belief for so long that it **feels** like a fact? It's like advertising: After a while, you start to believe it. Is this belief something that you have been in the habit of telling yourself for a long time?*

3. In what ways is your Stuck Point not including all of the information?

   *Is it **possible** that your Stuck Point is unrealistic or not **completely** accurate or not **completely** true? Does your belief reflect all the facts of the situation? Remember the context of the trauma.*

4. Does your Stuck Point include all-or-none terms?

   Does your Stuck Point reflect all-or-none, black-and-white categories? Are things all good or all bad? Are you missing the gray areas in between? Example: If your performance falls short of perfect, you see yourself as a failure.

5. Does the Stuck Point include words or phrases that are extreme or exaggerated (such as "always," "forever," "never," "need," "should," "must," "can't," and "every time")?

   These words or phrases may be hidden. Example: "Men can't be trusted" is actually "All men can't be trusted."

(continued)

6. In what way is your Stuck Point focused on just one piece of the story?

   This question is about deciding that one piece of information from the event caused the event to happen. Then, you use this one aspect to create your Stuck Point. Example: "If I had been stronger, then this wouldn't have happened." Now think about drawing a pie chart and showing one small slice of that pie as the one aspect you are focusing on. You are probably assigning 100% of the "blame" or "cause" to this "slice" and discounting all the remaining factors (other slices) in the rest of the pie. Other slices might include that you were outnumbered, the perpetrator had a weapon, you were taken by surprise, there were no other options at the time, or similar factors. Why are these other factors/slices not considered here as contributory? Are you discounting them and only focusing on the one factor/slice?

7. Where did this Stuck Point come from? Is this a dependable source of information on this Stuck Point?

   Think about the time period when the event happened. Who were you at the time (a scared 20-year-old in combat, a child victimized by an adult, etc.)? Your Stuck Point may be based on a thought that you developed when you were scared or very young. You have retained that Stuck Point all these years, based on how you thought at the time. Or think about the enemy/perpetrator/other sources: Are these people reliable? Can they be trusted to make judgments about the event (or you)? Your Stuck Point might be a statement told to you by a perpetrator. Is a perpetrator to be trusted (reliable) to make this statement? Would we expect that a perpetrator is truthful? Consider your source.

8. How is your Stuck Point confusing something that is possible with something that is likely?

   *This question is best for a Stuck Point that is focused on the present or the future. It asks you, "What is the likelihood or percentage/chance that the Stuck Point will happen again?" An example of a present or future-oriented Stuck Point would be "If I trust others, then I'll get hurt." It may actually be a low probability, but you are living your life as if it is a certainty. Yes, it **could** happen, but are you living as if it **will** happen? Of course, in a dangerous environment, you may have to consider everything as a high probability, because the consequences (death or injury) are great. But are you taking into consideration that you don't need to hold this same degree of probability in **all** environments? In other words, are you applying the Stuck Point as if it has a high probability (a certainty) of happening again in **all** situations now? For example, think about driving. We all know that many people die every year in car accidents, yet we still drive. We do this because although we are aware that we could die in a car accident, we don't live as if it **will** happen.*

9. In what ways is your Stuck Point based on feelings rather than facts?

   *This question represents the idea that if you **feel** something is true, then it must be. For example, think about hypervigilance: Because you **feel** uncomfortable or under threat in a crowd, you assume (or develop the belief) that it is dangerous. This becomes "I don't like crowds," which translates into the Stuck Point "I am never safe in a crowd," or "If I am in a crowd, then I will be harmed." Another example is that if you **feel** guilty, then you assume you must be at fault.*

10. In what ways is this Stuck Point focused on unrelated parts of the story?

    This question is about focusing the cause or blame on something that had nothing to do with the event's happening. For example, "I wore a red dress; therefore, I was assaulted." This is different from question 6 because it is about something that was irrelevant, whereas in question 6 the factor may have contributed to the event but is not wholly to blame. However, even in question 6, the piece may be incorrect rather than factual.

Practice Assignment after Session 4 of CPT

Please choose one Stuck Point each day, and then answer the questions on the Challenging Questions Worksheet (Handout 7.2) with regard to this Stuck Point. Please work on Stuck Points related directly to the trauma first (e.g., "It is my fault," "I could have prevented it," or "If I had done *X*, it would not have happened"). Your therapist will give you extra copies of the Challenging Questions Worksheets, so you can work on multiple Stuck Points. Completed examples of this worksheet are provided as Handouts 7.2a and 7.2b, and a Guide to the Challenging Questions Worksheet (Handout 7.3) is also available.

Patterns of Problematic Thinking Worksheet

Date: _____   Client: _____

Listed below are several different patterns of problematic thinking that people use in different life situations. These patterns often become automatic, habitual thoughts that cause people to engage in self-defeating behavior. Considering your own Stuck Points, or samples from your everyday thinking, find examples for each of these patterns. Write in the Stuck Point or typical thought under the appropriate pattern, and describe how it fits that pattern. Think about how that pattern affects you.

1. **Jumping to conclusions** or predicting the future.

2. **Exaggerating or minimizing** a situation (blowing things way out of proportion or shrinking their importance inappropriately).

3. **Ignoring important parts** of a situation.

4. **Oversimplifying** things as "good–bad" or "right–wrong."

5. **Overgeneralizing** from a single incident (e.g., a negative event is seen as a never-ending pattern).

6. **Mind reading** (assuming that people are thinking negatively of you when there is no definite evidence for this).

7. **Emotional reasoning** (using your emotions as proof—e.g., "I feel fear, so I must be in danger").

Sample Patterns of Problematic Thinking Worksheet

Date: _____   Client: _____

Listed below are several different patterns of problematic thinking that people use in different life situations. These patterns often become automatic, habitual thoughts that cause people to engage in self-defeating behavior. Considering your own Stuck Points, or samples from your everyday thinking, find examples for each of these patterns. Write in the Stuck Point or typical thought under the appropriate pattern, and describe how it fits that pattern. Think about how that pattern affects you.

1. **Jumping to conclusions** or predicting the future.

   [Victim of childhood sexual abuse:] *If a man is alone with a child, then the man will hurt the child. But I know my husband will not hurt my kids so this belief is causing problems in my marriage*

2. **Exaggerating or minimizing** a situation (blowing things way out of proportion or shrinking their importance inappropriately).

   [Traveler:] *I saw a dead body and riots, but I didn't get hurt and others saw worse, so my reaction to the situation was wrong. I was weak.*

3. **Ignoring important parts** of a situation.

   [Robbery victim:] *I keep forgetting the fact that the perpetrator had a gun, which is important information about how much control I had.*

4. **Oversimplifying** things as "good–bad" or "right–wrong."

   [Police officer:] *Not everyone is all good or all bad. I may have done some things in my life that were not that good, but that does not make me a bad person.*

5. **Overgeneralizing** from a single incident (e.g., a negative event is seen as a never-ending pattern).

   [Adult rape victim:] *I was raped by a man, so all men are dangerous. Maybe I am using this belief to stay away from men?*

6. **Mind reading** (in particular, assuming that people are thinking negatively of you when there is no definite evidence for this).

   [Victim of childhood physical abuse:] *My dad yells now, so I assume he must be angry. But it's not true a lot of the times, because he yells sometimes because he is deaf in one ear and going deaf in another. He yells because he doesn't know he is yelling.*

7. **Emotional reasoning** (using your emotions as proof—e.g., "I feel fear, so I must be in danger").

   [Survivor of a traumatic bereavement:] *I feel guilt over my friend's death, so I must have done something wrong.*

Practice Assignment after Session 5 of CPT

Your practice assignment is to consider your Stuck Points, as well as some examples of your everyday thinking, and to find ones that fit into each relevant thinking pattern on the Patterns of Problematic Thinking Worksheet (Handout 7.5). Each day, list a Stuck Point or example of everyday thinking under each pattern, and think about ways in which your reactions to the traumatic event may be affected by these habitual patterns. A completed example of this worksheet is provided as Handout 7.5a.

8

Learning to Self-Challenge

Sessions 6 and 7

Goals for Sessions 6 and 7

The first goal for Sessions 6 and 7 is to continue teaching clients to become their own cognitive therapists by initially asking themselves questions with the Patterns of Problematic Thinking Worksheet, which helps clients identify their characteristic patterns of interpreting events. Clients are then introduced to the final cognitive worksheet, the Challenging Beliefs Worksheet, which brings together all the worksheets that the client has been taught and introduces the development of alternative thoughts and related feelings. The Challenging Beliefs Worksheet is used throughout the rest of the CPT protocol.

Session 6: Patterns of Problematic Thinking Worksheet and Introduction to Challenging Beliefs Worksheet

---

Procedures for Session 6

1. Review the client's scores on the self-report objective measures, and conduct a mid-protocol assessment of the client's treatment response to this point.
2. Review the client's Pattern of Problematic Thinking Worksheet.

3. Introduce the Challenging Beliefs Worksheet, and have the client practice completing it with a trauma example.

4. Give the new practice assignment.

5. Check the client's reactions to the session and the practice assignment.

Conducting a Midprotocol Assessment of Treatment Response

Given that Session 6 marks the halfway point in the typical CPT protocol, the client's scores on the PCL-5 or other PTSD self-report scale being used should be significantly decreased. If it is not, this probably indicates that assimilated thoughts have not been successfully addressed. As stressed in the "Case Conceptualization" section of Chapter 3 and in the preceding chapters of Part III outlining the CPT protocol, the therapist should continue to focus these sessions on the index event and assimilated thoughts. It is also possible that the client may have other traumatic events with related assimilated Stuck Points that need to be targeted. It is our experience that assimilated thoughts about thematically similar traumas (e.g., interpersonal violence, military experiences) tend to be addressed through a focus on the index trauma. For example, if a client has identified an adult rape as her index trauma, but also has a history of childhood sexual abuse, the accommodated beliefs she develops about her and her perpetrator's role in the rape are likely to generalize to her beliefs about her childhood sexual abuse experiences (e.g., "I'm not to blame for my perpetrator's taking sexual advantage of me"). Conversely, if a core belief is identified ("People will always betray me"), it may have originated with the childhood abuse and then may have been activated with the adult trauma.

Other traumatic experiences that are not as similar to the index event may need to be specifically addressed. For example, one of us had a client who identified her index event as her child's drowning, but had also experienced a robbery. With greater accommodation of her beliefs about her child's death, the therapist was able to focus on assimilated beliefs related to the robbery to facilitate even greater improvements in her PTSD symptoms. It is also possible that a client is leaving out an important part of the index trauma, either because of shame or because the client is protecting a more important Stuck Point (e.g., "If it isn't my fault that the incest happened, then that means that my father didn't love me. If my own father didn't love me enough to protect me, then no one will").

The therapist should also closely review item-level responses to the PTSD self-report scale, to determine the symptoms that are still problematic. If the client is still avoiding thinking about the event or feeling natural emotions about it, the therapist should help the client challenge this avoidance. This process may include identifying Stuck Points the client has about facing the event and/or experiencing emotions, and using the cognitive worksheets to challenge these Stuck Points. If the client reports continued nightmares or flashbacks, the therapist should inquire about the content. The content is likely to give clues to the part of the event in which the client is still stuck. It is also important to check that the client is anchoring his or her report of symptoms to the index event, and not responding to the measure in terms of general stress.

It is also important to review the results of any self-report measures of relevant comorbid conditions (e.g., the PHQ-9), to determine how those conditions are responding to treatment. If, for example, there are no decreases in the quantity or frequency of substance use, this issue will need to be addressed so that substance misuse is not interfering with treatment. Likewise, maintenance of or increases in dissociation should be addressed to decrease its likelihood of impeding treatment progress.

Reviewing the Patterns of Problematic Thinking Worksheet

This session should focus on a review of the client's Patterns of Problematic Thinking Worksheet. The therapist should determine whether the client has had any difficulties identifying these patterns and understanding the problems with the statements. The therapist should discuss with the client how these patterns may have affected the client's reactions to the traumatic event(s) or developed in reaction to the event(s). Several problematic thinking patterns are seen frequently within this population. For example, a client who habitually jumps to the conclusion that negative outcomes are his or her fault may increase the likelihood of self-blame after the event. Mind reading is also very common: The client assumes that other people think and feel the same way the client does and reacts as if this were the case, resulting in alienation from others. Emotional reasoning about fear, shame, and guilt are frequently observed as well: A client who feels these emotions may regard them as proof that he or she must have done something wrong. Overgeneralizing from a single incident, and extreme, black-and-white thinking, are also very common.

Even if a client does not initially believe a more balanced thought, working with the client to modify his or her language can have an immediate effect on the magnitude of manufactured emotions. Once the therapist can point out, for example, that perhaps some people (even one person) can be trusted in some way, then the therapist can continue to remind the client that "No one can be trusted" is inaccurate. When the client starts to say, "Some people cannot be trusted," the accompanying emotions are less intense than when the client was saying "No one." Because some of a client's patterns of problematic thinking may represent automatic core beliefs, the therapist might wonder with the client where the thoughts originated. Some of them may have stemmed from early childhood maltreatment and have become core beliefs or schemas—thoughts that are automatic and deeply held.

Introducing the Challenging Beliefs Worksheet with a Trauma Example

After the review of the Patterns of Problematic Thinking Worksheet, the therapist introduces the Challenging Beliefs Worksheet (Handout 8.1). The therapist should take care in introducing this worksheet not to overwhelm the client, since it may be perceived at first as too complex. A good way to begin is by saying that the worksheet brings together all the skills the client has already learned through using the prior worksheets. The only new elements of the Challenging Beliefs Worksheet are the introduction of alternative thoughts and feelings, and the ratings of the believability of thoughts and intensity of emotions. The Challenging Beliefs Worksheet is used throughout the rest of the CPT sessions.

The therapist should point out that the ABC Worksheet is found in the two sections on the left (A and B), and can cover the rest of the new worksheet with a piece of paper to highlight this). In section B of the Challenging Beliefs Worksheet, however, the client is asked to add a rating of the extent to which he or she believes each thought or Stuck Point (0–100%); in section C, the client is asked to rate how strong the resulting emotions are (0–100%). The rationale for introducing these ratings at this point in the therapy is that at the beginning of CPT, the client is likely to perceive these thoughts as facts to be believed 100%, and the related emotions as either "on" or "off." With more practice, the client is likely to perceive greater variation in the strength of thoughts and feelings.

The next two sections (D and E) contain prompts from the Challenging Questions and Patterns of Problematic Thinking Worksheets to help the client challenge the identified thought. As a reminder, not every challenging question or pattern may be relevant for a given noticed thought. In the beginning, the client may have to pull out one or both of the two earlier worksheets to see what the prompts in the columns are referring to. Finally, for the first time, the client is asked to generate another thought that is more balanced and evidence-based (section F); to re-rate his or her level of belief in the original Stuck Point after generating the new thought (section G); and to monitor changes in related feelings (section H).

It is important for the therapist to emphasize that the goal of the Challenging Beliefs Worksheet is not necessarily to return the client to his or her prior beliefs, because the client may have held unrealistic beliefs prior to the trauma (e.g., "I can predict and control bad things from happening to me" or "No one can be trusted"). The goal is for the client to develop balanced, adaptive, and realistic beliefs. To use "No one can be trusted" as an example, the client is likely to be using the traumatic event as evidence supporting that belief. The goal is for the client to arrive at a more flexible and nuanced belief, such as "Some people can be trusted about some things, to varying degrees." Or a client may have had the pretrauma belief "It is always important to shut down my emotions. The therapist will not want to help the client return to that earlier belief. Clients with a long history of trauma, particularly those whose trauma began in early childhood, are prone to extreme beliefs that can become very entrenched. If the client has difficulty generating a more balanced thought, the "evidence against" the Stuck Point in section D may provide some ideas.

The therapist and client should fully complete at least one Challenging Beliefs Worksheet in this session, to ensure that the client understands the worksheet and to enhance the likelihood that it will be completed daily after this session. As a reminder, the therapist should continue to prioritize assimilated thoughts about the traumatic event in order to be most efficient in achieving outcomes. The therapist and client may want to review the Stuck Point Log, in order to cross off any Stuck Points that the client no longer believes and to pick out the ones that need more work. Those that reflect an underlying core belief (e.g., "If something bad happens, it is my fault") may take many worksheets to resolve. Core beliefs may be about overaccommodated concepts, but they can also emanate from clients' frequently being blamed by abusive parents for the abuse or being told that traumas happened to them because they were worthless or stupid. These automatic assumptions may take a number of worksheets on various traumas or everyday events to fall under the weight of the disputation and more balanced alternative thoughts.

Giving the New Practice Assignment

The practice assignment subsequent to this session is for the client to challenge Stuck Points with the Challenging Beliefs Worksheet. The therapist should help the client choose Stuck Points from the Stuck Point Log that that are in need of continued attention, and write these down on copies of the Challenging Beliefs Worksheet. This will increase the likelihood that the client will complete these worksheets outside the session. Examples of completed Challenging Beliefs Worksheets, and especially those most relevant to the client's own situation, should be provided to facilitate the client's understanding of the worksheet (see Handouts 8.1a–8.1e). One Challenging Belief Worksheet per day should be completed (see Handout 8.2).

Checking the Client's Reactions to the Session and the Practice Assignment

As usual, the therapist should conclude Session 6 by eliciting the client's reactions to the session and asking whether the client has any questions about the session content or the new practice assignment. The therapist should reinforce any important ideas or discoveries made in the session, and should note the important take-home messages that the client offers.

Session 7: Challenging Beliefs Worksheets and Introduction to Modules

Procedures for Session 7

1. Review the client's scores on the self-report objective measures. (See the discussions of this review for Sessions 2 and 3 in Chapter 6.)
2. Review the client's Challenging Beliefs Worksheets, to determine whether the client understands the worksheet and has successfully challenged some trauma-related Stuck Points.
3. Provide an overview of the five specific themes/modules that will be discussed in the remaining five sessions.
4. Introduce Safety, the first of these themes.
5. Give the new practice assignment.
6. Check the client's reactions to the session and the practice assignment.

Reviewing the Client's Challenging Beliefs Worksheets

After reviewing the client's scores on the self-report objective measures as usual, the therapist should review with the client the Challenging Beliefs Worksheets that he or she has completed since Session 6. Special attention should be paid to discussing the client's successes or problems in changing cognitions (and subsequent emotions) by using this worksheet. The therapist and client should use the Challenging Questions in section D of the worksheet to help the client confront cognitions that are still problematic. For example, one client had been in an elevator that fell 20 floors and then stopped just as it reached the bottom. Aside from having nightmares and flashbacks, he found himself unable to get into an elevator again. His thoughts were "Elevators are unsafe" and "The next time, I am going to die." On the worksheet, the client stated that the evidence was correct that elevators were unsafe, and that he knew he would die the next time because he had survived this time. He did not see that he was exaggerating or drawing conclusions when evidence was lacking, nor did he report engaging in emotional reasoning. At the end of the worksheet, his ratings did not change. This was an opportunity for the therapist to revert to Socratic dialogue for 10–15 minutes and then start again with the worksheet. The therapist reminded the client of the determinations they had made in prior sessions about the probability that the client would die the next time or that elevators would suddenly drop 20 floors.

   It is important to note that some clients initially struggle with this worksheet, but that most are able to generate alternatives and change their emotions, with the help of the foundation laid in the Challenging Questions Worksheet and the Patterns of Problematic Thinking Worksheet. The therapist should act as a coach, gently correcting worksheets in order for the client to obtain the maximum benefit from their use. The therapist should also prioritize review of any assimilated Stuck Points that the client is continuing to challenge. A number of similarly phrased Stuck Points may need to be assigned, to give the client sufficient practice in alternative ways of thinking. For example, a sexual assault victim was assigned the Stuck Points "I should have fought back harder," "I knew I shouldn't have trusted him," "I shouldn't have flirted with him," and "If I just hadn't frozen, I wouldn't have been raped." All of these thoughts represented assimilated thoughts aimed at changing the outcome of what happened at the time and forgetting the context of the event. Progress made on similar assimilated Stuck Points should generalize to other Stuck Points and help make new, healthier ways of thinking more routine for the client.

It is not unusual at this point in therapy for the client to say something like this: "I hear what you are saying, and it makes sense, but I don't feel that way." When this occurs, the therapist can congratulate the client on the progress he or she has made: "In the beginning, you were convinced that your thought was true. Sometimes it takes your feelings a little longer to catch up with your thoughts." Or the therapist can say something like this: "You have been thinking the other way for a long time, and it is a habit. The new way of thinking is not as comfortable and doesn't yet feel true. With more practice, this new, more balanced way of thinking about the event will become a new habit, and feeling better won't seem so strange."

Providing an Overview of the Five Themes

The therapist should now orient the client to the five themes that will be consecutively discussed over the five final sessions of the therapy. As discussed in Chapter 3 regarding case conceptualization, these themes represent important negative core beliefs or schemas that can be seemingly confirmed by a traumatic event or can change as a result of a traumatic event. The topics are Safety, Trust, Power/Control, Esteem, and Intimacy, presented in this order because they represent a hierarchy from more basic to complex human needs. Moreover, each theme is presented as it relates to self- and other-dimensions (e.g., beliefs about the ability to keep oneself safe and the perceived safety of others). Here is an example of how the five themes may be presented to a client:

"For the next five sessions, we will begin considering specific themes that may be areas or beliefs in your life that were affected by your trauma. At each session, I will be asking you to consider what your beliefs were prior to the event, and how your trauma has affected them and been affected by those prior beliefs. If we decide together that any of these themes bring up Stuck Points for you, I will be asking you to complete worksheets on them, in order for you to begin changing what you are saying to yourself. The five general themes are Safety, Trust, Power/Control, Esteem, and Intimacy. Each of these themes can be considered from two directions: how you view yourself and how you view others."

It is important for the clinician to present each of the topics in the ensuing sessions, to ensure that any Stuck Points in the various areas can be identified. However, in keeping with the individual approach to case conceptualization emphasized in this book, Stuck Points that are key to a given client's recovery should be prioritized. In particular, any lingering assimilated Stuck Points should be emphasized, because resolution of these Stuck Points has implications for the overaccommodated beliefs addressed in these five topics. For instance, one of our clients addressed her Stuck Point that she could have prevented a bank robbery from occurring; she came to believe that "I couldn't have controlled the robbers' doing what they did." She then began to articulate overgeneralized beliefs about her ability to keep herself safe and to exert power/control in her work setting. As this example shows, changing specific trauma appraisals can have downstream effects on overaccommodated beliefs. The overall goal of these later sessions is thus to help the client develop balanced and multidimensional beliefs in each of these five areas.

Introducing the Safety Theme

As mentioned above, the first theme the clinician presents is Safety (with regard to self and others). This topic may be introduced to the client as follows:

"The first topic we will discuss is Safety. If prior to your index traumatic event you thought that you were quite safe, that others were not dangerous, and that you could protect yourself, these beliefs are likely to have been disrupted by the event. On the other hand, if you had prior experiences that left you thinking others were dangerous or likely to harm you, or believing that you were unable to protect yourself, then the event would have served to confirm or strengthen those beliefs. When you were growing up, did you have any experiences that left you believing you were unsafe or at risk? Were you sheltered? Did you believe you were invulnerable to traumatic events?"

After the client describes his or her prior beliefs, the therapist should help the client to determine whether prior beliefs were disrupted or seemingly reinforced by the traumatic event(s). The therapist and client should determine whether the client continues to have negative beliefs about the relative safety of others or the client's ability to protect him- or herself from harm. If so, they should discuss how these negative beliefs elicit anxiety reactions (e.g., "Something bad will happen to me if I go out alone in my car"). The client also needs to recognize how these beliefs and emotions affect behavior (e.g., avoidance, social withdrawal).

Overgeneralized fears may lead some clients to avoid entire groups of people. For example, Vietnam veterans may report that they are always uncomfortable around Asian people, while Iraq veterans may say that they are always on guard near someone who looks Middle Eastern. Rape victims often want to avoid men. In all these cases, the clients have learned to be leery of most people they encounter who remind them in any way of their experiences. At the beginning of therapy, they may see no difference between low-probability and high-probability events and believe that they are at equal risk in various settings. Any possibility of harm may be too much to tolerate.

Therapists may need to help such clients differentiate prudent safety practices from fear-based avoidance, either at the end of this session or during the next session. Clients can reduce the probability of being victimized through increased safety practices (e.g., locking doors, but not repeatedly checking them), without feeling fearful and panicky or engaging in excessive avoidance behavior. However, some events are so unpredictable and unavoidable (e.g., the World Trade Center attack) that there is no way to decrease risk. If a therapist recognizes that a client has been engaging in high-risk behaviors, this should not be addressed at the beginning of treatment, because the client is likely to assume that the therapist is blaming him or her for the event. The therapist should wait until the Safety module to discuss risk reduction strategies.

Generalized fears and related safety obsessions will not prevent traumatic events; they will only serve to prevent recovery. Along these lines, some clients have focused so much attention on some factor or factors associated with the trauma that they focus their safety planning on those factors, to the exclusion of other, higher-risk sources of danger. For example, one client who had been attacked in her home spent years and a great deal of money on alarm systems, new windows, and constant changes to the locks on her home doors. In contrast, she was going out to bars and getting inebriated with friends on a regular basis. She was even the victim of a "date-rape drug" slipped into one of her drinks. Still, she focused only on the likelihood of being attacked in her home, while ignoring higher risks elsewhere.

Therapists should help clients recognize problematic self-statements about safety and begin to introduce alternative, more moderate, less fear-producing self-statements (e.g., to replace "I'm sure it's going to happen again" with "It's unlikely to happen again"). Some clients believe that if an event happens once, it will happen again. Therapists may need to encourage such clients to seek out probability statistics, and may need to use Socratic dialogue to "right-size" how often these events occur, even in high-risk situations (e.g., military deployment). Although therapists cannot promise that traumatic events will not occur again, they can help clients stop behaving as if they are high-frequency events, especially in certain contexts. Moreover, therapists should promote healthy self-statements about clients' abilities to tolerate (and perhaps be more resilient in facing) another traumatic event, based on their recovery efforts and skills learned through CPT.

Giving the New Practice Assignment

The client should be given the Safety Issues Module (Handout 8.3) to reinforce the psychoeducation provided about the Safety theme in this session. If safety issues related to self or others are evident in the client's statements or behavior, he or she should complete at least one Challenging Beliefs Worksheet on safety before the next session. Otherwise, the client should be encouraged to complete copies of this worksheet on other identified Stuck Points and recent trauma-related events that have been distressing. One Challenging Beliefs Worksheet per day should be completed (see Handout 8.4).

Checking the Client's Reactions to the Session and the Practice Assignment

As usual, the therapist should conclude Session 7 by eliciting the client's reactions to the session and asking whether the client has any questions about the content or the new practice assignment. The therapist should reinforce any important ideas or discoveries made in the session, and should note the important take-home messages that the client offers.

Challenging Beliefs Worksheet

Date: _____   Client: _____

A. Situation	B. Thought/Stuck Point	D. Challenging Thoughts	E. Problematic Patterns	F. Alternative Thought(s)
Describe the event, thought, or belief leading to the unpleasant emotion(s).	Write thought/Stuck Point related to situation in section A. Rate your belief in this thought/Stuck Point from 0 to 100%. (How much do you believe this thought?)	Use **Challenging Questions** to examine your automatic thought from section B. Consider whether the thought is balanced and factual, or extreme.	Use the **Patterns of Problematic Thinking Worksheet** to decide whether this is one of your problematic patterns of thinking.	What else can I say instead of the thought in section B? How else can I interpret the event instead of this thought? Rate your belief in the alternative thought(s) from 0 to 100%.
		Evidence for?	Jumping to conclusions:	
		Evidence against?		
		Habit or fact?	Exaggerating or minimizing:	
		Not including all information?	Ignoring important parts:	
		All-or-none?		
		Extreme or exaggerated?	Oversimplifying:	
		Focused on just one piece?	Overgeneralizing:	**G. Re-Rate Old Thought/ Stuck Point** Re-rate how much you now believe the thought/Stuck Point in section B, from 0 to 100%.
	C. Emotion(s) Specify your emotion(s) (sad, angry, etc.), and rate how strongly you feel each emotion from 0 to 100%.	Source dependable?	Mind reading:	**H. Emotion(s)** Now what do you feel? Rate it from 0 to 100%.
		Confusing possible with likely?		
		Based on feelings or facts?	Emotional reasoning:	
		Focused on unrelated parts?		

HANDOUT 8.1A
Sample Challenging Beliefs Worksheet

A. Situation	B. Thought/Stuck Point	D. Challenging Thoughts	E. Problematic Patterns	F. Alternative Thought(s)
Describe the event, thought, or belief leading to the unpleasant emotion(s).	Write thought/Stuck Point related to situation in section A. Rate your belief in this thought/Stuck Point from 0 to 100%. (How much do you believe this thought?)	Use Challenging Questions to examine your automatic thought from section B. Consider whether the thought is balanced and factual, or extreme.	Use the Patterns of Problematic Thinking Worksheet to decide whether this is one of your problematic patterns of thinking.	What else can I say instead of the thought in section B? How else can I interpret the event instead of this thought? Rate your belief in the alternative thought(s) from 0 to 100%.
I have to ride on a plane.	*Air travel is dangerous.—75%*	*Evidence for? People have been killed.*	Jumping to conclusions: *Yes, I assume that if I fly, the plane will crash.*	*The chances are very small that I will be killed or hurt while flying.—95%*
		Evidence against? Airport security has been increased.		*Even if the plane blew up, I could not do anything about it.—80%*
		Habit or fact? It is a habit.	Exaggerating or minimizing: *I am exaggerating the possibility.*	
		Not including all information? The fact that planes fly every day and nothing happens to them.		
		All-or-none? Yes, I am making a statement that all flights are dangerous.	Ignoring important parts: *All the thousands of planes that fly every day and don't crash.*	
		Extreme or exaggerated? Yes. I am exaggerating the risk.		
		Focused on just one piece? I notice in the news when there is a crash, but I don't pay attention to all of the flights that travel safely every day.	Oversimplifying:	**G. Re-Rate Old Thought/ Stuck Point**
		Source dependable? No, I misinterpreted turbulence.	Overgeneralizing:	Re-rate how much you now believe the thought/Stuck Point in section B, from 0 to 100%.
	C. Emotion(s)	*Confusing possible with likely? Yes, I have been saying that it is likely that the plane will crash.*		*15%*
	Specify your emotion(s) (sad, angry, etc.), and rate how strongly you feel each emotion from 0 to 100%.		Mind reading:	**H. Emotion(s)**
	Afraid—100%	*Based on feelings or facts? I am letting myself believe this because I feel scared and not because it is realistic.*		Now what do you feel? Rate it from 0 to 100%.
	Helpless—75%		Emotional reasoning: *Just because I am anxious on flights doesn't mean that flying is dangerous*	*Afraid—40%*
	Anxious—75%	*Focused on unrelated parts? Many people I know have flown and haven't crashed.*		*Helpless—5%*
				Anxious—10%

Sample Challenging Beliefs Worksheet

A. Situation	B. Thought/Stuck Point	C. Emotion(s)	D. Challenging Thoughts	E. Problematic Patterns	F. Alternative Thought(s)	G. Re-Rate Old Thought/Stuck Point	H. Emotion(s)
Describe the event, thought, or belief leading to the unpleasant emotion(s).	Write thought/Stuck Point related to situation in section A. Rate your belief in this thought/Stuck Point from 0 to 100%. (How much do you believe this thought?)	Specify your emotion(s) (sad, angry, etc.), and rate how strongly you feel each emotion from 0 to 100%.	Use Challenging Questions to examine your automatic thought from section B. Consider whether the thought is balanced and factual, or extreme.	Use the Patterns of Problematic Thinking Worksheet to decide whether this is one of your problematic patterns of thinking.	What else can I say instead of the thought in section B? How else can I interpret the event instead of this thought? Rate your belief in the alternative thought(s) from 0 to 100%.	Re-rate how much you now believe the thought/Stuck Point in section B, from 0 to 100%.	Now what do you feel? Rate it from 0 to 100%.
I led my company into an ambush, and many of my men were killed.	I should have prevented it.—100%	Guilty—100% Helpless—100% Anxious—75%	Evidence for? People were killed. Evidence against? There was no way to know that there was going to be an ambush—that's the nature of an ambush. To think I should have known it was coming is to ignore the fact that it was an ambush. Habit or fact? A habit. I have been saying this for years. Not including all information? It was an ambush. We had no intel that there were insurgents in that area. All-or-none? No one else would have led their company into an ambush. Extreme or exaggerated? Extreme to say I should have prevented it when I didn't know. Focused on just one piece? That I am responsible for my men. Source dependable? I am the source of the self-blame. No one else blamed me. Confusing possible with likely? Based on feelings or facts? Feelings. Focused on unrelated parts? That I was their leader. I couldn't predict the future.	Jumping to conclusions: That I could have prevented it. Exaggerating or minimizing: Exaggerating my control in the situation. Ignoring important parts: I haven't been paying attention to the fact that it was an ambush. There was no way I could have known. Oversimplifying: Overgeneralizing: Mind reading: Emotional reasoning: Because I feel guilty, I am guilty.	There was no way to see it coming at the time.—85% I did the best I could, given the circumstances.—90%	10%	Guilty—40% Helpless—80% Anxious—40%

Sample Challenging Beliefs Worksheet

A. Situation	B. Thought/Stuck Point	D. Challenging Thoughts	E. Problematic Patterns	F. Alternative Thought(s)
Describe the event, thought, or belief leading to the unpleasant emotion(s).	Write thought/Stuck Point related to situation in section A. Rate your belief in this thought/Stuck Point from 0 to 100%. (How much do you believe this thought?)	Use **Challenging Questions** to examine your automatic thought from section B. Consider whether the thought is balanced and factual, or extreme.	Use the **Patterns of Problematic Thinking Worksheet** to decide whether this is one of your problematic patterns of thinking.	What else can I say instead of the thought in section B? How else can I interpret the event instead of this thought? Rate your belief in the alternative thought(s) from 0 to 100%.
I am putting off doing my therapy practice assignment.	If I let myself feel angry, I'll be out of control.—50%	Evidence for? I have acted aggressively in the past when I felt angry.	Jumping to conclusions: I am jumping to conclusions to assume that I will have no control if I feel my feelings.	Anger can be expressed without aggression.—60% Anger is an emotion (like sadness). I can let myself feel that and still maintain control over my behaviors.—60%
		Evidence against? I have never been really destructive when I was angry. It is my choice how I act when I feel angry. I can always take a break or leave the situation.	Exaggerating or minimizing: I am equating anger with rage instead of what it is—unpleasant.	
		Habit or fact? Habit.	Ignoring important parts: I am disregarding the times I have felt angry and maintained control.	
		Not including all information? That I am not totally out of control. I am still making choices on how to behave.		
		All-or-none? Yes, no control.	Oversimplifying: Yes, feeling angry is bad.	
		Extreme or exaggerated? It is exaggerated to say that I would be out of control, I have some control.	Overgeneralizing: Just because I have been aggressive in the past doesn't mean I will do it with a worksheet.	
		Focused on just one piece? That if I do my out-of-session therapy assignment, I will be angry and out of control.	Mind reading:	G. Re-Rate Old Thought/ Stuck Point
		Source dependable? No, my assumption.		Re-rate how much you now believe the thought/Stuck Point in section B, from 0 to 100%.
		Confusing possible with likely? Not likely I will lose control just from filling out a worksheet.	Emotional reasoning: Anger always leads to aggression.	20%
	C. Emotion(s)	Based on feelings or facts? Feelings.		H. Emotion(s)
	Specify your emotion(s) (sad, angry, etc.), and rate how strongly you feel each emotion from 0 to 100%. Angry—50% Afraid—95%	Focused on unrelated parts? It's just a worksheet, not the trauma.		Now what do you feel? Rate it from 0 to 100%. Angry—30% Afraid—35%

178

HANDOUT 8.1D
Sample Challenging Beliefs Worksheet

A. Situation	B. Thought/Stuck Point	C. Emotion(s)	D. Challenging Thoughts	E. Problematic Patterns	F. Alternative Thought(s)
Describe the event, thought, or belief leading to the unpleasant emotion(s).	Write thought/Stuck Point related to situation in section A. Rate your belief in this thought/Stuck Point from 0 to 100%. (How much do you believe this thought?)		Use **Challenging Questions** to examine your automatic thought from section B. Consider whether the thought is balanced and factual, or extreme.	Use the **Patterns of Problematic Thinking Worksheet** to decide whether this is one of your problematic patterns of thinking.	What else can I say instead of the thought in section B? How else can I interpret the event instead of this thought? Rate your belief in the alternative thought(s) from 0 to 100%.
A friend wants to set me up for a date with someone she knows.	I can't get involved with anyone and let anyone close enough to see how restricted my life has become.—75%		Evidence for? One person I told about the assault while we were dating was very supportive at the time, but became more and more distant after that and finally stopped calling altogether.	Jumping to conclusions: Yes, assuming that it will go badly.	~~A date could tell me they don't want anything to do with me because I am dealing with having been assaulted.~~—60
			Evidence against? My friends and family have been supportive.	Exaggerating or minimizing: Because one date may have had problems, this doesn't mean that others will.	Some people have been very supportive.—70%
			Habit or fact? Habit.	Ignoring important parts: That person was not healthy or secure.	
			Not including all information? My friend wouldn't set me up with a mean person.		
			All-or-none? Most healthy people would not run from a relationship.	Oversimplifying: If I tell someone who can't deal with it, it is not necessarily bad, because I could find out something important about the relationship.	
			Extreme or exaggerated? I am making assumptions about how other people will react.		
	C. Emotion(s)		Focused on just one piece? That he will judge me.	Overgeneralizing: Same as above. One bad experience doesn't mean that everyone is the same. I don't have to talk about my restricted life.	**G. Re-Rate Old Thought/ Stuck Point**
	Specify your emotion(s) (sad, angry, etc.), and rate how strongly you feel each emotion from 0 to 100%.		Source dependable? Coming from past negative experience and from an unhealthy person.		Re-rate how much you now believe the thought/Stuck Point in section B, from 0 to 100%.
	Fearful—50%		Confusing possible with likely? It is possible that he won't like me, but it is possible I won't like him either.	Mind reading: Yes, I am assuming what he thinks, and I haven't even met him yet.	50%
	Sad—80%		Based on feelings or facts? Feelings.		
	Angry—50%		Focused on unrelated parts? Just because I was a victim before doesn't mean that everyone will judge me. Maybe they would judge the rapist.	Emotional reasoning: Because I am scared, I assume that it will go badly.	**H. Emotion(s)**
					Now what do you feel? Rate it from 0 to 100%.
					Fearful—25%
					Sad—40%
					Angry—10%

Sample Challenging Beliefs Worksheet

A. Situation	B. Thought/Stuck Point	D. Challenging Thoughts	E. Problematic Patterns	F. Alternative Thought(s)
Describe the event, thought, or belief leading to the unpleasant emotion(s).	Write thought/Stuck Point related to situation in section A. Rate your belief in this thought/Stuck Point from 0 to 100%. (How much do you believe this thought?)	Use Challenging Questions to examine your automatic thought from section B. Consider whether the thought is balanced and factual, or extreme.	Use the Patterns of Problematic Thinking Worksheet to decide whether this is one of your problematic patterns of thinking.	What else can I say instead of the thought in section B? How else can I interpret the event instead of this thought? Rate your belief in the alternative thought(s) from 0 to 100%.
My lieutenant sent us down a road that he knew was filled with insurgents. Four friends were killed because of him.	He got them killed.—100%	Evidence for? They are dead! Evidence against? He was probably given an order to send us there because they needed the supplies. Habit or fact? He didn't actually kill them. Not including all information? Insurgents killed them. All-or-none? Yes. Extreme or exaggerated? I guess. The order didn't seem to make sense, though—why did we have to go then? And there was a pretty good chance we all could have made it. Focused on just one piece? I guess I don't know if he had pressure (orders) to send us there right then.	Jumping to conclusions: I guess I don't know what he was thinking when he ordered us there. Exaggerating or minimizing: Yes. Ignoring important parts: I don't really know why he made that call. Oversimplifying: We had made the run before there, even though it was really dangerous. Overgeneralizing:	I hate that my friends died, and although it didn't seem critical to make that run, I don't know what the lieutenant was thinking or responding to.—95% It was really risky, but we had made it safely four times previously.—90%
	C. Emotion(s)			**G. Re-Rate Old Thought/ Stuck Point**
	Specify your emotion(s) (sad, angry, etc.), and rate how strongly you feel each emotion from 0 to 100%.	Source dependable? My assumption. Confusing possible with likely?	Mind reading: I am mind-reading his intentions.	Re-rate how much you now believe the thought/Stuck Point in section B, from 0 to 100%. 40%
	Angry—100%	Based on feelings or facts? Outrage at not understanding why he made that call. Focused on unrelated parts? That it was his fault. He didn't intend for them to get killed.	Emotional reasoning: I was angry and blamed him.	**H. Emotion(s)** Now what do you feel? Rate it from 0 to 100%. Relieved, not as angry—60%

Practice Assignment after Session 6 of CPT

Use the Challenging Beliefs Worksheets (Handout 8.1) to analyze and confront at least one of your Stuck Points each day. You can also use the Challenging Beliefs Worksheets to challenge any negative or problematic thoughts and related emotions you may have about day-to-day events.

Safety Issues Module

Safety Beliefs Related to SELF: The belief that you can protect yourself from harm and have some control over events.

PRIOR EXPERIENCE

Negative	Positive
If you repeatedly experienced dangerous and uncontrollable life situations, you may have developed negative beliefs about your ability to protect yourself from harm. A new traumatic event may seem to confirm those beliefs.	If you have had positive prior experiences, you may develop the belief that you have control over most events and can protect yourself from harm. The traumatic event may have shattered this belief.
Symptoms Associated with Negative Safety Beliefs about the Self	
<ul><li>Chronic and persistent anxiety</li><li>Intrusive thoughts about themes of danger</li><li>Irritability</li><li>Startled responses or physical arousal</li><li>Intense fears related to future victimization</li></ul>	
Examples of Possible Stuck Points	
"I can't protect myself from danger." "If I go out, I will be hurt." "When I feel fear, that means I am in danger."	

POSSIBLE RESOLUTIONS

If you previously believed that . . .	A possible alternative thought may be . . .
"It can't happen to me," then you will need to resolve the conflict between this belief and the traumatic event.	"It is unlikely to happen again, but the possibility exists. Even if it does, I have more skills I can use to manage my reactions."
"I can protect myself from any harm," then you will need to resolve the conflict between your prior beliefs and the traumatic event.	"I do not have control over everything that happens to me, but I can take precautions to reduce the risk of future traumatic events."
"I cannot protect myself," then the new traumatic event will seem to confirm these beliefs. New beliefs must be developed that are more balanced regarding your ability to keep yourself safe.	"I do have some ability to keep myself safe, and I can take steps to protect myself from harm."

(continued)

Safety Beliefs Related to OTHERS: Beliefs about the dangerousness of other people and expectancies about the intent of others to cause harm, injury, or loss.

PRIOR EXPERIENCE

Negative	Positive
If you experienced people as dangerous in early life, or if you believed violence to be a normal way of relating, the new traumatic event will seem to confirm these beliefs.	If you experienced people as safe in early life, you may expect others to keep you safe and not cause harm, injury, or loss. The traumatic event may have caused a disruption in this belief.
Symptoms Associated with Negative Safety Beliefs about Others	
• Avoidant or phobic responses • Social withdrawal	
Examples of Possible Stuck Points	
"The world is very dangerous everywhere." "People will always try to harm me." "There is nowhere safe to be."	

POSSIBLE RESOLUTIONS

If you previously believed that . . .	Possible alternative thoughts may be . . .
"Others are out to harm me and most people will hurt me if they can," then you will need to modify this belief, or it will be impossible to have trusting, happy relationships with others.	"There are some people out there who are dangerous, but not everyone is out to harm me in some way."
"I will never be hurt by others," then you will need to resolve the conflict between this belief and the victimization.	"There may be some people who will try to harm me, but not everyone I meet will hurt me. I can take precautions to reduce the likelihood that others can hurt me."

Practice Assignment after Session 7 of CPT

Use the Challenging Beliefs Worksheets (Handout 8.1) to analyze and confront at least one of your Stuck Points each day. Also,
please read over the Safety Issues Module (Handout 8.3), and think
about how your prior beliefs were affected by your trauma. If you
have safety issues related to yourself or others, complete at least
one worksheet to confront those beliefs. Use the remaining sheets
for other Stuck Points on your Stuck Point Log (Handout 6.1) or for
distressing events that have occurred recently.

9

Trauma Themes—Safety, Trust, and Power/Control

Sessions 8–10

Goals for Sessions 8, 9, and 10

The primary goals for the sessions on the Safety, Trust, and Power/Control themes (Sessions 8–10) are very similar, with the therapist and the client reviewing the Challenging Beliefs Worksheets related to the respective trauma themes. In addition, if the client has any unresolved assimilated Stuck Points, or Stuck Points regarding another trauma, those should be integrated into the weekly sessions and the continued practice assignments. Session 10 includes two additional behavioral assignments designed to enhance self- and other-esteem.

Session 8: Processing Safety and Introducing Trust

Procedures for Session 8

1. Review the client's scores on the self-report objective measures. (See the discussions of this review for Sessions 2 and 3 in Chapter 6.)
2. Review the client's Challenging Beliefs Worksheets related to the Safety theme and to other Stuck Points.

3. Introduce the Trust theme.
4. Give the new practice assignment.
5. Check the client's reactions to the session and the practice assignment.

Reviewing the Client's Challenging Beliefs Worksheets

Session 8 should begin with the therapist and client's reviewing the client's completed Challenging Beliefs Worksheets and discussing the client's success or problems in changing Stuck Points (and subsequent emotions). Ideally, the client will have completed at least one worksheet on safety issues relating to self or others, and the therapist should make sure to focus on reviewing the safety worksheets and any sheets that are addressing unresolved assimilated Stuck Points before going on to review any additional sheets. Whatever is not covered in the session will need to be reviewed before the next session, so it is important not to become too focused on one sheet unless the client is really struggling with that Stuck Point.

Safety issues most often center on probabilities. One common safety Stuck Point for clients is that a traumatic event will happen again. Rape survivors may say, "All men are rapists"; military personnel or veterans may say, "I know I am going to die in combat," or "The world is so dangerous that I don't want my family to go out without me." These types of Stuck Points will significantly restrict these individuals from living complete lives. The rape survivors may fear dating, going to parties, or even being in public, and the military personnel may experience great difficulty if they are still on active duty and facing deployment, or interacting with society when they feel at risk.

When therapists are helping clients with Challenging Beliefs Worksheets, it is important that the therapists prompt the clients to edit the sheets during the session, so that the clients have new and improved sheets to review when they are at home. Also, we find that clients can become so entrenched in their beliefs that they have great difficulty seeing things another way, even at this point in the therapy. For clients who are having difficulty addressing their safety-related overaccommodated Stuck Points, therapists may choose a number of options to help get the clients unstuck. For instance, a therapist may help a client focus on the likelihood of a traumatic event's happening again. The therapist may ask the client to look up the actual probabilities of different events' happening, in order to help the client see that in day-to-day living, the likelihood of experiencing a significant traumatic event is actually quite low. But if the client's Stuck Point here is "It *will* happen again," it shapes the way the client acts in daily life and causes him or her to avoid situations that in the past might have been embraced.

Here are some specific examples of this approach. If someone says that going to a large store is too dangerous, it might be possible to have the client look up the crime rate for that store. For a rape survivor, a therapist might ask the following questions:

"How many men are in the world? Of these 3.6 billion men, how many do you think you have encountered? Of those, how many have tried to rape you? Do you know any men who have actually tried to help you or been kind to you? So, actually, is it more likely that you will meet someone who is kind, or that you will meet someone who will try to rape you?"

For a car accident victim who is afraid to drive again, the therapist might ask how many times the client had driven in the past and been injured in a car accident, as in the following exchange:

THERAPIST: How many times have you been injured before in a car accident?

CLIENT: None. But I see them reported on the news all the time.

THERAPIST: Did you notice them being reported on the news before you had the accident?

CLIENT: Not particularly.

THERAPIST: This is what we call "selective attention." You are selecting to pay attention, or noticing something now that you didn't pay attention to before, because now it has happened to you. But what evidence do you have that the accident rate has increased, or that you are more likely to be in an accident?

CLIENT: I don't have any evidence. I'm just more aware that it could happen.

THERAPIST: So, in fact, you might be a more careful driver in the future?

CLIENT: Probably. I sure won't text and drive again.

The therapist noted that the client himself did not know that he "would" be in an accident, and asked him how he felt when he said that it "could" happen versus that it "will" happen. The client was able to acknowledge that the two statements felt somewhat different, and that "could" was different from "will" in terms of probability (100% for the latter and something less for the former). Instead of pushing him further on this topic in this session, the therapist assigned him to work on this with more Challenging Beliefs Worksheets. The Stuck Point they wrote down was "If I drive, I will be in an accident."

Once a client has completed a Challenging Beliefs Worksheet that successfully challenges a Stuck Point, the client should be encouraged to reread the worksheet regularly so that the reasoning becomes comfortable. This is why it is critical that the therapist and client continually focus on writing on the worksheets and not just talking things through, so that the client has something helpful to read between sessions.

Introducing the Trust Theme

During the final third of the session, the therapist introduces the Trust theme. The therapist and client should briefly go over the Trust Issues Module (Handout 9.1). Here is an example of how this module can be presented to the client:

"The idea of self-trust involves the belief that people trust their own thoughts, perceptions, or judgments. After a traumatic event, many people begin to second-guess themselves and to question many aspects of the trauma. They may question their own judgment about being in the situation that led to the event, their behaviors during the event, or their ability to judge character—particularly if, in the case of an assault, the perpetrator was an acquaintance.

"Conversely, trust in others involves a person's ability to have a balanced sense of trust with other people. Other-focused trust is also frequently disrupted following traumatic events. In addition to the sense of betrayal that occurs when traumatic events are caused intentionally by people clients thought they could trust, sometimes clients feel betrayed by the people they turned to for help or support during or after the event. For example, if a soldier thought that a commanding officer made a blame-worthy mistake during battle, the soldier might decide, 'I cannot trust anyone to keep me safe under any circumstances.' Or if a child was assaulted by a parent, the child may come to believe as an adult that 'No one can be trusted.' Sometimes clients carry that belief for decades without actually knowing whether the other person or group in fact betrayed them, or whether there might be an alternative explanation for their behavior—for example, the military intelligence was wrong, or the nonperpetrating parent didn't know about the other parent's abuse."

Giving the New Practice Assignment

The client should be given the Trust Issues Module (Handout 9.1) to reinforce the psychoeducation provided about trust in this session. If issues involving trust of self or others are evident in the client's statements, behaviors, and Stuck Point Log, the client should complete at least one worksheet on trust before the next session. Otherwise, the client should be encouraged to complete worksheets on other identified Stuck Points and recent trauma-related events that have been distressing. One Challenging Belief Worksheet per day should be completed (see Handout 9.2).

Checking the Client's Reactions to the Session and the Practice Assignment

As usual, the therapist should conclude Session 8 by eliciting the client's reactions to the session and asking whether the client has any questions about the session content or the new practice assignment. The therapist should reinforce any important ideas or discoveries made in the session, and should note the important take-home messages that the client offers.

Session 9: Processing Trust and Introducing Power/Control

Procedures for Session 9

1. Review the client's scores on the self-report objective measures. (See the discussions of this review for Sessions 2 and 3 in Chapter 6.)
2. Review the client's Challenging Beliefs Worksheets related to the Trust theme and to other Stuck Points.
3. Introduce the Power/Control theme.
4. Give the new practice assignment.
5. Check the client's reactions to the session and the practice assignment.

Reviewing the Client's Challenging Beliefs Worksheets

Session 9 should begin with the therapist and client's reviewing the Challenging Beliefs Worksheets and addressing Stuck Points related to trust. The therapist should continue to use Socratic dialogue as needed to generate alternative ways of thinking, which, again, should be recorded on the worksheets throughout the session. Sometimes clients will identify new assimilated Stuck Points or Stuck Points related to topics other than the theme of the session. This is why the therapist should review as many of the problematic sheets as possible in session, to make sure that the client has provided reasonable challenges to the Stuck Points.

For many trauma survivors, trust becomes an either–or concept, rather than falling on a continuum. Therefore, other people are either given too much trust up front (e.g., "All people my age can be trusted") or are not trusted at all unless there is overwhelming evidence to the contrary. As a result, trauma survivors tend either to withdraw from relationships or to engage in unhealthy, unbalanced relationships. It can be helpful for a therapist and client to describe different kinds of trust, so that the client can see that there are many kinds of trust and that some are more important than others (e.g., trust with secrets; trust in the competence of a doctor or pilot; fidelity; reliability; not using information against the client).

The therapist can help the client explore the idea that trust falls on a continuum and is multidimensional, with different types/levels of trust for different people, through Socratic dialogue. An example of such a dialogue follows:

CLIENT: My Stuck Point is that if I trust someone, I will be hurt.

THERAPIST: First, what do you mean by "hurt"?

CLIENT: Well, they might physically hurt me or reject me.

THERAPIST: So there are different ways to be hurt? What do you mean by "trust"? It is a very big word.

CLIENT: What do you mean? You trust people or you don't.

THERAPIST: It might be helpful to think of trust has having different types and different levels. For example, do you know some people that you could trust with your dog, cat, or child, but you have no idea if you could trust them to pay back $100 if you loaned it to them?

CLIENT: Yes.

THERAPIST: What about trusting someone to save your life, but not being able to trust them to be on time for a movie?

CLIENT: I know someone like that.

THERAPIST: Doesn't it take time to get to know someone to figure out the areas you can and cannot trust them?

CLIENT: That's my point. It is safer just not to trust anyone!

THERAPIST: I understand your thinking, but are there any problems with thinking that way?

CLIENT: I don't know what you mean.

THERAPIST: Well, what if you do have people in your life who genuinely care for you? How long will they want to stick around if you always send a message that they cannot be trusted, even when they haven't done anything to prove that?

CLIENT: Probably not forever. I don't mean to hurt people's feelings.

THERAPIST: I guess you need to ask yourself, "When is it enough?" I remember our first session, when you said you were tired of being lonely.

CLIENT: But if I trust people from the start, I will get hurt.

THERAPIST: OK, that is the Stuck Point we can challenge. I agree, you *might* get hurt, and they *might* do things that violate your trust. But does running 20 minutes late for dinner with you equate to stealing $200 from you? Perhaps you can start in the middle with people and evaluate their behavior from that point.

CLIENT: What do you mean?

THERAPIST: Well, what if we called the middle point between total trust and total distrust 0, meaning "I don't have any information"? And rather than a single line with a middle point, we could think of trust as a star with many lines coming out in different directions to represent the different types and levels of trust you can have with different people. (*Shows the client Handouts 9.3 and 9.3a.*) Let's start completing this Trust Star Worksheet by listing different kinds of trust. Then let's pick one person in your life, and think about rating how much you trust that person on these different dimensions. In other words, you can trust [name of friend/relative] if you lend them money, but you might trust other friends to watch your kids or share a secret. As you learn more about a person, you might find that you can trust the person more deeply with more things. It is OK not to trust all people the same way in all areas. For example, you might trust your mechanic to fix your car, but not to walk your dog. Knowing someone's limitations allows you to decide what type of friendship you have and not to have unrealistic expectations that can lead you to feeling hurt when they let you down.

CLIENT: I get that, but I don't want to get hurt again.

THERAPIST: I don't think anyone wants to get hurt, and the best way to reduce the possibility of that happening is to start slow and only with small things until people have earned your trust in some ways. Also, see how much they are sharing with you. If they are not sharing their secrets with you, that tells you a lot about their own trust in you.

CLIENT: OK, I get that.

THERAPIST: The other way to tell in which ways you can trust someone is to watch how they treat other people, whether you like their friends and family, and how they behave in different kinds of situations. Do you have to trust someone with your life to play on a basketball team with them? All right, let's take a look at the Challenging Beliefs Worksheet you did, and look more closely at the evidence against the idea that you *will* be hurt if you trust someone.

It is important for therapists to make sure that clients have looked for Stuck Points related to trust of self and others, because assimilated Stuck Points regarding self-blame can lead to Stuck Points regarding an inability to trust. Often self-trust Stuck Points revolve around clients' doubt in their ability to make good decisions, due to their belief that the trauma happened because of something they did or did not do, or that they "should have known" the traumatic event was going to occur. This hindsight bias and outcome-based reasoning allows the clients to beat themselves up for what happened based on the information they know now, instead of only looking at the facts as they were at the time of the event. The Challenging Beliefs Worksheet will allow such clients to look objectively at the facts at the time, and to break apart some of the inaccurate conclusions. Here is an example:

THERAPIST: So what evidence do you have that you always make bad decisions?

CLIENT: Well, I made a bad decision when I walked down that street.

THERAPIST: I thought we had determined that you had no reason to believe that it was not going to be safe that night, and that you had walked down that street every day from the bus stop?

CLIENT: Well, I guess that is not "evidence for." [See the first Challenging Question in section D of the Challenging Beliefs Worksheet.]

THERAPIST: How many bad decisions did you make this week that you knew were dangerous?

CLIENT: Well, if you put it that way, none. I don't intentionally make bad decisions.

THERAPIST: So could that be evidence against the idea that you can't trust your decisions?

CLIENT: Hmm . . . yeah.

THERAPIST: And is it a habit of thinking, or a fact, that you make bad decisions?

CLIENT: Habit.

Finally, it may be necessary to help some clients consider why some of their friends or family members may have withdrawn from them initially after hearing about the traumatic event. It can be difficult for some clients to see this as anything beyond blame or betrayal of themselves. With the Challenging Beliefs Worksheet, they can be helped to consider that their loved ones' behaviors may have been their own reactions of helplessness and vulnerability. Or the loved ones may simply have been unable to find an appropriate way to respond to the clients' trauma. It may help these clients to understand that other people may also be suffering because of the traumatic event, and that the other people's reactions may be their own ways of managing their feelings. Alternatively, examining others' reactions may reveal that a friend or family member is not a trusted other, at least in this domain, and perhaps is not someone to whom a client should confide sensitive information.

As a client works through trust-related Stuck Points, it can be helpful to ask about the costs and benefits of holding onto these overaccommodated Stuck Points that likely grew out of self-blame Stuck Points. The client will often respond that self-blame and future self-doubt provide protection from other traumatic events and gives the client control over the future. This can provide a nice segue into introducing the next theme, that of Power/Control.

Introducing the Power/Control Theme

The Power/Control theme is introduced as the topic for the next practice assignment. The client is given the Power/Control Issues Module (Handout 9.4) to read after the session, to help with identifying additional Stuck Points the client should challenge before the next session. The concept of power or control in relation to the self refers to a person's belief in his or her ability to manage problems and take on new challenges.

Traumatic events are often largely out of survivors' control, so in response, they attempt to take complete control of all aspects of their lives in an attempt to remove the possibility that any future traumatic events will happen. When this happens, they can become very intolerant of other people's making mistakes as well. Conversely, sometimes clients will overgeneralize from the traumatic event and believe that they are now powerless and have no control over anything. This may cause them to doubt themselves and abdicate decision making to others.

Like the other themes, Power/Control resides on a continuum and is multidimensional (e.g., self-control over emotions, behaviors, urges). By using Socratic dialogue, the therapist can help the client consider that things do not have to be all-or-nothing, black-and-white. Thus it would be appropriate for a therapist to ask any of the following types of questions: "Control with regard to what? Your emotions? Getting dressed each day? Your children?" It is common for individuals with PTSD to believe that they also have to control their emotions, because if they do not they "will not be able to handle it" or "will lose control completely." Women who have been victimized by their partners emotionally as well as physically may come to believe that they are unable to take care of themselves and are helpless to leave their abusive relationships. They may have been brainwashed by their partners into believing in their own incompetence and powerlessness.

Power with regard to others involves the clients' beliefs about the power of others and about their own ability to control outcomes in interpersonal relationships. Many trauma survivors will attempt to control all aspects of their relationships in an attempt to feel safe and secure, and they may have difficulty letting other people have any control. This can be very disruptive for previously existing relationships and will make it very difficult to form new, healthy relationships. It is important for a therapist to look for changes in a client's relationships if the traumatic event(s) occurred in adulthood. If the index event occurred in childhood, it may be helpful to ask about longer-standing relationship patterns more generally, in an attempt to find power/control Stuck Points. Some people have Stuck Points with regard to the amount of control that others have over them, and their inability to tolerate having others tell them what to do (i.e., they have authority issues). They may have overaccommodated Stuck Points that they are helpless, or that others are always trying to control them or have power in their lives. Sometimes in severe PTSD, the other-control issues may come across as near-paranoid fears that people are trying to control them or have power over them.

Giving the New Practice Assignment

For the new practice assignment, the client should be asked to complete a Trust Star Worksheet (Handout 9.3) about someone in his or her life if this was not done in session, and to read over the Power/Control Issues Module (Handout 9.4) to reinforce the psychoeducation provided about this theme in the session. If power/control issues related to self or others are evident in the client's statements or behavior, the client should complete at least one worksheet on power/control before the next session. Otherwise, the client should be encouraged to complete worksheets on other identified Stuck Points and recent trauma-related events that have been distressing. One Challenging Belief Worksheet per day should be completed (see Handout 9.5).

Checking the Client's Reactions to the Session and the Practice Assignment

As usual, the therapist should conclude Session 9 by eliciting the client's reactions to the session and asking whether the client has any questions about the session content or the new practice assignment. The therapist should reinforce any important ideas or discoveries made in the session, and should note the important take-home messages that the client offers.

Session 10: Processing Power/Control and Introducing Esteem

Procedures for Session 10

1. Review the client's self-report objective measures. (See the discussions of this review for Sessions 2 and 3 in Chapter 6.)
2. Review the client's Trust Star Worksheet, as well as the Challenging Beliefs Worksheets related to the Power/Control theme and to other Stuck Points.
3. Introduce the Esteem theme.
4. Give the new practice assignment.
5. Check the client's reactions to the session and the practice assignment.

Reviewing the Client's Trust Star Worksheet and Challenging Beliefs Worksheets

Session 10 should begin with a review of the completed Trust Star Worksheet (Handout 9.3), to see whether the client can see how someone can be in his or her life without having to be trusted in all possible ways. If the client only wrote down a few kinds of trust that he or she positively knows about a friend or family member, the therapist should ask, "Would you trust this person to cut your hair, repair your car, or pull your tooth?" Alternatively, if the client has identified no or only minimal ways that he or she can trust friends or family members positively, the therapist should ask whether there are any ways in which the client can trust them. It can be difficult for some trauma survivors to identify any ways in which they can trust, so using the most basic ways of trusting should be considered (e.g., taking the client to the hospital, not poisoning the client's food, caring for the client's pet).

The focus then turns to the client's attempts to change Stuck Points regarding power/control through using the Challenging Beliefs Worksheets. It is very important for the client to have a balanced view of power/control, because many trauma survivors believe that they have no power, and they often believe they must always be in control. For many people, the dialectic of feeling powerless, but simultaneously needing to be in control, is the source of much confusion or anxiety, and the subsequent behaviors in which these clients engage can often be very destructive to their working and social relationships. Realistically, no one has complete control over all events that happen around him or her, or the behavior of other people. But on the other hand, people are not completely helpless responders to the world. They have the ability to influence the course of events, and they can typically control their own reactions to those events.

If clients state that they have no control over their lives, therapists may walk them through a typical day, focusing on all the decisions the clients made. Usually, by the time this review is completed, the clients realize how many hundreds of decisions they make in a day (from what time to get up, to what to wear and eat, whether or not to obey traffic laws, etc.). Although some clients may try to dismiss these decisions as irrelevant, it is important for therapists to help them take credit for making these decisions each day. Clients often blame some small everyday decision for putting them in the location and circumstances of a traumatic event. Therapists can ask such clients whether, if the traumatic event had not happened, they would have remembered the decisions they made that day, or whether the decision under discussion was similar to many they had made just like it on earlier days. Only because the outcome was so catastrophic do people go back and try to question all the decisions they made that day, and mentally try to undo those decisions. This is entirely normal, because people want to believe they have complete control over their safety and the safety of loved ones around them. Thus individuals look for variables that they had control over, in an attempt to believe that both the traumatic event and all future situations can be controlled or prevented from happening. Just because a choice or decision was made before the traumatic event, this does not mean that the choice caused the event.

For example, a client one of us worked with believed that she was helpless and incompetent in most areas of her life, because of the helplessness she felt during the traumatic abuse she experienced as a child. As a result of feeling helpless, she did not assert herself at work or with friends, and she often gave in to pressure from others to do things that she did not want to do (e.g., drive friends places, loan people money). She believed, "If I stand up for myself, it will turn out badly, and people will leave me." This left her not only believing that she was stuck in an unsatisfying job, but also feeling helpless to assert herself against her employer's unreasonable demands for project deadlines and overtime hours.

When this client's therapist helped her use the Challenging Beliefs Worksheet to help her look at her options, she began to see that she was not totally helpless and that she did have some options. She reminded herself that several people had asked her to apply for jobs with their agencies, and she also realized that she had several blooming friendships that did not demand excessive amounts of her time. She eventually became more assertive with her boss, and he ended up promoting her, citing her ability to set boundaries and make tough decisions. Through these interactions, she was able to see that she could effect change in other people, and that if people did not treat her respectfully, then perhaps they were not the right people to have in her life.

Some people go to the other extreme and engage in excessive controlling behaviors in an attempt to ensure that nothing bad will ever happen to them. This reaction is often due to the clients' assuming the assimilated belief "I could have prevented the traumatic event from happening," and overgeneralizing it to the overaccommodated belief "If something bad happens, it is my fault." Again, this is one of the important reasons why assimilated Stuck Points are targeted initially: Clients will use the assimilated Stuck Points as evidence for the overaccommodated Stuck Points when they try to challenge these.

Often power/control issues can be identified by asking about how much clients engage in compulsive behaviors (checking and rechecking locks, compulsive neatness, bingeing and purging, drinking, etc.). Although these compulsions may be ways for the clients to believe that they are in control of the world around them, the compulsions can also serve as escape from or avoidance of feeling their emotions. Over time, some clients may begin to feel controlled by their compulsions rather than the other way around. Reframing compulsive behaviors as out of control may help such clients to shift their thinking about the effectiveness of these behaviors.

For some clients, the topic of power/control leads to a discussion of anger and their concern that their anger responses are out of their control. It may be helpful to remind them of some of the basic biological information introduced in Session 1: Therapists can note that some anger may be related to the hyperarousal symptoms of PTSD, such as irritability from physiological arousal, lack of sleep, and frequent startle reactions. It can also be important to remind these clients that while fear is associated with the fight–flight–freeze response, so is anger. Therefore, trauma cues may cause a resurfacing of the anger associated with the fight response that clients have never fully processed. Over time, they may have grown to fear feeling this anger—not only because it reminds them of the trauma, but also because they believe they will do something violent in reaction.

Other trauma survivors will state that they did not feel anger during the event, but that anger emerged afterward. However, because the person or persons who harmed them may not be available for them to express their anger toward (or are too dangerous to express anger toward), the anger is sometimes left without a target and is experienced as helpless anger. This causes some survivors to turn their anger on family members and friends around them. Unfortunately, because many people have never been taught how to discriminate between anger and aggression or how to handle their feelings of anger appropriately, they believe that aggression equals anger.

Some clients state that they feel as if they have no choice but to become angry, even over little things that do not mean much in hindsight. In some cases, they will direct their anger outward toward anyone they perceive to have taken away their control and created feelings of helplessness. Anger may also be directed at society in general, "the government" or government agencies at various levels, or other groups or individuals whom a client may be holding responsible for not preventing the event in some way (e.g., a mother's not preventing child abuse by a stepfather). As in the case of guilt, it may be necessary for a therapist to help such a client discriminate among the unforeseeable, responsibility, and intentionality. Only an intentional perpetrator of an event should be blamed. Other people may be responsible for setting the stage or inadvertently increasing risk to the client, but they should not have an equal share of the blame and anger.

In contrast, some clients' anger is directed inward: The clients focus on not only all the things they "should" have done to prevent a traumatic event or defend themselves, but all the things they are continuing to do wrong in their present lives. Once these clients are able to see that a change in their behavior may not have prevented the event, or may have in fact worsened the outcome, they often feel better.

Each client should be given the Ways of Giving and Taking Power Handout (Handout 9.6). We recommend introducing this handout as follows:

"There are many ways people give and take power. You can do this appropriately or inappropriately, and this handout offers some examples. For example, if you tell your partner you will not have sex unless he or she does *XYZ*, you are taking power in a negative way. Or, if you base your actions or behaviors solely on the reactions you expect from others, you are giving your power away. If, on the other hand, you do something (or do not do something) because you want to and it makes you feel good, you are taking your power appropriately.

"Can you give me an example of things that you do that fit in each of the categories below? Are these behaviors that you would like to change? What Stuck Points keep you from making the changes you would like to make?"

Handout 9.6 should be used to generate additional power/control Stuck Points that can be challenged during the session on the Challenging Beliefs Worksheet or assigned to the client as part of the practice assignment.

Introducing the Esteem Theme

The remainder of Session 10 should focus on the introduction of the next theme, Esteem. The therapist briefly introduces this topic with the client and describes how self-esteem and esteem for others can both be disrupted by traumatic events. If the trauma occurred in adulthood, the client's self-esteem before the event should be explored. If the trauma occurred in childhood, it can be useful to help the client see how his or her self-esteem was shaped by the event(s) without being given a chance to develop in a safe and healthy environment.

At this point in therapy, two new behavioral assignments are given to the client: practice in giving and receiving compliments, and doing at least one nice thing for him- or herself each day without any conditions or strings attached (e.g., exercising, reading a magazine, calling a friend to chat). As an alternative, the client may choose to do something worthwhile for the community (e.g., volunteer work) that may help raise the client's self esteem. These assignments are designed to help the client build self-esteem by helping him or her become more comfortable with the idea that "I am worthy of compliments and pleasant events without having to earn them or disown them." The assignments also help the client connect socially with others, because those with PTSD tend to isolate themselves. Because compliments may have bounced off or were distorted to fit in with prior beliefs in the past, the therapist may need to teach the client how to respond ("Thank you") rather than making deflecting statements. Reconnecting with pleasant or worthwhile events helps a client to break out of this isolation and (ideally) begin to connect with other people. Clients with PTSD who have been avoidant and isolated may have stopped doing activities that they enjoyed doing before the traumatic event, and may need to consider how they will move back into their community.

Giving the New Practice Assignment

The client should be given the Esteem Issues Module (Handout 9.7) and practice assignment (Handout 9.8) to reinforce the psychoeducation provided about esteem in this session. If self- or other-esteem issues are evident in the client's statements or behavior, the client should complete at least one worksheet on esteem before the next session. Otherwise, the client should be encouraged to complete worksheets on other identified Stuck Points and recent trauma-related events that have been distressing. One Challenging Belief Worksheet per day should be completed.

Checking the Client's Reactions to the Session and the Practice Assignment

As usual, the therapist should conclude Session 10 by eliciting the client's reactions to the session and asking whether the client has any questions about the session content or the new practice assignment. The therapist should reinforce any important ideas or discoveries made in the session, and should note the important take-home messages that the client offers.

Trust Issues Module

Trust Beliefs Related to SELF: The belief that you can trust or rely on your own judgments and decisions. Trusting yourself is an important building block for developing healthy, trusting relationships with others

PRIOR EXPERIENCE

Negative	Positive
If you had prior experiences where you were blamed for negative events, you may have developed negative beliefs about your ability to make decisions or judgments about situations or people. A new traumatic event may seem to confirm these beliefs.	If you had prior experiences that led you to believe that you had great judgment, the traumatic event may have undercut this belief.
Symptoms Associated with Negative Trust Beliefs about the Self	
<ul><li>Feelings of self-betrayal</li><li>Anxiety</li><li>Confusion</li><li>Excessive caution</li><li>Inability to make decisions</li><li>Self-doubt and excessive self-criticism</li></ul>	
Examples of Possible Stuck Points	
"I can't make good decisions, so I let others make decisions for me." "Because I am a poor judge of character, I can't tell who can be trusted." "If I make choices, then they never work out."	

POSSIBLE RESOLUTIONS

If you previously believed that . . .	A possible alternative thought may be . . .
"I cannot trust my judgment" or "I have bad judgment," the recent traumatic event may have reinforced these beliefs. It is important to understand that the traumatic event was not your fault and that your decisions did not cause the traumatic event.	"I can still trust my judgment even though it's not perfect." "Even if I misjudged this person or situation, I realize that I cannot always realistically predict what others will do or how a situation may turn out."

(continued)

If you previously believed that . . .	A possible alternative thought may be . . .
"I have perfect judgment, and I never make bad decisions," then the traumatic event may have shattered this belief. New beliefs need to reflect the possibilities that you can make mistakes but still have good judgment, and that mistakes in judgment cannot always be blamed as the reason why traumatic events occur.	"No one has perfect judgment. I did the best I could in an unpredictable situation, and I can still trust my ability to make decisions even though it is not perfect." "My bad decision did not cause the event to happen."

Trust Beliefs Related to OTHERS: Beliefs that the promises of other people or groups can be relied on with regard to future behavior. One of the earliest tasks of childhood development involves trust versus mistrust: A person needs to learn a healthy balance of trust and mistrust, and to learn when each is appropriate.

PRIOR EXPERIENCE

Negative	Positive
If you were betrayed in early life, you may have developed the generalized belief that "No one can be trusted." A new traumatic event may serve to confirm this belief, especially if you were hurt by an acquaintance.	If you had particularly good experiences growing up, you may have developed the belief that "All people can be trusted." The traumatic event may have shattered this belief.

POSTTRAUMATIC EXPERIENCE

If the people you knew and trusted, or people in positions of authority, were blaming, distant, or unsupportive after the traumatic event, your belief in their trustworthiness may have been shattered.

Symptoms Associated with Negative Trust Beliefs about Others
• Pervasive sense of disillusionment and disappointment in others. • Fear of betrayal or abandonment. • Anger and rage at betrayers. • After repeated betrayals, negative beliefs so rigid that even people who are trustworthy may be viewed with suspicion. • Fear of close relationships; particularly when trust is beginning to develop, active anxiety and fear of being betrayed.

(continued)

Examples of Possible Stuck Points
"No one can be trusted."
"People in authority will always take advantage of you."
"If I trust someone, they will hurt me."
"If I get close to someone, they will leave."

POSSIBLE RESOLUTIONS

If you previously believed that . . .	Possible alternative thoughts may be . . .
"No one can be trusted," which was seemingly confirmed by the traumatic event, then you need to adopt new beliefs that will allow you to enter into new relationships from a neutral position that allows you to see whether various kinds of trust can be built.	"Although I may find some people to be untrustworthy in some ways, I cannot assume that everyone is always untrustworthy." "Trusting another involves some risk, but I can protect myself by developing trust slowly and including what I learn about that person as I get to know him or her."
"Everyone can be trusted," then the traumatic event will have shattered this belief. To avoid becoming suspicious of the trustworthiness of others, including those you used to trust, you will need to understand that trust is not an either–or matter.	"I may not be able to trust everyone in every way, but that doesn't mean I have to stop trusting the people I used to trust."
"I can trust my family and friends," then the traumatic event may have shattered your beliefs about the trustworthiness of your support system when these persons did not act the way you wanted them to after they learned about the traumatic event. Before you assume that you cannot trust anyone in your support system, it is important to consider why these people may have reacted the way they did. Many people do not know how to respond when someone they care about is traumatized, and they may have been reacting out of ignorance. Some people may have responded out of fear or denial, because what has happened to you made them feel vulnerable and may have affected their own beliefs.	"Trust is not an all-or-none concept. Some people may be more trustworthy than others." "It may help to tell others what I need from them and then see if they do a better job of meeting my needs. I can use this as a way to assess their trustworthiness." If you find that others continue to be unsupportive about the trauma, but kind to you in other ways, you may choose to adopt a statement such as "There are some people I cannot talk to about the traumatic event, but there are other areas of my life where I can trust them." If a person continues to be negative or make blaming statements toward you, you might want to tell yourself, "This person is not trustworthy, and it is not healthy for me to have the person in my life at this time."

Practice Assignment after Session 8 of CPT

Use the Challenging Beliefs Worksheets (Handout 8.1) to analyze and confront at least one of your Stuck Points each day. Also, please read over the Trust Issues Module (Handout 9.1), and think about how your prior beliefs about trust were affected by your trauma. If you have trust issues, Stuck Points, related to yourself or others, complete at least one worksheet to examine those beliefs. Use the remaining sheets for other Stuck Points on your Stuck Point Log (Handout 6.1) or for distressing events that have occurred recently.

Trust Star Worksheet

Date: _____   Client: _____

There are many different types of trust (such as keeping secrets and being reliable). Below, in the lines down the left side of the page, list all the different types of trust you can think of. Then think about one particular person. Write in your relationship with this person here: _____. If you cannot think of a family member or friend, then think of someone in which you must place your trust, such as a doctor, mechanic, or bus driver. Put a star by the most important types of trust for this person. Then fill in the Trust Star graphic by writing a type of trust on each line, and putting an × on the line to indicate how much you trust this person with that type of trust. The plus sign at one end of each line means maximum trust; the minus sign means no trust at all. If you don't know how much you trust the person in this way, put the × just inside the "No information" circle. Does this person need to be trustworthy in *every* way? What about the most important ways? Would you trust this person to pull your tooth, cut your hair, or fix your car?

TYPES OF TRUST

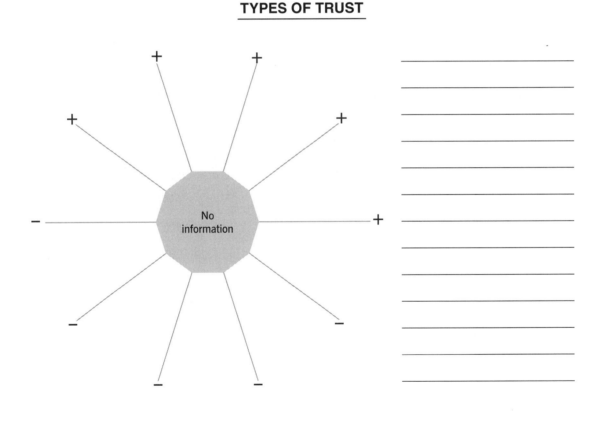

Sample Trust Star Worksheet

There are many different types of trust (such as keeping secrets and being reliable). Below, in the lines down the left side of the page, list all the different types of trust you can think of. Then think about one particular person. Write in your relationship with this person here: _____*friend*_____. If you cannot think of a family member or friend, then think of someone in which you must place your trust, such as a doctor, mechanic, or bus driver. Put a star by the most important types of trust for this person. Then fill in the Trust Star graphic by writing a type of trust on each line, and putting an × on the line to indicate how much you trust this person with that type of trust. The plus sign at one end of each line means maximum trust; the minus sign means no trust at all. If you don't know how much you trust the person in this way, put the × just inside the "No information" circle. Does this person need to be trustworthy in *every* way? What about the most important ways? Would you trust this person to pull your tooth, cut your hair, or fix your car?

TYPES OF TRUST

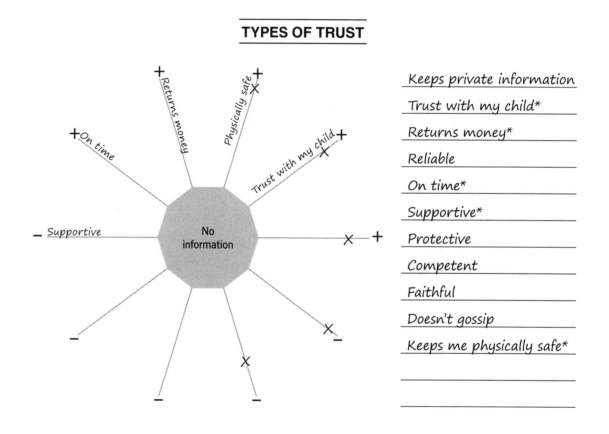

Keeps private information

Trust with my child*

Returns money*

Reliable

On time*

Supportive*

Protective

Competent

Faithful

Doesn't gossip

Keeps me physically safe*

Power/Control Issues Module

Power and Control Beliefs Related to SELF: Beliefs that you can solve problems and meet challenges that you may face.

PRIOR EXPERIENCE

Negative	Positive
If you grew up experiencing repeated negative events, you may have developed the belief that you cannot control events or solve problems even if they are controllable/solvable. A new traumatic event may seem to confirm prior beliefs about helplessness.	If you grew up believing that you had control over events and could solve problems, the traumatic event may have disrupted those beliefs.
Symptoms Associated with Negative Power/Control Beliefs about the Self	
<ul><li>Numbing of feelings</li><li>Avoidance of emotions</li><li>Chronic passivity</li><li>Hopelessness and depression</li><li>Self-destructive patterns</li><li>Outrage when you are faced with events that are out of your control, or with people who do not behave as you would like</li></ul>	
Examples of Possible Stuck Points	
"Because I can't be completely in control, I might as well be out of control." "The traumatic event wouldn't have happened if I had had better control over it." "I need to be perfect to be in control." "If I lose complete control over my emotions, something bad will happen."	

POSSIBLE RESOLUTIONS

If you previously believed that . . .	A possible alternative thought may be . . .
"I have control over everything that I do and say, as well as over the actions of others," then it will be important to realize that none of us can have complete control over our emotions or behavior at all times. Although you may be able to influence many external events, it is impossible to control all events or all behaviors of other people. Neither of these	"I do not have total control over my reactions, other people, or events at all times. However, I am able to have some control over my reactions to events, and to influence some behaviors of others or the outcomes of some events." "Bad things do not always happen when I am not in control."

(continued)

If you previously believed that . . .	A possible alternative thought may be . . .
facts is a sign of weakness, but only an understanding that you are human and can admit that you are not in control of everything that happens to you or your reactions.	
"I am helpless or powerless to control myself or others," then you will need to work on developing a sense of control to decrease the symptoms of depression and low self-esteem that often go along with believing you are helpless. It may help to look at your actual ability to control some events in your life.	"I cannot control all events outside myself, but I do have some control over what happens to me and my reactions to events." "I can try to notice all the little things I have control over in my life, and I can practice taking control over more things in my life that are important to me."

Power and Control Beliefs Related to OTHERS: Beliefs that you can control others or future events related to others (including people in power).

PRIOR EXPERIENCE

Negative	Positive
If you had prior experiences with others that led you to believe that you had no control in your relationships with others, or that you had no power in relation to powerful others, the traumatic event will seem to confirm those beliefs.	If you had prior positive experiences in your relationships with others and in relation to powerful others, you may have come to believe that you could influence others. The traumatic event may shatter this belief because you were unable to exert enough control, despite your best efforts, to prevent the event.
Symptoms Associated with Negative Power/Control Beliefs about Others	
<ul><li>Passivity</li><li>Submissiveness</li><li>Lack of assertiveness that can generalize to all relationships</li><li>Inability to maintain relationships, because you do not allow the other persons to exert any control in the relationships (including becoming enraged if the other persons try to exert even a minimal amount of control)</li></ul>	
Examples of Possible Stuck Points	
"People will always try to control you." "There is no point in even trying to fight against authority." "This event just proves that people have too much power over me."	

(continued)

POSSIBLE RESOLUTIONS

If you previously believed that . . .	Possible alternative thoughts may be . . .
"I am powerless and have no control in relationships," then you will need to learn ways that it is safe and appropriate for you to exert control over yourself, others, and events.	"Even though I cannot always get everything I want in a relationship, I do have the ability to influence others by standing up assertively for my rights and asking for what I want."
"I have to control everything in the lives of people I care about, or they will be hurt," then the traumatic event may have further reinforced this belief. It will be important for you to realize that healthy relationships involve sharing power and control, and that relationships in which one person has all the power can be abusive (even if you are the one with all the power). It may also be helpful to realize that it can be relaxing to give up some of the power, and freeing to let others make decisions some of the time.	"Even though I may not get everything I want or need out of a relationship, I can assert myself and ask for it. A good relationship is one in which power is balanced between both people. If I am not allowed any control, I can exert my control in this relationship by ending it, if necessary." "I can learn to let others have some of the power in a relationship, and even enjoy having others take responsibility for some of the things that need to be done."

Practice Assignment after Session 9 of CPT

Use the Challenging Beliefs Worksheets (Handout 8.1) to analyze and confront at least one of your Stuck Points each day. Also, if not completed in session, complete the trust star example (Handout 9.3). Please read over the Power/Control Issues Module (Handout 9.4), and think about how your prior beliefs about power/control were affected by your trauma. If you have power/control Stuck Points related to yourself or others, complete at least one worksheet to examine those beliefs. Use the remaining sheets for other Stuck Points on your Stuck Point Log (Handout 6.1) or for distressing events that have occurred recently.

Ways of Giving and Taking Power Handout

Giving Power	Taking Power
Positive	
• Being altruistic (helping others without expecting anything in return) • Helping others in need or crisis • Sharing yourself with another person as part of the give-and-take in relationships **Example**: You are on your way to the store when a friend asks for a ride to the doctor, and you decide to help your friend.	• Being assertive • Setting limits and boundaries with others • Being honest with yourself and others **Example**: You tell a friend you cannot help him or her now, but you schedule a time to meet later when it fits into your schedule.
Negative	
• Basing your actions or behaviors solely on the reactions you expect from others • Always placing the needs of others above your own • Allowing others easy access to your "hot buttons," to get you emotionally upset **Example**: You have a strong negative reaction to someone who is clearly manipulating you to feel that way.	• Giving ultimatums • Testing limits • Intentionally upsetting others for personal gain • Behaving aggressively **Example:** You tell your partner, "I will not have sex with you until you do what I want."

Esteem Issues Module

Esteem Beliefs Related to SELF: Beliefs in your own worth. Such beliefs are a basic human need. Being understood, respected, and taken seriously is basic to the development of self-esteem.

PRIOR EXPERIENCE

Negative	Positive
If you had prior experiences that made you doubt your own worth, a new traumatic event will seem to confirm these negative beliefs about your self-worth. Some life experiences that can lead to negative beliefs about the self include these: • Believing other people's negative statements about you • Receiving little caring or support from others • Being criticized or blamed by others, even when things were not your fault	If you had prior experiences that were positive and built up your beliefs in your own worth, the traumatic event may have disrupted those beliefs and lowered your self-esteem. Your self-confidence in making decisions and your faith in your opinions may be decreased.
Symptoms Associated with Negative Esteem Beliefs about the Self	
• Depression • Guilt • Shame • Possible self-destructive behavior	
Examples of Possible Stuck Points	
"I am bad, destructive, or evil." "I am responsible for bad, destructive, or evil acts." "I am basically damaged or flawed." "Because I am worthless, I deserve unhappiness and suffering."	

POSSIBLE RESOLUTIONS

If you previously believed that . . .	A possible alternative thought may be . . .
"I am worthless" (or any of the beliefs listed above) because of prior experiences, then the traumatic event may seem to confirm this	"Sometimes bad things happen to good people. Just because someone says something bad about me, that does not make

(continued)

If you previously believed that . . .	A possible alternative thought may be . . .
belief. If you received poor social support after the event, this may also confirm negatives beliefs about yourself. To improve your self-esteem, it may help to reevaluate your beliefs about your self-worth and replace maladaptive beliefs with more realistic, positive ones.	it true. No one deserves this, and that includes me. Even if I have made mistakes in the past, that does not make me a bad person deserving of unhappiness or suffering (including the traumatic event)."
"Bad things will not happen to me because I am a good person," then the event may have disrupted such beliefs, and you may wonder what you did to deserve the event (e.g., "Maybe I was being punished for something I had done, or because I am actually a bad person"). To regain your prior positive beliefs about your self-worth, you will need to look carefully at the situation, so that your sense of worth is not disrupted every time something unexpected and bad happens to you. When you can accept that bad things might happen to you (as they happen to everybody from time to time), you will let go of blaming yourself for events that you did not cause.	"Sometimes bad things happen to good people. If something bad happens to me, it is not necessarily because I did something to cause it or because I deserved it. Sometimes there is not a good explanation for why bad things happen. I might have been the occasion, but not the cause of the event."

Esteem Beliefs Related to OTHERS: Beliefs about how much you value other people. Realistic views of others are important to psychological health. In less psychologically healthy people, these beliefs are stereotyped, rigid, and relatively unchanged by new information.

PRIOR EXPERIENCE

Negative	Positive
If you had many bad experiences with people in the past, you may have concluded that other people are not good or not to be trusted. You may have developed this belief about everyone (even those who are basically good and have your best interests at heart). The traumatic event may seem to confirm these beliefs about people. In addition, negative experiences may make it difficult to respect people in authority, especially if your trauma involved someone in a position of power.	If your prior experiences with people were positive, and if negative events in the world did not seem to have an impact on you, the traumatic event was probably belief-shattering. Prior beliefs in the basic goodness of other people may have been particularly disrupted if people who were assumed to be supportive were not there for you after the event.

(continued)

Symptoms Associated with Negative Esteem Beliefs about Others
• Chronic anger • Contempt • Bitterness • Cynicism • Disbelief when treated with genuine caring compassion ("What do they really want?") • Isolation or withdrawal from others • Antisocial behavior, justified by the belief that people are only out for themselves
Examples of Possible Stuck Points
"People are basically uncaring, indifferent, and only out for themselves." "People are bad, evil, or malicious." "Large parts of the human race [e.g., all men, all government officials] are bad, evil, or malicious."

POSSIBLE RESOLUTIONS

If you previously believed that . . .	Possible self-statements may be . . .
"All people are no good," then it will be important for you to reconsider the automatic conclusion that all people (or at least all people from a particular group) are no good, and consider how that belief has affected your behavior and social life in general. When you first meet someone, it is important that you do not make decisions based on stereotypes, which are not generally true for the majority of people you will meet. It is better and more accurate to adopt a "wait-and-see" attitude, which will allow you time to develop your beliefs about the other person without automatically judging the person you are trying to get to know.	"While some [members of a particular group] do bad things, not all [members of this group] are out to hurt me." "While some people in power will abuse their power, not all people in power are out to hurt others."
"I need to put up with other people's behavior, even if it makes me uncomfortable," you need to keep in mind that if over time a person makes you uncomfortable, or does things that may hurt you, you are free to stop trying to develop the relationship. It is important to remember, however, that all people make mistakes, and you need to consider your ground rules for friendships or intimate relationships ahead of time. If you confront the person with a request to stop doing	"Although there are people I do not respect and do not wish to know, I cannot assume this about every new person I meet. I may come to this conclusion later, but it will be after I have learned more about this person."

(continued)

If you previously believed that . . .	Possible self-statements may be . . .
something that makes you uncomfortable, you can use that person's reaction to your request to help you decide if the person is going to be good for you to have in your life. That is, if the person is apologetic and makes a genuine effort to avoid making the same mistake, then you might want to continue getting to know this person. If the person is insensitive to your request or belittles you in some way, then you may want to get out of this relationship. The important point about esteem of others is like the point about trust of others: You need time to get to know people and form an opinion of them. It is important that you adopt a view of others that is balanced and allows for changes.	
"People I expect to support me will always let me down," it will be important not to drop relationships immediately, even if those you expected support from let you down. Talk to them about how you feel and what you want from them. Use their reactions to your request as a way of evaluating where you want these relationships to go.	"People sometimes make mistakes. I will try to find out whether they understand it was a mistake or whether it reflects a negative pattern that will continue from that person. At that point, I can end the relationship if it is something I cannot accept."

Practice Assignment after Session 10 of CPT

Use the Challenging Beliefs Worksheets (Handout 8.1) to analyze and confront at least one of your Stuck Points each day. Also, please read over the Esteem Issues Module (Handout 9.7) and think about how your prior beliefs about esteem were affected by your trauma. If you have esteem Stuck Points related to yourself or others, complete at least one worksheet to examine those beliefs. Use the remaining sheets for other Stuck Points on your Stuck Point Log (Handout 6.1) or for distressing events that have occurred recently.

Also, each day before the next session, do one nice thing for yourself "just because," not because you achieved something. Also, practice giving one compliment and receiving one compliment each day. Write the nice things you did for yourself, and the names of the persons whom you complimented and who complimented you, on this sheet. It is better to compliment people for something they did rather than how they look. If any of these assignments result in Stuck Points, please complete a Challenging Beliefs Worksheet on them.

10

Esteem, Intimacy, and Facing the Future

Session 11, Session 12, and Aftercare

Goals for Sessions 11 and 12

Although the goals for the sessions on the Esteem and Intimacy themes (Sessions 11 and 12) are very similar to the goals for the preceding three sessions, with the therapist and client reviewing the Challenging Beliefs Worksheets related to both of these themes, both sessions include additional activities. Session 11 includes a review of the two behavioral practice assignments from Session 10, and Session 12 involves revisiting the client's perception of the impact of the trauma.

Session 11: Review of Esteem and Introducing Intimacy

Procedures for Session 11

1. Review the client's scores on the self-report objective measures. (See the discussions of this review for Sessions 2 and 3 in Chapter 6.)
2. Review the Challenging Beliefs Worksheets related to the Esteem theme and to other Stuck Points.

3. Review the assignments regarding compliments and nice/worthwhile things that the client has completed.
4. Discuss therapy termination.
5. Introduce the Intimacy theme.
6. Give the new practice assignment.
7. Check the client's reactions to the session and the practice assignment.

Reviewing the Client's Challenging Beliefs Worksheets

After the usual review of the client's scores on the self-report measures, Session 11 should begin with the therapist and client's reviewing the Challenging Beliefs Worksheets on esteem. Clients will often have very strong beliefs about their own worth and capabilities. They may state that they are damaged because of their traumatic events; they may view their PTSD symptoms as evidence that they are weak, crazy, or permanently changed in some negative way. Or they may infer from the trauma that their judgment is impaired, or they may believe that others blame them for things they did or did not do during the events. These beliefs can erode the clients' beliefs about themselves related to the events, and then in turn eat away at their global perception of self-esteem. When a trauma is interpersonal in nature (e.g., rape, child abuse, or military sexual trauma), a client may also assume, "There was something wrong with me in the first place, or I would not have been the target of this type of trauma." When the client makes global negative comments about the self, the therapist can help him or her by identifying any new Stuck Points and then examining the specific nature of the self-criticism through Socratic dialogue. Like the other themes, the Esteem theme is a global multidimensional concept that should allow for flexibility in the ways in which the client views the self and others.

Often this is the point in the therapy when it is most helpful to address the client's beliefs about perfectionism and concerns that all mistakes will lead to horrific outcomes. This can become a debilitating cycle in which the client engages in undue self-blame for any mistakes he or she made, which fuels the belief that all mistakes are unacceptable. The client may reinforce this line of thinking by believing that he or she made mistakes before or during the traumatic event that caused the event to happen. Sometimes it can help to ask the client, "What would you think of a teacher who announced that a 100% was an A and a 99% was an F?" When the client says that this would be unfair, the therapist can ask, "So why are you being unfair to yourself?" It is also helpful to ask the client, "Do you know any perfect people? Perhaps 'good enough' is a more reasonable goal."

It can be helpful to use Challenging Beliefs Worksheets to explore the basic unfairness a client is practicing with him- or herself. For example, the client in the following example had made a mistake at work that resulted in her having to stay late to fix the problem.

THERAPIST: So with the Stuck Point "If I make a mistake, I am a failure," we need to look at the evidence against this Stuck Point. Did you do anything else that day at work?

CLIENT: Sure, lots of things.

THERAPIST: And, did those turn out all right?

CLIENT: I guess so, but I might find out otherwise later.

THERAPIST: OK, so in addition to work, how many things did you do yesterday? How many decisions did you make? What percentage correct did you have for the day?

CLIENT: Well, when you put it that way . . . I guess I did OK. But lots of the things I did yesterday don't matter as much as the mistake I made at work.

THERAPIST: That makes sense. Not everything has the same importance. But some of what you did involved taking care of your kids, right? So what was the most important thing you did all day?

CLIENT: Well, making sure my kids were safe and fed and stuff.

THERAPIST: OK, so in the scheme of yesterday, you did lots of other things well other than the mistake at work, right?

CLIENT: I guess.

THERAPIST: Did you have any important things happen at work in the past week?

CLIENT: Sure. I finished the big project I was working on and turned it in on Monday.

THERAPIST: And did that go well?

CLIENT: My boss said I did a great job.

THERAPIST: So what could we put on this sheet as evidence against your Stuck Point that "If I make a mistake, I am a failure"?

CLIENT: Well, I guess I could say that I did my project well, and I do try to take care of my kids.

THERAPIST: Great. Now let's use that information to fill in the rest of section D on the worksheet.

In looking at esteem as it relates to others, it is important to identify ways in which the client may overgeneralize attributes associated with the perpetrator or combat enemy to an entire group of people (e.g., all men, all Iraqis, all Asians). When this happens, it will be important to help the client see people as individuals and not lump everyone into a stereotype. One way to do this is to use the Challenging Belief Worksheets to help the client see that these stereotypes not only are unfair to members of the stigmatized group(s), but can have a strong negative impact on the client's own daily living (avoiding gas stations owned by members of certain groups, not dating members of those groups, etc.). The client may need help identifying how and why these overgeneralized thoughts are being maintained.

For clients who served in the military, another area where they may develop over-accommodated Stuck Points is their view of the "government." As with other concepts discussed throughout this book, "government" is an overly general term that can mean a great number of things. Many of these clients will use their thoughts about the government to help them stay angry and thus avoid feeling their other emotions, such as sad-ness or grief related to their traumatic events. Although it is important for clients to feel heard by their therapists, allowing them to rant about the government will not help them get better. Instead, it may help such a client to encourage a focus on the traumatic event that is behind the government blaming, or to ask questions such as "What do you mean by 'government'? A particular President? The military? The mayor? We the people?" In addition, if the client's focus is on the government's not being trustworthy, the therapist can ask questions such as "So you mean no one answers when you call 911? You never receive your mail?", or can give other examples where the "government" or govern-ment agencies do typically work efficiently. Through Socratic dialogue, the therapist can help the client begin to see that there are different types of "government" and different degrees to which each type can be trusted. Although at first this may seem like an exer-cise in semantics to the therapist, the client, or both, the ability to see things in shades of gray allows the client to feel more empowered and to begin decreasing hairtrigger reactions to ambiguous situations, especially those involving the government.

Reviewing the Assignments on Giving and Receiving Compliments/Behavioral Activation

The therapist should also make time to ask the client about how the assignments to give and receive compliments and to do nice things for him- or herself went. It can be helpful to ask whether the client was able to hear a compliment without immedi-ately rejecting it, and to encourage just saying "Thank you," even if this might feel uncomfortable at first because of the client's negative esteem cognitions. If any Stuck Points emerge in the process of receiving compliments, the client should add them to the Stuck Point Log and complete a Challenging Beliefs Worksheet on each of them. In addition, it is helpful to ask the client what happened when he or she gave compli-ments, including how the recipient responded and whether this was different from prior interactions with similar people.

Next, the therapist should ask how the client felt when doing nice things for him- or herself, and whether this triggered any new Stuck Points (e.g., "I don't deserve nice things," or "I am not honoring my lost combat buddy when I feel happy"). It is important that the therapist make sure that the client is not making him- or herself have to "earn" the nice things, because this defeats the purpose of having nice things without a price attached. For practice until the next session, the client should be encouraged to con-tinue to do nice or worthwhile things for him- or herself, practice giving and receiving compliments daily, and practice enjoying all of them. The therapist should continue to help the client identify esteem-related Stuck Points and generate some positive self-esteem-enhancing alternatives if the client tends to make disparaging comments about the self. The therapist can also say that this is a "practice assignment for life."

Discussing Therapy Termination

If therapists have not already done so in an earlier session, it may be helpful to ask clients whether they are experiencing any concerns or strong feelings related to the end of therapy. We have found that many clients, especially those who have been in long-term therapy prior to CPT, have Stuck Points about ending therapy (e.g., "I cannot manage my life without a therapist," or "If I don't have a therapist, everything will go back to the way it was"). Asking such clients to challenge these Stuck Points on Challenging Beliefs Worksheets can often help them to see how much progress they have made in treatment, and to realize that they have the tools they need to maintain more balanced and healthy views of themselves and others around them. In addition, it can be helpful for therapists to remind these clients that booster sessions can be arranged if these are ever needed in the future.

Introducing the Intimacy Theme

As in the prior sessions, the new theme (this time, the theme of Intimacy) is introduced toward the end of the session, and a therapist and client briefly discuss how the client's relationships may have been affected by the trauma(s). Intimacy is a natural progression from self-esteem, since it includes a strong sense of self-efficacy and comfort with one's own company. The Stuck Points related to intimacy can be either nonsexual or sexual in nature and can include the full range of possible relationships. Initially, the therapist may find that problems with intimacy related to others are easier to identify than difficulties with intimacy related to the self. Intimacy with others often involves Stuck Points such as "If I get close to someone, they will die," "Men only want me for sex," or "If I let someone get to know all of me, they will leave." Intimacy with the self, on the other hand, will often include Stuck Points such as "I cannot handle being alone," "I cannot meet my own needs," or "I don't know how I want to spend my time without PTSD." Self-intimacy goes beyond self-esteem and includes self-awareness, knowledge of one's own values/tastes, and decisions about future interests/activities. In other words, the goal with regard to self-intimacy by the end of the therapy is for the client to begin to catch up with his or her developmental peer group, whether in making early adulthood career and relationship decisions, or in deciding on a retirement identity and activities.

For a client traumatized in adulthood, it may be helpful to encourage the client to remember how intimacy with self and others was before the event and how it was affected by the event. The therapist should remember to check with the client regarding any continued problems with inappropriate attempts to self-soothe (via alcohol or other substance use, overeating, overspending, etc.); such attempts have probably been addressed earlier in the therapy, but may need to be discussed again to identify any lingering Stuck Points on self-care. For the practice assignment, the client should be asked to use the Challenging Beliefs Worksheets to confront maladaptive statements related to intimacy, any other unresolved or lingering Stuck Points, and Stuck Points related to the termination of treatment, and to generate more adaptive statements.

Giving the New Practice Assignment

In addition to reading the Intimacy Issues Module (Handout 10.1) and completing Challenging Beliefs Worksheets that include at least one worksheet on intimacy issues, the client is asked to write a new Impact Statement that addresses what it *now* means to him or her that the traumatic event(s) occurred, and what the client's current beliefs are in regard to the five topics of safety, trust, power/control, esteem, and intimacy (see Handout 10.2). This new Impact Statement will allow the client to see clearly how his or her beliefs have changed since the beginning of therapy, so it is important that the therapist stresses the need to focus on how the client is thinking and feeling now, not when the treatment started. Finally, the client is asked to continue to do nice/worthwhile things for him- or herself and to continue to practice giving and receiving compliments, in addition to completing daily Challenging Beliefs Worksheets.

Checking the Client's Reactions to the Session and the Practice Assignment

As usual, the therapist should conclude Session 11 by eliciting the client's reactions to the session and asking whether the client has any questions about the session content or the next practice assignment. The therapist should reinforce any important ideas or discoveries made in the session, and should note the important take-home messages that the client offers.

Session 12: Processing Intimacy and the Final Impact Statement

Procedures for Session 12

1. Review the client's scores on the self-report objective measures. (See the discussions of this review for Sessions 2 and 3 in Chapter 6.)
2. Review the client's Challenging Beliefs Worksheets related to the Intimacy theme and to other Stuck Points.

3. Review the client's original and new Impact Statements.
4. Review the course of treatment and the client's progress.
5. Identify the client's goals for the future.

Reviewing the Client's Challenging Beliefs Worksheets

In Session 12, the final session of CPT, the therapist and client review the client's Challenging Beliefs Worksheets on intimacy and any additional worksheets the client may have completed since the last session. For many of our clients with PTSD, intimacy problems often have caused them to become so dependent on others that they do not think they have the ability to care for themselves. We even see this in some of our male veterans, who need their wives or partners to drive them to every physical or mental health appointment, for fear that they will fall apart if the women are not there to soothe them as they wait for these appointments. Many clients only focus on physical intimacy or intimacy with others for their practice assignment, and do not focus on self-intimacy. It may be helpful to remind such a client that self-intimacy involves the ability to cope, maintain self-control, and provide appropriate self-comforting without needing to rely on other people or unhealthy behaviors to manage one's own behaviors and feelings. Self-intimacy also includes self-knowledge—coming to an understanding of one's tastes and values in the process of recovering from PTSD. Stuck Points that interfere with return to the client's appropriate developmental level should be added to the ongoing Stuck Point log.

As suggested in the Session 11 discussion above, a common indicator of a client's difficulty with self-intimacy is engaging in excessive behaviors—for example, substance abuse, overeating, compulsive spending/gambling, or even behaviors that may appear healthy but may not be if carried to extremes (e.g., working out). One client who completed CPT stated in Session 1 that in order to complete his first Impact Statement, he would "need to get drunk." The therapist quickly realized that the client probably had difficulty with self-soothing, and the two worked together to identify Stuck Points related to self-care and the client's ability to talk about his reactions to the trauma (e.g., "The only way to handle my trauma memories is if I am drunk"). The therapist continued to check in on this issue throughout therapy, to ensure that the client was not drinking before, during, or after sessions or homework. In the final two sessions of CPT, however, greater emphasis is placed on developing additional, potentially healthier means of self-coping. One way to do this is to encourage clients to complete Challenging Beliefs Worksheets instead of immediately eating, smoking, drinking, or shopping when they are upset, to allow them to see what thoughts are driving the emotional distress they are trying to avoid. Ideally, this will then give them time to challenge the disruptive cognitions and allow them to decrease the stressful emotions that cause them to engage in potentially unhealthy behaviors.

This is also a key time for therapists to check on how clients are continuing to do on giving and receiving compliments and on doing nice/worthwhile things for them-selves. Many clients are surprised by how much enjoyment they feel even after doing little things for themselves, without having to earn them, please everyone else first, or ask someone's permission. It can be important to help different clients explore different options, but a few of the common ideas we propose are taking a walk, drinking a cup of tea, phoning a friend, working out, gardening, or starting a new hobby. Clients often realize that they if they engage in one of these activities when they are starting to become emotional, they can interrupt the old cycle of negative thinking, painful emotions, and destructive behaviors.

Clients often report having difficulties in intimacy related to others in two ways: emotional closeness with friends/family, and sexual intimacy. Clients who experience trauma for the first time in adulthood may find themselves withdrawing from close friends and family and avoiding making new friends as a way of protecting themselves from possible rejection, blame, or further harm, which they believe (often inaccu-rately) that others may inflict on them. For example, many trauma survivors misin-terpret the well-meaning but fumbling attempts at support from family members and friends as their being judgmental, blaming them, or suggesting that they should "just get over it." Survivors also often assume that others will blame them if they find out the "whole story" of what happened during the traumatic events. Thus clients often distance themselves from others who could have been sources of support; as a conse-quence, their relationships/friendships often begin to disintegrate. Furthermore, cli-ents typically avoid establishing new relationships for fear of being hurt or abandoned. Eventually, many such clients feel isolated and alone, and have little faith that they can have healthy relationships in the future. Common Stuck Points are "No one will ever love me," "If people know what happened in my past, they will know what a terrible person I am," and "Everyone will leave me."

Conversely, clients whose traumatic experiences started in childhood will often stay in unhealthy relationships, because they have come to believe on the basis of their past experiences that they are incapable of having or deserving any other type of relationship. These clients may routinely accept poor treatment from friends and family members, and will often blame themselves for the way others misuse them. It is very important for therapists to find these underlying Stuck Points (which may be core beliefs) related to other-intimacy, if they have not done so in earlier sessions of CPT. Examples include "I do not deserve to be loved," "A bad relationship is the best I can ever hope for," and "I cause other people to treat me badly." It is important to help these clients see that the PTSD has probably kept them from making new friends who could be sources of support, often by causing them to ignore gestures by others who have tried to reach out in the past. This often makes it difficult for the clients to identify evidence to use when challenging their destructive thoughts about others, and therapists will often need to do extra questioning to find key "evidence against," as the clients may have great difficulty identifying any at first.

Although sexual intimacy can be a particular problem for sexual assault survivors, we have found that sexual functioning can be negatively affected by other kinds of trauma as well. Often the symptoms of PTSD and depression can interfere with sexual desire and performance, and it can be important to normalize these reactions for clients who assume that this is just another example of how they are "broken." Sometimes when clients with PTSD experience guilt or grief for friends who have died, they may believe that they do not deserve to be happy in any way, including sexual intimacy.

For sexual assault survivors, being intimate with others can be particularly challenging—not only because they have difficulty feeling the trust and vulnerability that are typically necessary for sexual intimacy, but because being sexual has often become a triggering cue associated with the assault. These intimacy issues have often been addressed earlier in therapy during the review of a client's trust issues, but a therapist should look for any unresolved Stuck Points in this area and work on these during this final session. Although CPT is not a sex therapy, it can be useful in identifying and correcting problematic beliefs that may interfere with sexual functioning, because it is a form of cognitive therapy. However, more serious or enduring forms of sexual dysfunction should be treated with other therapy protocols designed specifically for that purpose (e.g., Haines, 1999).

Reviewing the Client's Original and New Impact Statements

A client and therapist often find that reading and discussing the client's new Impact Statement about the meaning of the event is a wonderful way to bring the entire course of therapy together. The client should first read the new Impact Statement to the therapist, and this should be followed by the therapist's reading the original Impact Statement from Session 2 (or a subsequent session, if this statement was not brought to the second session). This allows the client to hear how much change has taken place in a rather short period. Usually there are significant changes from the first to the second Impact Statement, with the client typically remarking, "Did I really think that?" or "I cannot believe I talked like that to myself." The client and therapist should then highlight all of the key ways in which the client has changed and make note of any remaining problematic beliefs that the client should continue to work on after therapy ends. For clients who have not shown a drastic change from the first to the second Impact Statement, it may be helpful to ask the clients to identify cognitive and behavioral changes they have made with regard to each of the five themes (Safety, Trust, Power/Control, Esteem, and Intimacy). It can also be helpful to note any extreme thinking such clients are still engaging in, and to capture any relevant Stuck Points for them to work on after therapy has concluded.

Reviewing the Course of Treatment and the Client's Progress

Most of the rest of this final session should focus on a brief review of the concepts and skills introduced during CPT. The client should be reminded that continued success will largely depend on how much he or she continues to use the new skills and resists giving in to the old avoidance behaviors. The client should also be encouraged to take credit for facing and dealing with the traumatic event(s) and for doing the work required to get better. If the client brings up any additional Stuck Points during this part of therapy, these should be written on the Stuck Point Log, and the client should be given additional Challenging Beliefs Worksheets for addressing these Stuck Points and any other problematic beliefs that may arise as the client moves on with life.

Identifying the Client's Goals for the Future

The therapist should make sure that goals for the future are discussed as well. For some clients, issues of grief or traumatic bereavement cannot be expected to be resolved in 12 sessions, and therapists should encourage these clients to pursue the process of rebuilding their lives, while also giving themselves time to grieve for their losses. If clients should encounter something that triggers a flashback, a nightmare, or a sudden memory they do not remember having before, these do not mean that their PTSD is coming back. In response to a strong enough trigger, most people will have a reaction to a traumatic event that happened to them in the past. If clients find they are not able to get back to their previous level of functioning fairly rapidly, they should be encouraged to feel their natural emotions and to check their thoughts to make sure that these are not extreme. They should then complete worksheets to address any disruptive thoughts that are driving unpleasant emotions.

For many clients who have suffered from PTSD for decades, this question often emerges at some point in therapy: "Who will I be when I no longer have PTSD?" PTSD can have such an all-consuming influence on an individual's life that it can be difficult to imagine making a decision or taking an action without worrying about managing flashbacks or other symptoms. For some older clients, we have discussed the idea of "retiring from PTSD"; for some younger clients, we have talked about "graduating from PTSD." We remind clients that all people change their roles and identities over time, whether by getting married, having children, graduating from college, or retiring from a long career. Each of these changes brings many questions and uncertainties about personal roles, obligations, connections with other people, and ways to spend time. Therapists should help normalize this process for clients and encourage them to find thoughtful answers for each of the questions they have, instead of viewing all change with dread. In particular, the clients now have choices about how to spend their time, instead of having it largely controlled by PTSD as it has been in the past.

Therapists should guide clients to see these new changes in a positive light and should encourage them to explore all their options.

A Note on Aftercare

We recommend that after a client has completed the CPT protocol, whether it has been conducted weekly or twice a week, the therapist should set up a follow-up appointment for a month or two in the future. The client should be encouraged to continue completing Challenging Beliefs Worksheets for any remaining Stuck Points. The follow-up session should include the same assessment measures that were used during treatment, and it can be used either to get the client back on track or to reinforce gains. Such a session is also helpful in instilling in clients the notion of "episodes of care." They are encouraged to work as their own cognitive therapists on their Stuck Points and daily events that arise, and then to present for a booster session if they have difficulty resolving a Stuck Point or recent event. A specific goal-oriented piece of work can be done, and then they are encouraged to continue using the skills they have developed in the course of therapy.

Several outpatient programs we know of have instituted aftercare programs for clients who have completed CPT. This program can be conducted in a monthly group format and is typically intended for those clients who have a great deal of upheaval remaining in their lives or for those whose scores have not decreased as much as the clients and their individual therapists would like. Such a group is considered time-limited, and clients must be prepared to discuss worksheets they have completed for practice during each session. Typically these groups have been set up in a drop-in format, and clients may attend for one session or several, depending on what they are working on. The facilitators of these groups have reported to us that the groups have been very helpful in maintaining gains and giving the clients a place to continue their work on Stuck Points without needing to return to more formal therapy.

Intimacy Issues Module

Intimacy Beliefs Related to SELF: Beliefs that you can take care of your own emotional needs. An important part of healthy living is the ability to soothe and calm oneself. Part of self-intimacy is the ability to be alone without feeling lonely or empty.

PRIOR EXPERIENCE

Negative	Positive
If you had prior experiences (or poor role models) that led you to believe that you are unable to cope with negative life events, you may have reacted to the traumatic event with negative thoughts suggesting that you were unable to soothe, comfort, or nurture yourself.	If you previously had healthy, positive self-intimacy, you may be able to cope with a traumatic event because of the ability to use internal coping strategies. However, some traumatic events can create conflict; you may begin to doubt your ability to take care of your needs.
Symptoms Associated with Negative Intimacy Beliefs about the Self	
<ul><li>Inability to comfort and soothe the self</li><li>Fear of being alone</li><li>Experience of inner emptiness or deadness</li><li>Periods of great anxiety or panic if reminded of trauma when alone</li><li>Possibly looking to external sources of comfort—overeating, alcohol or other substance use, spending money, self-harm behaviors, or sex</li><li>Needy or demanding relationships</li></ul>	
Examples of Possible Stuck Points	
"If I get emotional, I will be out of control." "I can't tolerate being alone." "I can't handle my trauma symptoms by myself."	

POSSIBLE RESOLUTIONS

If you previously believed that . . .	A possible alternative thought may be . . .
"I can take care of myself, and other people's actions do not affect me," the traumatic event may have shaken this belief. It will be helpful for you to remember the ways that you have taken care of meeting your needs in the past,	"I will not suffer forever. I can soothe myself and use the skills I have learned to cope with these painful feelings. I may need help in dealing with my reactions, but that is normal." "The skills and abilities I am developing now

(continued)

If you previously believed that . . .	A possible alternative thought may be . . .
and how you were able not to make other people's crises your own. In addition, understanding the typical reactions to trauma may help you feel less panicky about what you are experiencing. When some people have a difficult time making themselves feel better, they may turn to unhealthy behaviors (substance abuse, overeating, gambling, etc.) that only mask the symptoms instead of helping with recovery. The painful thoughts and feelings do not go away, however, and these persons then have to deal with the consequences of the unhealthy behaviors, which usually compound the problems.	will help me to cope better with other stressful situations in the future."
"I cannot take care of myself; I must have other people to help me," the traumatic event may have reinforced this belief. You may have become convinced that you do not have any skills to help yourself or make yourself feel better. It will help for you to begin to identify the small ways that you take care of yourself every day and to build on these small wins. It is good to have others in your life that you can rely on, but there are times when others are not available.	"Although it may be hard at first, I can develop skills for taking care of myself, including practicing self-care by doing things that I enjoy doing." "It is healthy to ask others for help when I need it, but people are not always free immediately, and I can learn to take care of myself until they are available."

Intimacy Beliefs Related to OTHERS: Beliefs that you are capable of making different types of emotional connections with others. The desire for closeness is one of the most basic human needs. Intimate connections with others can be negatively affected by traumatic events or damaged by insensitive, hurtful, or unempathic responses from others.

PRIOR EXPERIENCE

Negative	Positive
Negative beliefs may have resulted from traumatic loss of intimate connections. The traumatic event may seem to confirm your belief in your inability to be close to another person.	If you previously had satisfying intimate relationships with others, you may find that the traumatic event (especially if it was an act committed by someone you knew) left you believing that you could never be close to anyone again.

(continued)

Posttraumatic Experience
You may also have experienced a disruption in your belief about your ability to be intimate with others if you were blamed or rejected by persons you thought would be supportive.

Symptoms Associated with Negative Esteem Beliefs about Others
• Pervasive loneliness • Emptiness or isolation • Failure to experience connectedness with others, even in relationships that are genuinely loving and intimate

Examples of Possible Stuck Points
"If I get close to someone, I will get hurt." "All anyone ever wants is sex." "I will always be taken advantage of in relationships."

POSSIBLE RESOLUTIONS

If you previously believed that . . .	Possible self-statements may be . . .
"I can depend on others and feel close and connected to them," the traumatic event may have had negative effects on your ability to feel intimate with others. It will be important for you to regain healthy beliefs about your ability to become close to others. To have intimate relationships with others again, you may need to adopt new, more adaptive beliefs about intimacy. Intimate relationships take time to develop and effort from both people. You are not solely responsible for the failure of prior or future relationships. The development of relationships involves risk taking, and it is possible that you may be hurt again. Staying away from relationships for this reason alone, however, is likely to leave you feeling empty and alone.	"Even though a past relationship did not work out, it does not mean that I cannot have satisfying intimate relationships in the future. Not everyone will betray me. I will need to take risks in developing relationships in the future, but if I take it slowly, I will have a better chance of telling whether this person can be trusted."
"I cannot be close to others, and everyone will hurt me," the trauma may have reinforced this belief. It will be important for you to begin slowly taking chances with some other people, and to learn that you can not only trust them but can also be intimate with them. If there are people who let you down or hurt you with their response after the event, you can attempt to improve your relationships with them by telling them what you need and	"I can still be close to people, but I may not be able (or may not want) to be intimate with everyone I meet. I may lose prior or future intimate relationships with others who cannot meet me halfway, but this is not my fault or due to the fact that I did not try."

(continued)

If you previously believed that . . .	Possible self-statements may be . . .
letting them know how you feel about what they said or did. If they are unable to adjust to your requests and are unable to give you what you need, you may decide that you can no longer be close to those people. You may find, however, that they responded as they did out of ignorance or fear. If you talk to them about this, your relationships with them may improve, and you may end up feeling closer to them than you did before the traumatic event.	
Remember, many people need the support of others to recover from a traumatic event.	

Practice Assignment after Session 11 of CPT

Read the Intimacy Issues Module (Handout 10.1), and use Challenging Beliefs Worksheets (Handout 8.1) to confront Stuck Points about intimacy related to yourself or others. Continue completing worksheets on previous topics that are still problematic, and/or any concerns you have about the ending of treatment.

Continue to practice doing nice/worthwhile things for yourself, and giving and receiving compliments.

Finally, please write at least one page on what you think *now* about why your traumatic event(s) occurred. Also, consider what you believe *now* about yourself, others, and the world in the following areas: safety, trust, power/control, esteem, and intimacy.

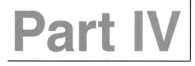

Part IV

Alternatives in Delivery and Special Considerations

11

Variations on CPT

CPT with Written Accounts, Variable-Length CPT, and CPT for Acute Stress Disorder

CPT with Written Accounts

The original version of CPT+A (Resick & Schnicke, 1992, 1993) included two written accounts of the index traumatic event within the 12-session protocol. Much of the early research was conducted on this version of the therapy, until the Resick et al. (2008) dismantling study found that the cognitive-therapy-only version of CPT did just as well without exposing clients to the distress of the accounts. Much of the research being conducted today is being done with CPT. However, in some cases, it may prove advantageous to include the written accounts. As discussed in Chapter 2, one study found that those with high levels of dissociation did better with CPT+A than with CPT, while those with medium and low levels of dissociation did better with CPT (Resick, Suvak, et al., 2012). In a related vein, examination of data from both the original study of CPT+A versus PE (Resick et al., 2002) and the dismantling study revealed that although severity or duration of child sexual abuse did not affect treatment outcomes with different types of CPT, frequency of such abuse did affect outcomes: Those who had experienced high-frequency abuse did better with CPT+A (Resick et al., 2014). In both cases, it is likely that it was not just the act of writing the accounts, but the combination of writing the accounts with cognitive processing, that made a difference. This group did not do better with either PE or written accounts only, so it is not just the repetition of the traumatic event recounting that matters. It is possible that these clients needed to reconstruct a fragmented set of memories into a coherent narrative in order to benefit from cognitive interventions.

In spite of the facts that CPT and CPT+A generally have similar outcomes by posttreatment, and that there has been no statistical difference in dropout rates between CPT (22%) and CPT+A (34%) (although the difference is probably clinically meaningful; Resick et al., 2008), some people may choose to do CPT+A because they want to write their accounts. We recommend that clients be given a choice of which therapy they wish to pursue.

Like CPT (which has been described in detail in Chapters 5–10), CPT+A is delivered in 12 sessions, but the order is a bit different from that in CPT. The CPT+A session topics are as follows:

1. Introduction and education
2. Meaning of the event (Impact Statement)
3. Identification of thoughts and feelings (ABC Worksheet)
4. Remembering traumatic events (first written account)
5. Remembering traumatic events (second written account)
6. Challenging Questions Worksheet
7. Patterns of Problematic Thinking Worksheet
8. Challenging Beliefs Worksheet and Safety Issues Module
9. Trust Issues Module
10. Power/Control Issues Module
11. Esteem Issues Module
12. Intimacy Issues Module and meaning of the event

The first three sessions of the two protocols are the same. It is not until the end of Session 3 that they diverge. Although CPT clients are assigned to write all of their ABC Worksheets on the traumatic event for Session 4, CPT+A clients are assigned to continue to complete ABC Worksheets, as well as to produce the first written account (see Handout 11.1). For the written account, the clients are assigned to handwrite what happened during the index trauma, from the time they realized they were in danger until the trauma was over. A handwritten account averages about eight pages long, but it may be longer or shorter depending on how long the incident lasted, whether the client has a complete memory of the event, and whether more than one incident was included. A single paragraph is not a trauma account. We do not instruct that the account should be written in the present tense (as is done in exposure therapy); in fact, we encourage the use of the past tense. We want each CPT-A client to recognize that an event is over and is just a memory.

If a client does not write the account, it is important for the therapist to ask the client whether he or she tried to write it, what the client felt, what Stuck Points he or she might have, and so forth. The therapist and client may want to do an ABC Worksheet on the client's thoughts (e.g., "If I write it down, that will make it real," "I was afraid that my emotions would overwhelm me or that I would have a flashback," "I don't want to think about it"). If the client has a Stuck Point about emotions' never ending or about fears of going crazy, the therapist and client can engage in some Socratic dialogue about the longest the client has cried (and then what happened, and then what happened, etc.), or about the differences between the time when the trauma happened and now. The therapist then asks the client to give the account orally in the session, and assigns the client to write it at home after the session. The therapist should *not* switch to CPT if the client has not written the account and has chosen to do CPT+A; such a change would reinforce avoidance.

In both of the trauma-processing sessions, if clients have written their accounts, they are first asked to read these aloud to their therapists. A client may initially balk at reading an account to the therapist or may try to hand it off to the therapist to read. The therapist needs to explain that it is the client's trauma account and that the therapist wants to listen to it first. If the therapist were to read it aloud, the client could engage in avoidance by thinking about other things or dissociating. The therapist can remind the client, "You have been living with the trauma memory for a long time, but not sharing the 'real PTSD' version of the story or allowing yourself to feel your natural emotions. Although it may have taken you a while or even days to write it, it will only take a few minutes to read it." After explaining again the importance of not avoiding the memory, the therapist should just sit quietly and wait for the client to begin.

It is the therapist's job not to interrupt the reading (or narrative) with questions or comforting statements. Interrupting the reading of the account is usually based on the therapist's own discomfort and does not benefit the client. It is important for the client to experience the natural emotions resulting from the trauma; any type of interruption will disrupt that potential and bring the focus to the therapist and back to the here-and-now. The only exception might be at the very beginning of the account, if the client is reading very quickly and clearly trying to avoid emotions. Then the therapist can stop and say, "I want you to have the opportunity to experience your natural emotions—the ones that you couldn't have at the time it happened. Why don't you start over and read more slowly, and allow yourself to remember what actually happened and how you felt?" If the client races through a second time, the therapist should not interrupt, but should save it for discussion later in the session.

Sometimes the client will interrupt the reading (i.e., avoidance), look up, and start talking to the therapist. Instead of saying anything, the therapist should look at the written account rather than the client, or point back to the written account. If the client continues to stay in a conversational mode or is elaborating on what he or she wrote, the therapist should say something simple like "We can talk afterwards. Please continue to read your account," and then look down again.

Therapists sometimes ask CPT+A trainers what they should be doing if they are not comforting clients or expressing empathy. The answer is twofold: First, therapists must not put themselves into the clients' shoes or try to imagine what they were experiencing. The traumatic experience and the consequent emotions are the clients', not the therapists'. The therapists cannot feel the clients' emotions for them. That said, therapists may have emotions about the event and may have some outward expressions of it (e.g., eyes welling up). Nevertheless, it is important for clients to know that their therapists can handle hearing their accounts. If a therapist reacts too much, a client may try to protect the therapist—or, worse, may decide that the trauma was too bad even for a therapist to hear about. Instead, the therapist should be thinking about the Stuck Points that have emerged in the Impact Statement and ABC Worksheets. Accordingly, the therapist should listen to the trauma account to hear about the context, the client's assumptions about what happened at the time, and the options the client actually had available at the time of the trauma, in order to frame questions such as these: When did the client decide that the event was his or her own fault and/or that the client should have done something different? If so, what would that something have been? In other words, the therapist should have some idea of where to begin the Socratic dialogue regarding assimilation when the time comes.

After the client stops reading the trauma account, the therapist should say nothing. If the client is feeling natural emotions, this should be allowed to continue. This may be the first time that the client has recalled the event in detail since it happened, and so this may be the first expression of natural affect. Typically, the affect is short-lived; the client will soon look up at the therapist, may take a tissue (a box of tissues should always be left within reach of clients), and may say something. At this point, the therapist's job is to amplify any natural emotions that the client is feeling. If no affect is apparent, and the client says that he or she is feeling "nothing," the therapist can ask whether this was how the client felt during the event. Sometimes clients went into "autopilot" during a traumatic event because of their training (e.g., military or first-responder training), or dissociated during the event and are experiencing the numbness or dissociative state upon reading the account for the first time. The therapist should then ask, "Did you feel emotions while you were writing the account at home or when you read it back to yourself?" It is not a requirement for clients to express emotions in the session. If they felt their emotions while writing or reading it to themselves, that is sufficient. If clients say they didn't feel any emotions in any of those circumstances and were just numb or being stoic, therapists can ask what the clients would feel if they were to allow themselves to feel emotions. Sometimes clients feel different emotions in having someone bear witness to their trauma. It is typical for those with self-conscious emotions such as shame or guilt to have more emotions upon reading their accounts out loud to therapists, even if that is not outwardly apparent. If so, this should be explored. They may also do one or more ABC Worksheets on any Stuck Points about feeling emotions (e.g., "They make me weak," "I will be vulnerable and unable to protect myself"). These clients should be encouraged to allow themselves to feel some emotions when writing or reading back the account during the week.

Before a therapist moves on to Socratic dialogue, the next step is to ask whether a client left out any important details. Some accounts sound like factual police records and include no sensory details, thoughts, or emotions. Other accounts are very detailed before and after the traumatic event, but the event itself is glossed over. If the client did not really write in any detail about what happened, or it is clear that the client is avoiding the most traumatic parts of the worst incident, the therapist should ask the client to fill in some more details and give him or her the opportunity to talk through what was avoided in writing. The client should then be assigned to include more details in the second account. The therapist should focus attention on the parts of the event that are relevant to the client's Stuck Points, but should not make assumptions about which parts of the event are associated with the PTSD symptoms and Stuck Points. A common therapist error is to focus attention on the parts of the event that the therapist finds particularly horrifying. However, those may not be the parts causing the client's actual Stuck Points; instead, the Stuck Points may be "I should have been able to prevent it," "If only I were there, my friend wouldn't have died," or the like. The violence and imagery may be distressing for the client, but may not be the reasons why the client has PTSD. Violation of the just-world myth, erroneous self- or other-blame, attempts to undo the event, and/or general lack of acceptance that the traumatic event actually happened are more likely to be the factor(s) keeping the client stuck.

Therapists new to CPT+A often wonder what to do if clients are overwhelmed with emotions. First, this is very rare. Typically, clients are very good at burying their true emotions; if there is large affect, it is most likely based on something that a client is thinking. In such a case, the therapist can ask what the client is thinking that goes with such big feelings. Again, clients are likely to say that the event was their fault or that they should have done something different. These kinds of statements can lead directly into the Socratic dialogue portion of the session. However, it is possible that if this is the first time a client has recounted the event, there could be strong natural emotions. If so, the therapist should just sit and not say anything. Normally, the client will stop the emotions within 5 minutes or so and will then look up at the therapist, say something, or take a tissue and pull the emotions back in. The therapist can ask what the client was feeling and whether the client has allowed him- or herself to feel that before. If this is a client who is fearful of emotions, the therapist can point out again that the client is dealing with a memory and the emotions are not as strong as when it was actually happening, or can note that nothing catastrophic has happened to the client as a result of experiencing these emotions.

Some clients may have a more angry presentation. This may be particularly true if there were other people with them or in their proximity whom they can blame (not the perpetrators), or if they cannot see that they made any mistakes. As discussed in earlier chapters, erroneous other-blame is another form of just-world thinking—one that focuses on how a traumatic event could have been averted by someone nearby. Examples described previously include military personnel who blame their commanders or unit leaders, while ignoring the people who set up an ambush or buried a mine; a child sexual abuse survivor who blames a nonoffending parent who actually did not know that the child was being abused; or a client who blames bystanders rather than the perpetrator of an event.

Once emotions have been labeled and any missing pieces have been added, it is time for the therapist to begin asking questions focused on the client's distorted (assimilated) thinking about the trauma. Because it does not take long to read a trauma account done at the beginning of the session, a large portion of Session 4 is spent in Socratic dialogue focused on trauma appraisals. Because there is no new worksheet to introduce for Session 5 in CPT+A, the therapist has more time in Session 4 to examine assimilated Stuck Points in depth. As the client reads the trauma account, the therapist can begin noticing any contradictions between this account and the client's Stuck Points from the Impact Statement, Stuck Point Log, and ABC Worksheets. Here is an example of a therapist–client dialogue following such an account:

THERAPIST: In your Impact Statement, we noticed and put onto the Stuck Point Log the statement that because of what happened, you can't trust anyone. Given that it was a stranger who attacked you, I am wondering what this has to do with trust. I listened to your account of the event, and I am a bit confused because you don't say you trusted the perpetrator. However, you also say that you should have known what he would do to you. If he was a stranger, how could you have known what he would do, and what does this have to do with trust?

CLIENT: I should have had my guard up sooner. I should have called out for help sooner or picked up that I was in a dangerous situation.

THERAPIST: What clues did you have that he was dangerous that you missed sooner?

CLIENT: As soon as I saw him, I should have crossed the street.

THERAPIST: But you have walked past people before on the sidewalk, and they didn't turn and pull a gun on you.

CLIENT: Sure, but I had a feeling.

THERAPIST: And when did you have this feeling? How far away was he?

CLIENT: A couple of feet. Actually when I think about it, I don't think I had that danger feeling until he moved closer to me on the sidewalk.

THERAPIST: And what were your options at that point?

CLIENT: I could have run.

THERAPIST: I thought you said he pulled out a gun.

CLIENT: Yes, as soon as he was close, he held up the gun and said that if I did what he said, I wouldn't get hurt.

THERAPIST: So your options were limited by the time you had the feeling.

CLIENT: Yes. When I saw the gun, I froze.

THERAPIST: Right. He shocked you and you just then realized what danger you were in.

CLIENT: Yes.

THERAPIST: So why do you think you should have crossed the street sooner or yelled or run before you saw the gun?

CLIENT: I don't know. I just wish I could have done something to stop it.

THERAPIST: That is not a Stuck Point. I wish it hadn't happened to you, either.

(*Pause*) But does saying "I wish it hadn't happened" feel different from "I should have done something sooner"? How much time did you really have to make a decision and react?

CLIENT: Seconds? If that.

THERAPIST: Right. You are being very hard on yourself for not being able to predict events before they happen. So now let's get this down on your Stuck Point Log, and I will want you to challenge the belief "I should have known sooner and stopped the assault." Next session, I am going to show you a new worksheet that I think you will like—one that helps you ask questions for yourself like I have been asking you. But before we do that, I think there is a Stuck Point we should get on the Log about trust. What does this stranger have to do with trusting people, or even trusting yourself?

If there is time in the session, the therapist may focus on another Stuck Point, but it should again be one about the causes of the trauma or an assimilated Stuck Point about erroneous self- or other-blame.

For the next session, the client is asked to write the account again with whatever details were left out last time, and to add parenthetical notations in places where he or she is feeling different emotions from those experienced since the writing of the first account (Handout 11.2). For example, the client may have written the first time, "He told me I was a slut, and I believed him. I felt such shame. (Now I am feeling angry. He just said that to justify what he did.)" Another example might be, "At the time I was convinced it was my fault that my friend died, and I would never stop feeling the guilt. (Now I don't feel so guilty, but I feel so sad.)" The client can also write new thoughts or feelings in the margins of the first account. Changes in feelings may indicate progress with thoughts and feelings. However, they may also reveal other Stuck Points, such as "I knew when it happened that I would never trust anyone in authority again. (I still feel betrayed by my mother, because she should have known what he was doing.)"

The client should again be encouraged to begin writing the account as soon as possible and to read it every day. The client should also record any new Stuck Points on the Stuck Point Log, and should continue to complete ABC Worksheets every day, especially about the trauma or the process of writing the account.

Session 5 of CPT+A is very similar to Session 4 of CPT: The client reads the new account, and the therapist and client continue to process any assimilated Stuck Points; the therapist also continues to encourage natural emotions. The client may remember parts of the event that were not revealed in the first account, and/or the second account may emphasize different parts of the event. After the client has finished reading the trauma account to the therapist, the therapist should again remain quiet if the client is experiencing natural emotions and should ask about their absence if not. If the client is steeling him- or herself not to feel emotions, the therapist and client should again do Socratic dialogue and ABC Worksheets about the potential outcomes of experiencing emotions, and the client should be encouraged to experience these. Furthermore, the client should be asked to continue to read the trauma account at home and to feel the natural emotions until they run their course. ABC Worksheets are also examined to see how well the client is doing with matching events, thoughts, and feelings. In both cases, the therapist asks questions about what emotions are associated with Stuck Points, as well as questions to help the client examine the evidence for and against the thoughts embodied in the Stuck Points. New Stuck Points that emerge from the second account should be added to the Stuck Point Log.

Several common therapist errors in CPT have been listed in Chapter 4, and these apply to CPT+A as well. However, there are also some common therapist errors that are specific to the written accounts in CPT+A. Sometimes a therapist fails to give an adequate rationale for writing the accounts of the index event. If the client starts with a less severe event, the client can finish those accounts and then continue to believe that he or she cannot tolerate thinking about the index event. If the client starts with the most difficult traumatic event, the other events are likely to have similar Stuck Points and underlying core beliefs, and can be more easily processed with worksheets after the index event is dealt with.

Therapists must also keep in mind that when they ask about the index trauma, clients may have in mind a bad life event, but not necessarily one associated with PTSD. For example, a client may rightfully say that the death of her mother from cancer when she was 10 years old changed the course of her life and was the worst event that she ever experienced. However, that event is more likely to be associated with grief or perhaps depression than with PTSD. The therapist, knowing that the client has also experienced Criterion A traumatic events, might review other events and ask which one is associated with the most intrusive memories, nightmares, and avoidance. Or therapists may ask clients if, before the first session, they hoped that they wouldn't have to talk about one particular event or that the therapists wouldn't ask them about all of their traumatic events. Even when there is serial trauma (as in child sexual or physical abuse, IPV, or combat), clients may initially say that the events were all the same, but after some questioning an index event may emerge. For example, for a child sexual abuse victim, the worst event might have been the first penetration after being groomed for a period of time. Another example might be when the victim tried to stop the abuse and the perpetrator threatened a younger sibling or other family members. Battered women often identify the worst event as occurring when they realized they could die, when the perpetrator began beating the children as well, or when there was marital/partner rape.

Another common therapist error in CPT+A is to allow the client to give a lot of details about the events leading up to the event, but then to gloss over the event itself. The therapist may have to ask a number of clarifying questions when the client is done reading the first account, in order to fill out the details that are associated with the PTSD Stuck Points. For the second writing assignment, the client should be encouraged to start at the point he or she recognized the danger; to continue the account until the event was over; and to give more detail about the worst parts of the trauma (the parts that have generated the most nightmares, intrusive thoughts, flashbacks, or Stuck Points).

Still another common therapist error is to forget to check on the daily reading of the second account, and especially whether the client has been avoiding the assignment or is still blocking any natural emotions. When a client asks whether he or she has to keep reading the account, the therapist should ask whether the client still feels numb, wants to avoid it, is still not feeling strong emotions, or continues to gloss over the difficult parts of the event. If the client says, "No, I am just bored reading it. I don't feel strongly about it anymore," then the therapist can say that the client can discontinue the reading. However, an important therapist error here would be to fail to differentiate avoidance from natural emotions that have run their course. The latter may not occur until several sessions later.

It is possible for a client to write accounts about another event in the background of the therapy, but the CPT+A protocol should proceed. The client should not write the second account about a different event. The second account should be about the same index event that the client wrote the first account about. If the client has another traumatic event with different Stuck Points, he or she should wait to write that account until after the first event has been processed. Even if the therapist discovers that another event was more traumatic, the processing of this event should still be postponed until the client has written two accounts about the first event. Any Stuck Points should be added to the Stuck Point Log and should become the topics of the next assignment with the Challenging Questions Worksheet.

In CPT+A, the Challenging Beliefs Worksheet and the Safety Issues Module are introduced in the same session (see Handout 11.3). The therapist introduces the worksheet to the client and points out that, except for the ratings of thoughts and emotions, the first four sections are the same as in other worksheets the client has completed; the purpose of the new sections (sections E–H) is to generate a more balanced statement after challenging the Stuck Point and then to re-rate the old thought and emotions, as well as any new emotions. The therapist and client then complete an example together in the session, using a safety-related Stuck Point from the Stuck Point Log, and the therapist gives the client the Safety Issues Module to read. The client is assigned to do at least one worksheet per day, and to complete worksheets on any Stuck Points related to safety. The remainder of the CPT+A protocol is the same as the CPT protocol in delivery.

Variable-Length CPT

As discussed in Chapter 2, there has been only one published study on variable-length CPT, which was conducted as CPT+A by Galovski et al. (2013). There are, however, two other studies (both using CPT) currently underway: one with active-duty military personnel (Resick, Wachen, & Peterson, in progress), and one in Germany with people with comorbid PTSD and borderline personality disorder (Bohus & Steil, in progress). In the latter two studies, CPT can extend up to 24 or 48 sessions, respectively. Furthermore, therapists often ask what to do if clients reach the end of 12 sessions but still have PTSD. Should they continue in CPT, or should they change to a different therapy? Galovski et al. (2013) allowed up to 18 sessions of CPT+A and found that the majority of clients stopped before 12 sessions with a good end state, but that some needed more sessions. By the 3-month follow-up, only 2 of the 50 treatment participants still met criteria for PTSD. Our advice is to continue with CPT, and below we offer advice about how this should be done.

Delayed Termination

The first rule for extending CPT is to adhere to the protocol for the first 12 sessions. The clients need the sequential skill building and focus on the index trauma that take place in the first half of the therapy, and the themes in the second half of treatment may reveal core beliefs that are very entrenched. If by Session 11 a client is still scoring above the threshold on objective measures of PTSD or depression, the client should not be assigned to write the final Impact Statement. Rather, the therapist should discuss continuing treatment for more sessions until the client reaches a better end state. They should also discuss why the client's PTSD scores are still high. For example, does the client need to work on a different trauma? Are there assimilated Stuck Points remaining from the index trauma that were not resolved? Are core beliefs still being activated regularly? Does the client have a deeper Stuck Point about letting go of some beliefs (e.g., "If I change my mind, that means I am weak," "If I don't have PTSD, I don't know what to think about or do anymore; who am I?", "If I let go of my guilt, that means that my friend died for no reason [or I am afraid I will forget my friend]").

For the remaining sessions, the therapist uses the Challenging Beliefs Worksheets and the Stuck Point Log to work on lingering assimilation or overaccommodation that is preventing full recovery. When the client reports reduced PTSD and depression, the therapist and client discuss whether it is time to stop treatment or whether there are other Stuck Points or core beliefs that need more work. Once they decide that the goals of therapy have been achieved, the next-to-last session includes the assignment to write the final Impact Statement. The last session includes a comparison of the new Impact Statement with the initial one, a review of the progress in therapy, suggestions for using the CPT skills in the future, and a strategy for dealing with any remaining Stuck Points.

Early Termination

In Galovski et al.'s (2013) study, 58% of participants reached a good end state in PTSD and depression before the completion of 12 sessions. This finding indicates that if clients drop out of treatment before 12 sessions, it may not necessarily mean that they are avoiding; it may mean that they have improved and do not believe they need more therapy. Therapists should assess PTSD and depression every week so that they can see when their clients "turn the corner" and start to resolve their major assimilated Stuck Points. It may well be possible to stop CPT before finishing the whole protocol.

When it looks as if clients may be candidates for early completion—that is, when the clients no longer meet criteria for PTSD and have low self-report scores (e.g., below 19 on the PCL-5 or 10 on the PHQ-9)—therapists can initiate a discussion regarding whether the clients have achieved their goals. Together, they may decide that a few more sessions dedicated to work on a particular topic, such as Stuck Points about self-esteem or intimacy, may be beneficial. There is not a requirement that clients stop treatment just because their scores are low. The ending of treatment should be a mutual decision between therapists and clients. If a client does decide to stop treatment before the CPT protocol has been completed, the therapist and client should review the Stuck Point Log for any remaining Stuck Points that need work; the final Impact Statement should be assigned; and the next session should be set as the final session. The therapist should also give the assignment that was originally due for the next session. If the client has not been given the entire set of materials for the therapy at the beginning of treatment, the therapist should give the client the remaining handouts to look over, to see whether there are any Stuck Points that should be added to the log or other topics for discussion.

If the client still has low PTSD and depression scores and is still happy with the decision to stop treatment, the therapist and client should begin the next session with the regular assignment and then move to the final Impact Statement. As in the full protocol, the client reads the new Impact Statement, and the therapist then reviews the original Impact Statement for comparison. The therapist notes any areas that still need work over time, and they review any modules and worksheets that the client has not reached thus far, so that they are available to the client if needed at some point. They finish by going through the Stuck Point Log and crossing off any Stuck Points the client no longer believes. Finally, they talk about the client's progress in therapy and plans for the future. It is advisable to set up a 1-month follow-up session to determine whether the client's gains have been maintained.

Continued Treatment of Nonresponding Clients

At this point, we do not know how many clients might still not be responding to treatment at the end of 24 or 48 sessions, depending on the population. There were very few such clients in Galovski et al.'s (2013) study. However, when looking at predictors of length of treatment, they found that men took a bit longer than women to respond, and that those with higher pretreatment depression took longer to respond. There is no evidence, one way or the other, that changing to another evidence-based treatment for PTSD will be effective for a client who does not respond to CPT. It is possible that the client has not been fully engaged in treatment (although engagement should have been attended to early in therapy); has been unwilling to change thoughts (i.e., has exhibited cognitive inflexibility), which might itself have constituted a Stuck Point; or has been poor at practice completion. On the other hand, some clients have not revealed their worst trauma to their therapists, due to their profound lack of trust or shame regarding the event. Therapists should be asking about therapy-interfering Stuck Points if at least some improvement is not evident by Session 6.

CPT and other cognitive therapies have been found to be effective for PTSD in spite of various comorbidities, such as psychosis (stabilized), bipolar disorders, personality disorders, traumatic brain injury, substance abuse, and depression. If clients take it upon themselves to remove themselves from medication suddenly and without the advice of a physician, it is possible that they could experience rebound effects affecting their PTSD treatment. One goal of the study of variable-length CPT with active-duty military personnel (Resick et al., in progress) will be to determine predictors of early, normal, and late treatment response versus nonresponse. Until that study is complete, we do not have informed advice to give about continued treatment of nonresponding clients.

CPT for Acute Stress Disorder

In the immediate aftermath of traumatic events, people with PTSD symptoms tend to hope that the symptoms will go away with time or distraction, and therefore often do not present themselves for therapy for many years. Those on active duty in the military may not have the opportunity to seek out therapy until their deployment has ended, and many others may have been exposed to stigma and beliefs that only weak people seek out treatment. Children or victims of IPV may not have the opportunity to receive treatment until they are safely out of their dangerous relationships or are old enough to decide for themselves that they need therapy for symptoms that do not abate. For research purposes, most studies have required a minimum period of time to have elapsed since the traumatic event—not because the therapy will not work in the early aftermath of such an event, but for the methodological reason that participants might have improved naturally over time and might not have developed PTSD.

At this point, there has only been one single-case study (Kaysen, Lostutter, & Goines, 2005) and a small pilot study (Nixon, 2012) using CPT+A for acute stress disorder. The Kaysen et al. (2005) case study is discussed in more detail in Chapter 14. Nixon (2012) implemented CPT+A across 6 weeks with one 90-minute session per week. Challenging Questions Worksheets were introduced at the first session, the trauma account was only written once, and the Patterns of Problematic Thinking Worksheet was eliminated. Although the sample size was too small to have sufficient power to detect statistical differences, at posttreatment only 8% ($n = 11$) of the intent-to-treat CPT sample met criteria for PTSD, compared with 36% ($n = 7$) of the supportive counseling group. Good end-state functioning was achieved by 50% ($n = 6$) of the CPT+A group and 9% ($n = 1$) of the supportive counseling group, with this difference being significant. This compares very favorably to the 55–77% of PTSD cases found in wait-list control conditions in other trials of treatment for acute stress disorder (Bryant et al., 2008; Foa, Hearst-Ikeda, & Perry, 1995; Foa, Zoellner, & Feeny, 2006; Shalev et al., 2012).

Practice Assignment after Session 3 of CPT+A

Please begin this assignment as soon as possible. Write a full account of the traumatic event, and include as many sensory details (sights, sounds, smells, etc.) as possible. Also include as many of your thoughts and feelings that you recall having during the event. Pick a time and place to write that will give you privacy and enough time to write this account. Do not stop yourself from feeling your emotions. If you need to stop writing at some point, please draw a line on the paper where you stop. Begin writing again when you can, and continue to write the account even if it takes several occasions.

Read the whole account to yourself every day until the next session. Allow yourself to feel your feelings. Bring your account to the next session.

Also, continue to work with the ABC Worksheets (Handout 6.3) every day. When you find Stuck Points, add them to your Stuck Point Log (Handout 6.1).

Practice Assignment after Session 4 of CPT+A

Write another account of the whole traumatic incident as soon as possible. If you were unable to complete the assignment the first time, please write more than you did last time. Add more sensory details, as well as more of your thoughts and feelings during the incident. Also, this time, write your *current* thoughts and feelings in parentheses—for instance, "(Right now I'm feeling very angry.)"

Remember to read over the new account every day before the next session.

Also, continue to work with the ABC Worksheets (Handout 6.3) every day.

Practice Assignment after Session 7 of CPT+A

Use the Challenging Beliefs Worksheets (Handout 8.1) to analyze and confront at least one of your Stuck Points each day. Also, please read over the Safety Issues Module (Handout 8.1), and think about how your prior beliefs about safety were affected by your traumatic event. If you have issues with safety pertaining to yourself or others, complete at least one Challenging Beliefs Worksheet to confront those issues. Use the remaining sheets for other Stuck Points on your Stuck Point Log (Handout 6.1) or for distressing events that have occurred recently.

12

Group CPT and CPT
for Sexual Abuse

The first goal of this chapter is to discuss specific issues that should be addressed when CPT is provided in groups or in a combined group and individual format. The second goal is to review CPT-SA, a CPT modification for childhood sexual abuse survivors. Although CPT is more widely known as an individual therapy, it originated as a group therapy, and significant research has shown group CPT to be effective either alone or in combination with individual therapy (see Chapter 2). Group CPT has been used to treat PTSD successfully in a variety of client populations, including rape victims, childhood sexual abuse survivors, combat veterans, and military sexual trauma victims. The group format also has been used in residential treatment programs in conjunction with other treatments (coping skills building, dialectical behavior therapy, and psychoeducation, to name a few).

Group CPT

Why Use Group CPT?

When both group and individual CPT are available, we typically suggest that a client be allowed to choose the format of treatment, because client choice has been linked to stronger outcomes in psychotherapy. However, we are aware that it is not always possible to offer individual therapy in all settings, and group CPT may be the only option for many clinics. Group CPT has been shown to be an effective treatment in its own right, and for many clients the group format helps them to address their traumatic memories through sharing their thoughts and feelings with other group members.

Other advantages of CPT groups include cost-effectiveness, the social support afforded by other group members, and the opportunities for clients to challenge each other's disruptive cognitions in a healthy and assertive manner. In addition, the group experience can facilitate a sense of normalization and universality regarding trauma-related symptoms by allowing clients to see that they are not "nuts" or "crazy," and that their thoughts and behaviors are very similar to those of others who have experienced traumatic events. Regardless of the population served or the setting where it is applied, therapists need to consider some general issues and make some decisions before using CPT in a group format.

Prescreening and Information Sessions

As in individual CPT, we encourage therapists conducting group CPT to complete a prescreening session with each client. This session serves several purposes. First, the therapist doing the screening should do a formal assessment for PTSD, to determine whether the client meets criteria for the disorder. Second, if the screening therapist is a group leader, this will allow the client and therapist the opportunity to talk about why the client wants to join the group, what the client hopes to get out of the group, any concerns the client has about participating in this group, and any prior experiences the client has had with groups. The therapist should also provide the client with a description of what CPT will involve (including practice assignments), and should discuss the CPT group format and indicate how it is similar or dissimilar to any previous groups the client has experienced. Third, as part of this screening session, the therapist can ask the client to give a 5-minute description of his or her most distressing traumatic event. We do not recommend discussing trauma details in the group sessions, because they can be unnecessarily distressing to other clients, but having each client retell this information in the screening session gives the leader more information regarding the types of trauma the clients will be working on for their practice assignments. Finally, the screening sessions allow the therapist time to gather psychosocial information that may help determine whether the client is not ready for group treatment at this time (e.g., unwillingness to talk in a group, a recent history of physical aggression toward others, or other symptoms that would preclude someone from starting trauma-focused treatment at this time; see Chapter 3 for more information).

For some clinics, it may be easier and more cost-efficient to offer a pretreatment information session in a group format for potential CPT clients. This session can include a review of PTSD symptoms, treatment options available in these clinics, the process of group therapy, and an overview of CPT. Many clinics have found this session to be useful for acclimating clients to the group CPT format before the protocol begins. The session serves as a neutral environment for presenting the structure of CPT (e.g., number of weeks, practice assignments, worksheets, stages of therapy, agenda, self-report measures); introducing cognitive theory (i.e., treatment rationale, purposes of assignments and worksheets); and discussing commitment to the therapy and attendance. At this point in the process, the clients may be less anxious and able to take in information more readily. The group prescreening session also gives clients the opportunity to ask questions and voice concerns about group therapy, the PTSD diagnosis, or CPT before they enter the protocol. Group leaders may want to consider holding this session in the same room and at the same time that the CPT group will be held, to help familiarize the clients with the clinic, the room, and the therapist(s) ahead of time. In addition, the group orientation format will allow clients to meet with other potential group members, which may make starting the group easier for some people.

Setting the Stage

The content of CPT is very similar, whether it is conducted with a group of clients or a single client, but group CPT includes several modifications to allow more effective delivery of the treatment in a group setting. In spite of its unique benefits, group CPT involves some challenges that therapists should be aware of. The most significant challenges are pragmatic issues, such as recruiting enough clients for a group, giving each member enough time and attention in sessions, and managing group members who may dominate the group or who have severe personality disorders. For these reasons, some clinicians choose to offer CPT in a combined group and individual format, in which practice assignments are given in the group but reviewed in individual sessions. The group can then be used to process members' reactions to their completed practice assignments, and to provide further practice with the worksheets. If it is not feasible to offer individual sessions throughout the duration of the group, the therapist may choose to conduct individual therapy only during the sessions on written accounts and introduction of the Challenging Questions Worksheet if CPT+A is being implemented (see Chapter 11). These sessions require the most one-on-one time with a therapist and allow the clients to feel safe in knowing that they will only share their traumatic material with one person. Clients in a group format may be less willing to ask questions when they are confused, so if an individual format is not available, the therapists will have to be more proactive to make sure that everyone understands the concepts and practice assignments. If group CPT is conducted without concurrent CPT individual therapy, the leaders should ensure during the prescreening process that all group members will be able to complete the practice assignments with little outside assistance, and that they are truly motivated for change.

Timing, Group Size, and Format

CPT group sessions typically last 90 minutes; individual sessions are 50 minutes long when they are part of the combined protocol. With a larger group (over 10 members), the therapist(s) may consider conducting the group for 120 minutes with a 10-minute break in the middle. But we have often found that it is hard to get a group reconvened in 10 minutes, or that the timing of the break interrupts the process flow in the group. Thus we recommend 90-minute groups in most cases.

We also recommend that CPT groups be "closed," meaning that once a group has started, no new members may join. The closed format is necessary because CPT was developed as a progressive therapy in which skills are taught in a particular order and build on one another. Ideally, groups should have between 6 and 9 members (although we know of some very talented therapists who can manage 10–12). We believe that 5 members is the minimum for starting group CPT (5 rather than 4, to avoid the pairing effect that can happen with 4), because if 1 or 2 people miss a session, then the group ceases to be a group and becomes individual therapy with several clients in attendance. With more than 9 members, the group may feel too large, especially for one therapist; there may not be enough time for the individual members to get their needs met; and the large size may inhibit individual disclosures.

Combining group and individual therapy can be done in two ways. In the first option, individual sessions are added (or offered in lieu of group sessions) in weeks 4 and 5, to allow the therapist and each client to focus more intently on the client's trauma-related Stuck Points; in the case of CPT+A, the client can read the trauma accounts and identify relevant Stuck Points related to the event privately with one of the therapists. In the second combined option, group and individual sessions occur each week (or even twice a week in residential programs), with the treatment rationale and practice assignments covered in group sessions and then reviewed in the individual sessions.

It is advisable to have as much time as possible between a group session and the following individual session, so that the client can practice the assignment at length before reviewing it in the individual session. For clients who travel a long way, it may be useful for them to complete their individual sessions right before the group session, so that they only need to come to the clinic once a week. This combined format is especially helpful in a number of other situations: (1) in residential programs where additional programming is desirable, to maximize the clients' benefits from their residential stays; (2) in working with clients who are insistent that they need individual time with their therapists; and (3) in training students, because the students can serve as coleaders of groups and can see some of the clients for their individual therapy sessions, allowing for more oversight of the students.

Cotherapists

Although one skilled CPT therapist can manage a group alone, we have found that having cotherapists is more effective for a number of reasons. First, when one therapist is on vacation, is taking a personal leave, or has an unplanned emergency, the group sessions do not need to be canceled, which can cause a loss of momentum and an increase in avoidance. Second, having cotherapists allows one therapist to stand at a whiteboard and lead the discussion while writing the information on the board. The other therapist can be watching the group interaction and noting clients who might need help in participating. In addition, if a group member becomes emotional or disruptive, one of the therapists can attend to that client's needs while the other therapist continues to lead the discussion. Finally, because of the number of practice assignments that will need to be reviewed and commented upon between sessions, having two therapists can make it easier to manage this workload. As noted above, many clinics have found it helpful to include student trainees as cotherapists; this is an excellent way for a student to learn CPT, with a more senior therapist as a model. We do not, however, support the use of three or more therapists, even for large groups of 12 clients, because this can lead to too much therapist involvement (as each therapist tries to contribute) and not enough time for the clients. If there are a number of dropouts or missed appointments and the group shrinks, there can be almost as many therapists in the room as clients.

Scheduling

Another concern when setting up a CPT group is what day and time the group sessions will be held. Although this may seem like a small issue, time of day can be a very important variable when therapists are dealing with clients' work or school schedules. Clients may not realize how emotional they may become during or after group sessions, and going straight to work or school may not be advisable. In addition, many clients may have difficulty taking time off from work to attend 12 sessions of group therapy, or they may be unable to arrange for child care during business hours, making evening groups a necessity. Second, if several national or religious holidays fall in the 12-week window when a group will run, it will also be important to consider avoiding those days, or the group may need to be extended beyond what members had planned for. Finally, if a group is going to be offered twice a week (e.g., on a military base, in a prison, or in a residential care program), we recommend offering the group on Mondays and Thursdays or Tuesdays and Fridays, to allow clients the maximum amount of time between sessions to complete their practice assignments.

Trauma History Considerations

It is also important to decide ahead of time whether or not a group will be homogenous with regard to the type of index trauma that participants have experienced, so that proper assessment and trauma screening can be conducted before the group begins. Although there are some advantages to running a group with members who share the same type of trauma, we have found that there are no significant difficulties with combining different trauma types in groups. When all group members share the same type of trauma, it can be easier for them to challenge each other's Stuck Points and point out problems in their thinking, because they share similar experiences and are likely to have very similar Stuck Points. But we have found that a majority of our clients have been multiply traumatized; even when all members have the same type of initially identified index trauma, many of them will have experienced other events that may in fact be more traumatic for them. Thus individuals with different traumas are likely to be the rule rather than the exception, and a mixed-trauma group is particularly useful in smaller clinics or cities where it can be difficult to find enough group members with the same type of trauma at the same time.

It is important to inform potential members of the group's constellation before they agree to participate, so that any of their concerns or questions can be addressed ahead of time. One Stuck Point that we often hear is that "Only other people like me can understand what I am going through" (e.g., other combat veterans, other sexual abuse survivors). This is actually a good place to start the discussion and identification of Stuck Points, because the clients may be applying this belief to their lives as a whole and thus greatly limiting the numbers and types of people they are willing to accept as friends.

Client Gender Considerations

Although it is possible to combine men and women in a group, it is very important that clients are carefully screened to make sure that this will not be triggering for any potential members. It can be helpful to ensure that the participants in a mixed-gender group have similar trauma histories (e.g., combat, natural disaster, child sexual abuse), to help them realize that they all have shared experiences and beliefs. The issue of client gender is also important in the choice of therapist(s). Although some female clients will not accept a male therapist and vice versa, we have often found that when clients are open to the possibility of having a male–female therapist team, this allows the clients to challenge their Stuck Points by using the gender of one therapist or the other as evidence against their beliefs.

Missed Sessions

Perhaps one of the most obvious concerns in doing group CPT is what to do about clients who miss sessions. We strongly recommend informing clients before starting the group that it is very important not to miss any sessions, and that they should not enroll in the group if they have issues or life circumstances that will interfere with attending the group sessions over the course of the therapy. At the same time, we acknowledge that unforeseen circumstances may keep a client from attending a group session. If the group is conducted in conjunction with individual therapy, the individual session following the missed session can be used to cover what was missed in group. If the group does not have adjunctive individual therapy, a group therapist can meet individually with the client during the week; can review in a phone call what was covered in the group; or, if necessary, can meet with the client just before the next group session. If none of these options can be arranged, the group members can be asked to provide a brief overview of what was covered in the prior week's session. Given that many people now have computers and email, especially younger clients, it may be possible to email the practice assignment to a group participant who has missed a session, so that the client can bring it to the next session. We typically suggest that if someone misses more than two group sessions, they should wait until the next group starts or continue their treatment in individual therapy.

Therapists' Role in Group Treatment

Group CPT, like individual CPT, is a collaborative process, and thus an important role for group therapists is structuring the sessions to allow all the clients to learn each new assignment and discuss their progress on the previous practice assignment. Thus, one of the most important jobs for the therapists is making sure that group members stay "on task," which can be particularly difficult when clients (and therapists!) are first learning to do group CPT. One common example of this is managing client avoidance. Avoidance symptoms often make clients want to avoid people, places, and things that will remind them of the index traumatic event, so it is no wonder that clients will try to avoid completing their assignments or processing their thoughts and feelings about the trauma. This is especially true in the early sessions of group CPT, before the clients have become more comfortable around each other and until they have learned that the memories will not harm them and that processing their thoughts and feelings will actually allow them to feel better.

In an effort to reduce avoidance, the therapists will discuss avoidance in the first session and ask the clients to share ways in which they might engage in avoidance (e.g., not doing assignments, missing group sessions, coming late to sessions, drinking/using drugs, gambling, shopping, putting other people's needs first). The therapists should also help the clients identify any fears and underlying thoughts that may be causing the avoidance. This discussion helps clients become more aware of all the behaviors that can constitute avoidance, and ideally it will help them limit the amount of avoidance they exhibit, both in and out of the group. The therapists should continue to address avoidance in the group whenever they notice group members engaging in behaviors that distance them from the group and the material.

Managing CPT in a Group Setting

Setting an Agenda

To keep the group on track, the therapist should provide structure for each session by setting an agenda at each session and letting the participants know what will be covered during that session. The agenda should include a brief check-in (no more than 5–10 minutes for the whole group) to see how everyone is feeling and to establish whether anyone will need help from the group to address a pressing issue that day. This check-in has a number of benefits, including allowing the therapists to take a quick "pulse reading" of the group members' emotional state that day; this can help to identify where individuals are in their progress toward changing maladaptive cognitions. In addition, the check-in empowers the clients to ask for help, teaches them to control their distress by asking them to determine whether they would like to discuss their issues at the beginning or end of the group session, and allows them to see healthy help seeking by other participants who ask for time from the group.

Problems with check-in can stem from therapists' not setting up the expectation from the beginning that the check-in should include just a *few words* describing each client's feelings and a request for assistance if needed. Some clients may use the check-in as an opportunity to avoid addressing their issues by derailing the focus of the group that day, or they may try to take over the group by jumping into a lengthy description of their difficult week. If a client does attempt to take over the group, a therapist will need to interrupt the client gently and get the group refocused. Although this can be uncomfortable for some therapists, it is critical that therapists not allow clients to digress for long, or this will send a message that all clients are supposed to spend a long time discussing their week—and this will not give the group members time to review the work they did over the prior week, or the therapists' time to introduce the next assignment.

The best way to keep digressions from happening is to make it clear from the beginning that the check-in should not be long or involve a recap of the week, but instead should focus on clients' feelings and needs from the group. But if a digression does occur, a therapist might ask the storytelling client, "Do you need time from the group?" and offer to come back to the client after the check-in is complete. If the client says "Yes," then when the therapist comes back to the client the therapist should not ask the client to return to the story, but should instead ask whether the client did any sheets for homework on the issue over the prior week. If the client says "Yes," those can be reviewed as a group on the board. If the client says "No," the therapist can excitedly note that this offers the group a great starting point to get to work on the most recent worksheet, and can begin doing so at the whiteboard.

By bringing the digressing client's experiences back to the worksheets, the therapist and group members will be role-playing how the clients can address the events of the week in real time with their CPT worksheets, and will show that the clients can obtain relief from their distressing thoughts and feelings when they engage in the therapy outside sessions. The therapist should remember to try to engage the other group members in this activity by asking if anyone else is sharing similar thoughts or had difficulty completing the practice assignment during the week.

Practice Assignment Completion

The monitoring of practice assignment completion is one of the most challenging issues in conducting CPT groups. For some of the more complex practice assignments, the leaders should leave 20–25 minutes to explain the assignment and to create one or more examples with the group. Once the ABC Worksheets are introduced, a therapist should spend a majority of the session using the whiteboard/flipchart to review the worksheets that clients had difficulty with over the week, or to process issues or concerns that the clients have brought to the session. Putting examples of worksheets up on the whiteboard or flipchart can enable the therapist to engage the entire group more easily and help them relate the examples to their own similar Stuck Points.

The Use of Bridging Questions and Common Stuck Points

One way to engage the group as a whole to participate in sessions is to use "bridging questions" to create links between members' experiences. These are important tools that can be used to get more members involved in the group and to make sure that some clients are not left out while others monopolize the discussions. For example, a therapist might ask, "What do others think/feel about this?" It is important for the therapist to encourage responses to such a question from more than one client, instead of stopping with the first person who answers.

Sometimes it is also helpful to suggest some commonly held Stuck Points as examples, in order for members to feel more of a connection with one another. Examples of Stuck Points that can be used in this way are "It is my fault," "If only I had done X, this would not have happened," "No place is safe," "People can't be trusted," and "Showing emotions is weakness." Once a Stuck Point is endorsed or independently verbalized by one group member, the therapist can ask, "Does anyone else share this Stuck Point?" or "Does this sound familiar to anyone else?"

Noncompletion of Practice Assignments

Because clients may not share their worksheets during a group session, the therapist may not know until after the session whether the participants completed the assignment at all or whether there was a conceptual problem with the assignment. Thus it is very important that the therapist check in with each group member (even via a show of hands) to see whether they completed the assignment or had difficulty with the assignment. Following the check-in, the therapist should ensure that a majority of the group time is spent reviewing several practice assignments from different clients, and avoid having the group get bogged down in a potentially unrelated discussion.

In individual CPT, clients who do not complete their Impact Statements, written accounts (in CPT+A), or various worksheets between sessions are asked to complete them orally in sessions, to acclimate them to the process. In CPT groups, we ask clients to focus on identifying Stuck Points related to their traumatic events, along with the other members of the group. We do not ask them to retell their Impact Statements (or trauma accounts), to avoid triggering other group members or taking too much time from the key process of identifying Stuck Points and beginning to challenge them. When clients do not complete their practice assignments, this is a good time to see whether several members did not complete worksheets and to identify any shared Stuck Points regarding the treatment, such as "This therapy will not help me," or "I don't have time to do any worksheets." At this point, a therapist should go to the whiteboard and complete a worksheet on the shared Stuck Point, using the most recently assigned sheet (i.e., the ABC Worksheet, the Challenging Questions Worksheet, or the

Challenging Beliefs Worksheet). Group members who have completed their home-work should be enlisted in helping to identify evidence against the Stuck Points and new, healthier alternative beliefs.

In CPT groups, it can be more difficult to convince clients that they can and should complete their practice assignments, because there is less time to focus on the individual group members each week. This is another reason why it is important for the therapist leading the group to ask for a show of hands regarding who completed the assignment, and then to ensure that different people are called upon to share their Stuck Points each week. Finally, the therapist should endeavor to enlist all group members in the discussion of each worksheet being completed on the whiteboard/flipchart, either by sharing their own similar thoughts or by helping to generate alternative evidence and beliefs.

One of the advantages of group treatment is that group members who may be reluctant to participate will be able to see that other group members, who are partici-pating and completing their practice assignments, are getting better. This will often motivate the hesitant members to better adherence with the assignments, especially if the group therapists highlight that doing the work is helping other people with their symptoms. For example, if a group member does not complete a worksheet assignment, the therapist leading the group should ask whether anyone else did not complete the assignment, and then lead the group in completing a worksheet on the shared beliefs that are preventing the clients from doing their practice assignment. Possible Stuck Points (in addition to the ones noted above) may include "I will never get better," and "I cannot tolerate writing about my thoughts." The leader should make sure to engage the entire group in this exercise by eliciting alternative thoughts, or evidence against these Stuck Points, from group members who have successfully completed the assignment.

There are several reasons why clients may not complete their practice assign-ments, and they are typically related to some type of avoidance. Many trauma survi-vors believe that if they write down the events, thoughts, or feelings related to their traumatic events, the memories will become too "real" and therefore too difficult to handle. Hearing that other people were able to identify and challenge their thoughts about their traumas (and to write details about their events, in the case of CPT+A) will often make it easier for clients who did not do the assignment the first time around. After this discussion on reasons for not completing practice, it is important that the therapist move forward with a discussion of the material scheduled for the day, even if several of the clients did not do the assignment. In addition, the next practice assign-ment should be introduced and assigned to the entire group. Those who did not do the prior assignment should be asked to complete that one as well.

Some clients may avoid completing the assignment because they have difficulty labeling their events as traumatic ("rape," "killing," etc.). Instead, they may label the events as "misunderstandings" or "accidents" and try to minimize the impact of the events or inaccurately represent the details (e.g., blaming themselves for their child abuse). To help challenge these cognitions, it may be helpful to point out the trauma symptoms that the clients reported on their pretreatment assessments and to describe those symptoms as evidence that the traumatic events actually did occur. In addition, it may be useful to remind the clients of the ways in which their identified symptoms are negatively affecting their lives (e.g., isolation, problems at work or school). For some clients, it can be helpful to ask them why they are coming to the group. The answers they give can point out the contradictory thoughts they are having: On the one hand, they may be misinterpreting (or minimizing) the details of the trauma, but on the other hand, they are experiencing distress in their lives and are seeking help.

In general, it is helpful for group leaders to inform clients at the beginning of therapy that they may have an urge to avoid doing their practice assignments or even coming to group sessions. This will help to normalize their reactions and facilitate greater openness among the clients about discussing their thoughts and feelings. It can even be beneficial to help the clients identify potential Stuck Points about the therapy. This will facilitate the normalization process and help clients become more comfortable with discussing their ambivalence or concerns about completing the treatment.

Phone List Assignment

To reinforce the positive social support that a group offers, we recommend the use of a phone list assignment during the week for clients who are being seen in an outpatient setting. All clients who are willing to participate place their first names and the phone numbers of their choice on the phone list. Each group member is then asked to call the person below him or her on the list before the next session, to check on practice assignment completion and provide support in doing the treatment. The following week, each client calls the person two places below him or her on the list, and so on, until finally everyone has called everyone else on the list. Clients are instructed that they should not talk about their trauma histories on the phone, but instead use these phone calls as opportunities to socialize or receive help in completing their practice assignments. These phone calls can also be used to have the callers give the assignment and explain what the recipients missed if the recipients did not attend the session. Clients are instructed not to use the phone calls as a way to begin socializing in pairs, but only to meet one another if the entire group is invited. We have commonly found that most people agree to participate, and that even when one individual declines at Session 1, they typically ask to join the list at Session 2 or 3.

Managing Group Conflict and Emotion

Whenever multiple people are brought together in a group, it increases the likelihood that conflict will develop between or among the group members. In addition, due to their abuse histories, many clients come to group treatment with problematic communication patterns that can make it difficult for them to manage their emotional and cognitive reactions during group sessions. Again, this highlights the need for thorough prescreening and education about the group process. It is important to highlight that we have typically not excluded clients because of personality disorder diagnoses, but we do acknowledge that some clients can be more difficult to manage in groups than others; in some cases, clients may have symptoms that are so disruptive that they need to be addressed in individual therapy or a treatment designed for personality disorders before these clients can engage in CPT. Symptoms that we have found to interfere with group CPT include high levels of dependence on others, an inordinately high sense of entitlement, excessive combativeness, and a significant stake in maintaining the "sick" or "patient with PTSD" role. Even when personality disorders are present, we have used group CPT successfully to treat individuals with borderline, histrionic, narcissistic, and antisocial personality disorders.

If the group loses focus during the session, one strategy to get the group back on track is to ask the client who is digressing to make the connection between what he or she is saying and the topic that the group was originally discussing. If the client appears to be avoiding the topic at hand, the therapist may want to use gentle confrontation, noting that the topic appears difficult for the client or that the client seems to be having a difficult time staying with his or her feelings about the topic. The therapist can then ask whether anyone else ever wanted to avoid a topic or stop feeling natural emotions in the group, and the rest of the group can normalize these reactions. This technique will build a bond among the clients and will allow the therapist to address the underlying fears that are causing the digressing client to avoid.

Many new therapists are also concerned about the amount of affect that might be generated in a trauma group. Just as in individual CPT, we have found that although some clients in group CPT do feel worse before they get better, the majority of our clients do not show a worsening of their symptoms during the group treatment. More often, the strong emotions seen during group sessions are related to clients' feeling free to experience their natural emotions related to the trauma for the first time. The group offers them a safe place to feel their emotions without judgment, and leaders should encourage the clients to share their feelings during the group without fear of recrimination. Group leaders also have the responsibility of guiding the clients through their feelings and helping them see that showing their emotions in an appropriate fashion often diffuses excessive emotional responses and disruptive group behaviors.

Two other client reactions that need to be monitored in a group are excessive dominance and excessive shyness. Dominant clients may tend to answer first, make absolute statements (e.g., "No one but another trauma survivor can understand me"), tell stories, or challenge a leader's role. These behaviors will often silence many of the group members (particularly the shy members) and may create hidden animosities in the group that affect future dynamics. In addition, members who are already struggling with avoidance will see other members' excessive dominance as sufficient reason for why they do not need to participate. The first step for the therapists is to identify the dominant and shy clients as early as possible. The therapists can then begin to loosely monitor and control the amount of time each client has to talk. One technique that may be effective is to propose to the members that those who are quick to respond should count to 10 before giving an answer, thus giving clients who are slower to respond an opportunity to voice their thoughts or feelings. Another option is to ask that once a person has participated in a session three times, this person wait until someone else has spoken on a topic before adding further to the discussion. By making these suggestions to the group as a whole, the therapists do not single out a particular client or make some clients feel embarrassed.

Some clients are much shyer or less expressive than others during group sessions. It is important to check in with these clients to determine whether their shyness is a personality trait, a response to their trauma, or a form of avoidance. It can be helpful for therapists to ask such clients privately whether they would like to be called upon during the group, so that they do not feel the pressure of jumping into the conversation at some point. It can also be effective to ask the entire group for their reactions or answers to a worksheet, and then for the therapist leading the group to check in with each member before moving on to the next part of the group agenda.

Conducting CPT+A in a Group Format

The greatest difference between group CPT and group CPT+A is in the management of the written accounts in group CPT+A. In individual CPT+A, clients are given an opportunity to experience their emotions in a one-on-one setting during sessions (in addition to experiencing the same between sessions). In group CPT+A, we strongly recommend that clients do *not* read their accounts out loud during therapy sessions. Although processing one's own traumatic event is important, hearing the graphic details of another person's experience can cause increased distress and a greater likelihood of treatment dropout for many clients.

Many mental health clinics have been using group formats for years, and thus many clients will be very familiar with a group format. However, these groups have often involved long-term supportive psychotherapy, with clients either telling extensive details about their traumas, avoiding the trauma events altogether, or focusing largely on venting about current problems in their lives. Although this type of treatment can be helpful or even normalizing for some clients, many others may feel triggered by hearing details of other clients' trauma accounts. Still other clients may attempt to tell "war stories" or engage in "one-upmanship" storytelling in an attempt to feel accepted by the other group members. This behavior may make other clients very hesitant about attending the group for fear of being pressured to tell their own stories. Thus CPT+A group leaders will need to establish rules very early in treatment (or even in the pre-screening session) that specify no detailed trauma storytelling in group sessions. If a client does begin to tell a detailed story in the group, a therapist should gently interrupt and remind the entire group of the no-trauma-account rule. It may also be helpful to ask the group about the reasons for this rule, which often stimulates one or more of the group members to answer that hearing other people's stories is distressing to them.

Instead of having clients read their impact statements or written accounts during group CPT+A sessions, therapists should explore the clients' reactions to writing about their events, in order both to normalize their emotions and to determine whether they wrote all of the details about the events. Specifically, group participants should be asked whether they included sensory details, thoughts, and feelings in their accounts, and whether they experienced strong emotions or recalled new memories while writing. If group members did not write their full accounts, or if they were unable to express their natural emotions while writing or reading the accounts, they are encouraged to take steps to increase their likelihood of successfully completing the assignment. The discussion about the writing assignment also focuses on Stuck Points that were identified and on evidence from the event that may refute those distorted beliefs and interpretations, not on the details of the event itself.

If one or more clients in group CPT+A do not write their accounts, the therapist leading the group should focus a few minutes on clients who have completed their accounts and may be showing some improvement. This will often help the clients who have not written accounts realize that they too can complete the assignments, and motivate them to do the assignment for the next group session. Following this discussion, the therapist collects the written accounts to read between sessions. While reading the accounts, the therapist searches for Stuck Points, which are usually indicated by points at which clients stopped writing and drew a line, or parts of the events that clients skip, gloss over, or report amnesia about. The therapist also makes note of whether an account has been written like a police report (without accompanying thoughts and feelings) or whether the full memory has been retrieved and activated. Encouragement, praise, and possible Stuck Points are recorded on the accounts before they are returned to the clients.

Aftercare Groups

As in individual CPT, we recommend that therapists follow up with clients who have successfully completed group CPT at a check-in meeting 2–3 months after the end of treatment. This follow-up can be conducted in an individual session or by reconvening the entire group. At this session, group members are asked to indicate how they have been doing in general, and to describe any problems they have encountered; they are encouraged to use the Challenging Beliefs Worksheets to address any continuing or new Stuck Points or difficult situations. This follow-up session should include the same assessment measures that were used during treatment, and it can be used to get the clients back on track or to reinforce gains.

Many clinics have opted to offer a CPT aftercare group that can be adapted to fit the needs of different clients coming from group or individual treatment at the same time. The group can be conducted once a week, twice a month, or once a month, depending on the clinic's goals and the clients' needs. Many clients who have been in trauma treatment for a long time may be fearful of stopping therapy altogether at the end of CPT. The aftercare group allows them to "step down" slowly from weekly group or individual therapy sessions, while continuing to address Stuck Points that may be making treatment termination more difficult. For clients who have shown strong improvement in either group or individual CPT, but perhaps could use a few more sessions to address Stuck Points in specific areas that the standard course of therapy has not resolved, the aftercare group allows these clients to continue using the CPT skills to manage these final issues. It is important for the leader(s) of the aftercare group to insist that attendees continue to bring in completed worksheets each time they come; the group sessions should focus on the review of these worksheets at the whiteboard. Finally, group members should be given a limit on how long they can stay in the aftercare group, to prevent them from creating an unhealthy dependence on this group instead of practicing their skills outside group sessions.

CPT for Sexual Abuse

As discussed in Chapter 2, one of the adaptations of CPT has been a manual for survivors of childhood sexual abuse (Chard, 2005). CPT-SA is 16 sessions long and is typically conducted as a combination of group and individual therapies, but it can be offered as either individual or group treatment alone. In addition, many clinicians have conducted CPT-SA without the trauma accounts for those clients who are not willing or able to discuss their trauma histories in great detail. Although several studies (described in Chapter 2) have shown that clients with histories of childhood sexual abuse do as well in CPT as those with only adulthood traumas do, some therapists and clients want the additional sessions that CPT-SA provides, to allow for additional time to work on other areas that are often affected by childhood trauma. Handout 12.1 provides an overview of CPT-SA for clients. (Note that this handout refers to several other handouts—the ones on developmental stages, assertiveness, communication, and social support—that are specific to CPT-SA and are not included in the present book. These may be obtained at *www.guilford.com/cpt-ptsd*.)

As shown in Handout 12.1, CPT-SA includes a new Session 2 assignment that asks clients to focus on their development, including any family "rules" that may have developed into core beliefs (e.g., "Children must do what adults say," "No one will ever protect me," or "When someone is drinking, you will get hurt"), before going on to the ABC Worksheets. As in CPT+A, each client is asked to write trauma accounts of the childhood sexual abuse experience that the client believes has had the strongest impact on him or her. For individuals who have experienced multiple types of trauma, CPT-SA includes additional sessions for writing about other traumatic events or focusing on identification of Stuck Points related to their complicated trauma histories. After the Esteem Issues Module, CPT-SA adds handouts on assertiveness and communication; these handouts are designed to help trauma survivors identify unhealthy ways they may be trying to get their needs met (e.g., aggression or passivity), as well as Stuck Points about communication with others. This session allows clients to develop healthier, more effective, and safer strategies for getting their needs met.

Cognitive Processing Therapy for Sexual Abuse (CPT-SA): Treatment Overview

CPT-SA is conducted in 16 sessions lasting 55 minutes each. Here is a general overview of the session content:

SESSION 1

Therapist provides introduction to CPT-SA and education about the treatment, symptom responses, social-cognitive theory, emotions, and Stuck Points.

Practice assignment: Read the handouts on Stuck Points and developmental stages.

SESSION 2

Review the Session 1 practice assignment. Discuss developmental issues and their impact on current beliefs and behaviors. Explore family dynamics.

Practice assignment: Write an Impact Statement on the ways in which the abuse has affected your beliefs about yourself, others, and the world.

SESSION 3

Review the Session 2 practice assignment. Begin examining connections between thoughts and feelings. Look over the ABC Worksheet.

Practice assignment: Complete ABC Worksheets.

SESSION 4

Review the Session 3 practice assignment. Look at links among thoughts, feelings, and behaviors.

Practice assignment: Write a full account of the index traumatic incident of childhood sexual abuse, and read it to yourself daily. Continue to complete ABC Worksheets.

SESSION 5

Review the Session 4 practice assignment. Read the written account in session, process emotions, and review the account for Stuck Points.

Practice assignment: Write a second account of the index traumatic incident of childhood sexual

(continued)

abuse, incorporating more sensory detail, and read it to yourself daily. Continue to complete ABC Worksheets.

SESSION 6

Review the Session 5 practice assignment. Read the second written account in session, process emotions, and review the account for Stuck Points.

Practice assignment: Write an account of the next most traumatic incident (if there is one), and read it to yourself daily. Continue to complete ABC Worksheets.

SESSION 7

Review the Session 6 practice assignment. Read the third written account, continuing to process emotions and looking for Stuck Points. Look over the Challenging Questions Worksheet.

Practice assignment: Challenge at least one Stuck Point related to the abuse, using a Challenging Questions Worksheet, and use additional copies of this sheet to challenge Stuck Points from your Stuck Point Log. If you wish, write another account of the second incident, or write about a third incident, and read the account to yourself daily.

SESSION 8

Review the Session 7 practice assignment. Read the most recent written account, and continue to process emotions and review the account for any additional Stuck Points. Review the Challenging Questions Worksheets. Look over the Patterns of Problematic Thinking Worksheet.

Practice assignment: Use the Patterns of Problematic Thinking Worksheet to identify such patterns as they relate to your Stuck Points. Challenge at least one rule with the Challenging Questions Worksheet. Continue to read account(s) daily.

SESSION 9

Review the Session 8 practice assignment. Review problematic thinking patterns, their development, and their impact. Look over the Challenging Beliefs Worksheet and the Safety Issues Module.

Practice assignment: Read the Safety Issues Module. Challenge Stuck Points (including ones on safety), using Challenging Beliefs Worksheets. Continue to read accounts.

SESSION 10

Review the Session 9 practice assignment. Discuss safety, and challenge Stuck Points related to safety. Look over the Trust Issues Module.

Practice assignment: Read the Trust Issues Module. Continue to challenge Stuck Points (including ones on trust), using Challenging Beliefs Worksheets.

(continued)

SESSION 11

Review the Session 10 practice assignment. Discuss trust, and challenge Stuck Points related to trust. Look over the Power/Control Issues Module.

Practice assignment: Read the Power/Control Issues Module. Continue to challenge Stuck Points (including ones on power/control), using Challenging Beliefs Worksheets.

SESSION 12

Review the Session 11 practice assignment. Discuss power/control, and challenge Stuck Points related to power/control. Look over the Esteem Issues Module.

Practice assignment: Read the Esteem Issues Module. Continue to challenge Stuck Points (including ones on esteem), using Challenging Beliefs Worksheets.

SESSION 13

Review the Session 12 practice assignment. Discuss esteem, and challenge Stuck Points related to esteem.

Practice assignment: Continue to challenge Stuck Points (including ones on esteem), using Challenging Beliefs Worksheets. Read handouts on assertiveness and communication.

SESSION 14

Review the Session 13 practice assignment. Continue to discuss esteem, and explore how assertiveness is tied to self-esteem. Look over the Intimacy Issues Module.

Practice assignment: Read the Intimacy Issues Module. Continue to challenge Stuck Points (including ones on intimacy), using Challenging Beliefs Worksheets.

SESSION 15

Review the Session 14 practice assignment. Continue to discuss intimacy, and challenge Stuck Points related to intimacy. Look over the Social Support Module.

Practice assignment: Read the Social Support Module, and continue to challenge Stuck Points (including ones on social support), using Challenging Beliefs Worksheets. Write a second Impact Statement.

SESSION 16

Review the Session 15 practice assignment. Read the new Impact Statement in session, discuss social support, and identify goals for the future.

13

Issues in Working with Different Trauma Types

The purpose of this chapter is to discuss specific issues or topics in therapy that may arise, depending upon the type of trauma a client has experienced. Some issues are specific to particular types of trauma. On the other hand, sometimes traumas blend together, because so many of our clients have experienced traumas across the lifespan. For example, a combat veteran who was shot by the enemy may say, "I don't trust anyone." The therapist may wonder aloud why trust was affected, when the enemy was not someone the veteran knew or trusted to begin with. It may turn out that there was abuse in the veteran's childhood, and that the veteran developed an early schema/core belief about trust that was activated with the later trauma. The client may not even realize that the statement about trust doesn't even make sense in the context of the trauma under discussion, but it may serve as a "red flag" to the therapist for other traumas that may need to be addressed during the course of treatment.

Combat and the Warrior Ethos

This section focuses on some of the areas for consideration when therapists are working with active-duty service members or veterans. Many former or current service members have developed overaccommodated views of the military or the government. These Stuck Points can arise in almost any part of the treatment, and thus they can be worked on either early or while focusing on a particular module such as Safety, Trust, or Esteem. Just as the word "trust" is an overly general term, so is a word like "government." We have even noted that some veterans with PTSD continue to manufacture their anger at the government as a way of avoiding the natural emotions resulting from their traumatic events. This can often be seen when a therapist asks a client to focus on specific thoughts related to the traumatic event, or asks the client to write the trauma accounts for CPT+A (see Chapter 11). Instead, the client typically attempts to move the discussion to politics or long diatribes about how the military/ government has failed the service members. The therapist will need to bring the focus of the discussion back to the index event, and not allow the client to dominate the session with a diatribe. It may be helpful to focus the client by using whatever worksheet is currently being discussed as a way to process these thoughts and help the client generate alternative thoughts. Here are some possible questions the therapist may use to facilitate the discussion: "What do you mean by 'government'? Do you mean the federal government? Do you mean the state or local government? Are they all the same? When you say that the government does not care, does this mean that when you call 911, no one answers the phone?" As with other overly vague terms, it is important for the client to move from seeing only one extreme to viewing the full continuum by admitting the existence of different types and categories that might in fact be judged in a more graded fashion. If the client has been using anger at the government as a way to avoid more healthy behaviors that would permit connections with others, then this topic should be approached very early in treatment. However, it may come up again in many of the later modules.

Similarly, in group settings, veterans and service members will often bring up their anger about the government, the VA (the Department of Veterans Affairs, which includes hospitals, benefits, and cemetery services, all of which are sometimes confusing to veterans), and the military in general or their particular branch of it. These can be very important topics for these clients to address, but they can also become a form of avoidance and can interrupt the process of the group. If clients believe that they were mistreated by the military, the government, or the VA, they may have difficulty identifying their underlying Stuck Points; instead, they may engage in impassioned speeches that will only further their avoidance. In addition, these speeches can cause other veterans to begin avoiding more, and they may even cause divisiveness in the group if some veterans do not agree and are in fact pro-government or pro-VA. It can be helpful for group leaders to establish a rule early that "political" discussions or lengthy discussions about the military or government should not be a part of group therapy. The therapists may also want to point out that groups that have included these types of discussions have historically not led to long-term improvements for the attendees, which is why many clients have ended up attending them for years with little change in their functioning. Another option would be asking whether overgeneralizing from a few "bad" people the clients have encountered within an organization to all people in that organization has caused them any problems with overreacting to situations where they had to communicate with people in the organization (e.g., the VA).

Other specific Stuck Points and clinical issues are frequently found among service members and veterans (Wachen et al., 2016). One issue is the youth of many people who join the military and take on the military ethos, which prepares them for combat but does not work in the civilian world. Because they are often taught while they are still in their formative years that "If we all do our jobs, we will all come home," "Never leave a soldier behind," and "You are responsible for your unit," they may take these lessons literally and experience great guilt or engage in erroneous other-blame when someone in their unit is killed or they cannot carry out these imperatives. Similarly, "Stay alert, stay alive" may be a slogan to keep people attentive in dangerous situations, but it may lead to PTSD hypervigilance upon return from deployment.

Because they are being trained to fight rather than flee, and trained repeatedly so that they can do their jobs automatically during combat, veterans who are returning to civilian life may have anger and aggressive responses out of proportion to most civilian situations when they are triggered, or may report to their therapists that they did not experience emotions during their traumatic incidents and have Stuck Points about the meaning of emotions (e.g., "Emotions mean I am weak and vulnerable," or "Emotions will never stop"). During CPT, therapists may have to help such clients to separate these well-learned core beliefs from more balanced beliefs that are more adaptive in a civilian world.

Military and veteran clients are also more likely to have issues with having killed or having witnessed the violent deaths of others than many other types of clients. Because of their warrior-trained beliefs, these clients often blame themselves or someone in their near proximity in their Impact Statements, rather than the person who buried the mine or shot the mortar into their base. Sometimes war veterans will avoid writing or talking about the index event in particular by just ascribing the cause to "It happened because we were at war." A therapist can agree with that, but can then ask about the cause of the specific index event. Sometimes the just-world myth is evident in statements like "But why was he killed? He was such a nice guy." The therapist can ask whether that person was targeted specifically because he was a nice guy or was targeted generally because he was a gunner in a truck. Seeing children killed often triggers another belief based on the just-world myth: "Children shouldn't die in war." Although we might all agree with the philosophy behind that statement, the fact is that children do die in war, and the therapists need to help these clients accept what they witnessed. Attempts by the clients to undo the event (e.g., "If only I had been earlier," or "He shouldn't have been shot until it was clear he had a bomb, even though he wouldn't stop running toward us") are common.

Some veterans isolate themselves from others because they have killed, label themselves as "murderers," and fear that they are at great risk of harming others because they have done it before. After affirming that these clients have not, in fact, killed anyone since returning from deployment, it is important for therapists to help the clients "right-size" the event by putting it into the context in which it occurred. As described in detail in Chapter 7, a therapist can draw a pie chart and ask a client to draw in slices of what else the client has done before and after the event, or what other roles the client plays in life, so that it becomes clear that having killed someone is not the client's entire identity.

Killing in war (and defending others) is different from murder. Sometimes in war, a client was actually trying *not* to kill—for instance, by ordering a person to stop driving through a checkpoint, shooting over the person's head as a warning, and then finally shooting into the vehicle when the person wouldn't stop. The client's intent was not to kill someone, but to protect the base. Context is everything. Even in the cases in which someone killed intentionally and perhaps killed a noncombatant, there is a context to consider, while accepting that the client did in fact commit an unsanctioned act. For example, we have heard of clients who were the only survivors of their entire units; everyone else was killed. They were not thinking, but just feeling, when they shot the next person they saw—who happened to be an unarmed villager. (See Chapter 1 on the reciprocal relationship between the prefrontal cortex and the amygdala.) While a therapist can agree that such a client did have intent and therefore guilt, the therapist can point out that in this context, the client was overwhelmed and horrified. The therapist can check whether the client ever killed anyone coldly before or after that incident, and can emphasize that the context needs to be taken into account. It is unlikely that a psychopath who enjoys killing is going to have PTSD or seek treatment for it, so it is not probable that the therapist will need to deal with that kind of person. The therapist and client can also discuss possible acts of restitution—not for the dead person (who may be unidentified) or the person's family, but for the client's community, so that the client has the opportunity to give back and feel worthwhile. When such clients are discussing the extra assignments to be done after Session 10, for example, they may discuss not just doing nice things for themselves but doing worthwhile things that help them feel better about themselves, such as volunteering at a shelter for homeless persons or some other agency that provides help for those in need.

Sexual Assault

This section discusses rape (including marital rape), child sexual abuse, and military sexual trauma (i.e., coercive or forced sexual contact or severe harassment in the context of military service). CPT was first developed with rape victims and clients of rape crisis centers in mind. It quickly became apparent in our first research projects that rape victims often had multiple rapes in their histories following childhood sexual abuse. In the Resick et al. (2002) study, although the index event among clients being recruited for treatment was completed rape (i.e., penetration of vaginal, oral, or anal orifices), 86% of the sample had at least one other traumatic event; 48% had at least one other rape; and 41% had genital-contact sexual abuse as children. They averaged six other criminal victimizations as adults. So it was rare to see someone in therapy who had experienced only one traumatic event. However, if the index event (the event with the most severe and frequent PTSD symptoms) is the one a therapist is going to start with, there is likely to be a pattern of Stuck Points to keep an eye out for.

Rape is rarely witnessed by people other than the victims and perpetrators. One of the issues that may arise for rape victims is whether they will be believed. Sometimes they are not, which can leave them wondering whether the event happened at all, whether it was really a rape, what they did to lead to such a "misunderstanding," and so forth. They may question their own judgment about themselves and other people. In other words, they are likely to be very self-focused in their causal attributions (e.g., "I am to blame for the rape"). We rarely see much anger in rape victims, and they tend to score at normal levels on anger scales because they look to themselves as the cause of the events (another example of the just-world myth—"Bad things happen to bad people") rather than the perpetrators. These thoughts often lead to strong feelings of guilt.

In addition, shame is a very common emotion in assault survivors. Guilt is about what someone has done; shame is about who someone is. Rape victims may feel shame because they believe that they are now permanently changed by such a personal invasion, or they may think that the assault must have happened because of something about bad about them as people. The sense of violation and the Stuck Points related to the thoughts about being permanently damaged are things therapists may need to start dealing with fairly early in treatment, even though these Stuck Points may arise later (in regard to the self) during the modules on Trust, Esteem, and Intimacy. Because shame is schema-level, it may take many worksheets and Socratic dialogues to help these clients realize that their events were not about them as people, but about the perpetrators as predators and their choice of convenient targets.

Clients' relationships with their perpetrators may be an issue if the perpetrators were not strangers (which is the case more often than not). The sense of betrayal is particularly shattering, and clients who have been raped may blame themselves for trusting the perpetrators, instead of blaming the persons who betrayed that trust. This issue crosses all types of sexual victimization. Victims of childhood sexual abuse are most likely to have been abused by family members or friends of their families. Marital rape victims have been betrayed and degraded by the persons they chose to spend their lives with—the persons who vowed to cherish and protect them. In military sexual trauma, the persons who are supposed to watch their backs in combat, or even their commanders, are the persons who have betrayed the trust. These situations are similar to those involving abuse by other people who should be assumed to be trusted, such as teachers, coaches, police officers, and religious leaders. The difference is that in many cases of child sexual abuse, marital rape, and military sexual trauma, the victims must live with the perpetrators, and the events may be a series of assaults over a period of time.

Unlike combat veterans, who are usually far away from the site of their trauma when they return from war, rape victims, of whatever type, continue to live in the "war zone." Children who are abused in their own homes may have to dissociate as the only means of coping when the fight–fight response is ineffective. Enough traumatic events, and enough dissociation, leave victims vulnerable to revictimization because dissociation becomes so automatic. Once they begin to dissociate, they lose the ability to solve problems effectively, and events may go on without them. Child sexual abuse often starts with a period of "grooming," in which the perpetrators slowly prepares the children to participate in the sexual abuse by showing the children special attention and affection, and slowly draw the children into their "special" relationship. Some children realize that there is something wrong, because the perpetrators tell them that it is "our secret" or threaten to hurt their family members if they tell anyone. Others may not realize that anything is wrong until they are older and they learn that sex between adults and children is wrong and illegal. In either case, the children are made to feel like participants rather than victims, and they carry guilt and negative schemas/core beliefs forward into their lives. Any other events are filtered through those childhood beliefs without alteration. Therapy will need to take account of the negative schemas that color even positive events, and the clients may need to complete many worksheets on specific events that regularly activate these schemas.

Developmental level at the time of the trauma may have a large effect on stuck points/schemas and how clients behave in therapy. It has been our observation that clients can become stuck developmentally at the time that their trauma occurred and they began to suffer from PTSD. The attention that would have been dedicated to cognitive, emotional, or social development is instead spent on avoiding memories of the trauma or coping in a violent environment. Those who are traumatized in adolescence may have particular problems with authority figures or with developing an independent identity, as we discuss later in this chapter. Those who were very young at the time of the trauma may develop problems with affect regulation, and may even have childlike temper tantrums or be mistaken for those with borderline personality disorder. They may have very simple black-and-white cognitive categories (e.g., "You are either my friend or my enemy"), because they have failed to develop the more nuanced thoughts that typical adults have developed. Because of such either–or thinking, it can be difficult for them to develop and maintain social relationships. Therapists should keep in mind the age at which their clients first developed PTSD, even if the first traumatic event is not the index event with which therapy begins, because developmental level may emerge in Stuck Points that do not exactly match the index event or may affect the client–therapist relationship.

Specific issues related to military sexual trauma include an inability to escape the environment, as well as the fact that the victims may be punished instead of the perpetrators; indeed, many women will lose their military careers if they report the abuse. In addition, if the perpetrators happen to be commanders, the victims may feel trapped and may not believe that they can report the abuse or seek help, especially if it has occurred in a war zone.

Intimate-Partner Violence

Victims of IPV are likely to experience a range of traumatic experiences over a period of time. In addition, much IPV is bidirectional in nature, meaning that each partner has committed acts of aggression toward the other. However, given the relative physical strength of men versus women (in heterosexual relationships), the aftereffects of IPV are generally greater for women than for men. This is not to say that men cannot be affected by IPV, but rather that the majority of IPV causing PTSD is found in women.

Given the likely chronicity of IPV, one typically occurring issue is difficulty in defining the index event. As in other types of chronic abuse, clinicians should help the clients determine whether there were instances that were particularly distressing by doing a fine-grained assessment of the clients' presenting PTSD symptoms (i.e., the content of intrusive and avoidance symptoms). Often there have been abuse experiences that were particularly distressing for victims—instances in which they were injured (or more severely so), children witnessed or heard the abuse, weapons were involved, or they were caught off guard by the violence. The most severe of these incidents should be used as the index event. If a client has a difficult time identifying a most traumatic event, a clinician should inquire about a typical pattern of abuse and use an incident emblematic of this pattern as the index event. One in which they thought that they or their children would be killed is a good candidate for the index event.

Another question that frequently arises with regard to PTSD resulting from IPV is when it is appropriate to begin PTSD treatment in cases where there is potential for ongoing IPV. In earlier treatment outcome trials, we did not include victims who were currently involved in violent relationships or were the victims of ongoing stalking behaviors. Given our subsequent clinical experience with victims of this type of abuse and military service members treated in combat theatres, as well as the research with participants in the Democratic Republic of Congo (see Chapter 2), we have come to recommend that victims of IPV be treated as soon as possible. We recognize that many such victims may choose to return to their perpetrators or may be at risk for retaliation by perpetrators if they leave. The goal of treatment is not to alleviate appropriate vigilance, but the *hyper*vigilance symptoms of PTSD, so that these victims can appraise risk as accurately as possible. Moreover, improving any comorbid depressive or dissociative symptoms may help these victims become more behaviorally activated or increase their level of consciousness and self-worth in general, to help protect them against further victimization or PTSD symptoms. Again, this is consistent with research reviewed in Chapter 2.

In work with victims at risk for current IPV, it is important to develop a standard safety plan that involves emergency contact numbers and other methods to contact and utilize naturally occurring supports in the victims' social network before CPT begins. Co-occurring case management services to help clients access necessary economic and social resources (e.g., housing, financial assistance, child care) are likely to be necessary in cases of more recent IPV, because if these more basic needs are not met, any psychosocial intervention will be difficult to deliver.

Disasters and Accidents

With regard to natural or technological disasters or accidents, such as motor vehicle accidents, it is important for clinicians to remember that accidents do happen in an uncertain world. Common Stuck Points include such notions as "Things are preventable, if one takes good precautions," or "My friend died in the car accident. I should have done something to prevent it." It is important to consider the difference among blameworthiness, responsibility, and the unforeseeable in these incidents (see Chapter 7). Blame is only appropriate when a combination of intentionality and some behavioral action or inaction caused the traumatic event.

Galovski and Resick (2008) presented a single case of a 63-year-old long-haul truck driver whose driving record was exemplary, and who was planning to drive for 17 more months and then retire, when he was involved in a severe accident. After the accident, he was unable to return to work and could barely tolerate being a passenger in a car, much less a truck driver. The limited disability payments he received did not replace what he would have earned either working or retired, and he agreed to therapy 4 months after the incident, in which a station wagon plunged across the median and into his truck. He swerved but could not avoid the crash. A 16-year-old girl was driving, and she, as well as the rest of her family of six, was killed; the only survivor was a baby. It was believed that everyone had fallen asleep. One of the truck driver's major Stuck Points was "I killed this family. That baby will never know her family." He responded early to CPT+A and was asymptomatic after six sessions. After he completed treatment at Session 7, he was able to return to work as well as feel closer to his family again.

One of us supervised a case involving a client who, in adolescence, had an older brother who died in a fire. The brother had put a cigarette lighter up to the gas tank in the family's lawn mower to see whether there was enough gas, and the tank exploded. He ran into the house ablaze, setting the house on fire, and died. The client thought she should have saved him, indicating, "If I had been smarter, my brother wouldn't had died." The contextual events were that she had just returned from her paper route to find the house on fire, and that she had done everything in her power to assist: She had called for help, gotten her other brother out, tried to use water and a fire extinguisher to put out the fire, and only left the house when she couldn't breathe. This case illustrates the importance of closely examining the context of all traumatic events and determining the preventability (or not) of such events.

Trauma among Clients with Brain Injuries, Low Intelligence, or Aging/Dementia

Many of the clients who have participated in our research studies and clinical programs have cognitive deficits stemming from a variety of factors, including developmental difficulties, organic brain damage, work or automotive accidents, and dementia. In addition, many service members and veterans who sustained traumatic brain injuries during their time in combat present for clinical care of PTSD. As discussed in Chapter 2, research on CPT suggests that a majority of clients with cognitive deficits respond well to the full protocol of CPT, and thus we recommend that therapists use the original worksheets until such clients begin to struggle with even basic comprehension of the current exercise. At that point, the clinicians may find it helpful to switch to one of the modified worksheets described below and included at the end of this chapter.

If clients are literate but have difficulty with the standard Challenging Questions Worksheet (Handout 7.2), we recommend using the Modified Challenging Questions Worksheet (Handout 13.1), which shortens that sheet to five questions. On this modified worksheet, all clients are asked a version of question 1 from the original worksheet, which focuses on the evidence for and against the belief; this information helps to set the stage for the later questions. Clients are then asked to choose among questions 3, 6, and 10 from the original worksheet (the context questions), because clients will often have an easier time comprehending one of these questions over the other two. Finally, the clients are asked to choose any three of the remaining questions that the clients find more comprehensible than the others.

After the Modified Challenging Questions Worksheet has been used, the Patterns of Problematic Thinking Worksheet is introduced at the usual time. Therapists should then see whether the clients can manage the Modified Challenging Beliefs Worksheet (Handout 13.2, a modification of Handout 8.1, with the same five items in section D as those selected for the Modified Challenging Questions Worksheet). If even the Modified Challenging Beliefs Worksheet is too difficult, therapists can use the Simplified Challenging Beliefs Worksheet (Handout 13.3), which combines aspects of the Challenging Questions and the Challenging Beliefs Worksheets. The rest of therapy will rely on the Simplified Challenging Beliefs Worksheet in place of the regular Challenging Beliefs Worksheet.

Please note that clients with cognitive challenges can be expected to have some confusion when they learn any new worksheet, but that this confusion typically lessens as they practice more both in the clinic and at home. Again, we only recommend the use of the modified/simplified versions if the clients not only are confused, but fail to comprehend the basic purpose of the original worksheets. Finally, the modified/simplified worksheets can be used in either individual or group treatment, and in either CPT or CPT+A. Clients should be encouraged to read over their successful worksheets every day in order to remember them. They can also post alternative thoughts on their mirror, refrigerator, or cell phone.

PTSD Complicated by Grief

Sometimes the primary trauma may be the violent death of someone close to a client, or the death may be in addition to or part of the client's own traumatic event. Grief may become so entangled with PTSD symptoms that clients are unwilling to let go of some of their PTSD reactions, such as anger, in order to avoid the grief response and the need to accept that the dead person is gone. In particular, it is not uncommon to hear veterans say, "If I give up my PTSD, then it means that my friend is really dead, or died in vain." Sometimes people are afraid of forgetting the person who died if they don't have their intrusive symptoms to keep him or her at the forefront of memory.

Usually these Stuck Points can be dispelled by asking clients about other memories of the person who died that are not involved in the death, and asking whether it would be better to remember how the person lived than how he or she died. The clients can add these Stuck Points to the Stuck Point Log and work on them as they arise, often after they have worked on the assimilation of the traumatic event. The therapist might ask why the clients fear forgetting the person if he or she was so important, and whether the clients have anything to remember the person by. Of course, it is always helpful to ask what the other person would want for the clients, or what the person would want if the situation were reversed: "Would your friend want you to have a miserable life, or would he want you to live well for both of you?" or "What would you want for her, if you had died? Would you want her to be suffering for the rest of her life?"

One of the differences between PTSD and complicated grief is the level of avoidance in PTSD—the attempts *not* to remember the trauma, versus an almost obsessional rumination in the case of complicated grief. People suffering from complicated grief build shrines to the victim, don't change anything in the victim's room for years at a time, or spend a great deal of time thinking about how they could have prevented the death. Although people with PTSD also spend much time wondering how they could have prevented the death, this rumination serves an avoidance function in PTSD: It prevents the clients from actually accepting the death and grieving. Anger and guilt are often more acceptable than grief as emotions, and because grief and sadness may last longer than other natural emotions, they can be much more daunting to clients. People may also feel helpless because there is nothing they can do to bring the person back, to change the relationship with the deceased, or to change what they might or might not have said the last time they saw the deceased. All of these may be Stuck Points that can be addressed with worksheets and Socratic dialogue.

Sometimes topics related to grief and mourning become Stuck Points that need to be resolved. In the past, people wore black clothing, black armbands, or other indicators of mourning, sometimes for an extended period of time. Although some people might not have wanted to follow strict guidelines on proper mourning, they were afforded recognition of their loss and were usually extended support. Because modern society does not recognize bereavement as a process and often expects people to return to work almost immediately without a word said, or because coworkers and friends lack knowledge of what to say or how to give ongoing support, clients often think that no matter what they do or feel, they must be "doing it wrong." There is no prescribed length of time in which one should feel sadness or loss. Indeed, when a death is seen as a relief because of prior treatment by the person who died (e.g., abuse), or because the deceased has been suffering greatly, one may not need to feel sad at all. In those cases, the client may have guilt and Stuck Points about not grieving. There are no rules and no norms at this point about when grief makes a transition into something pathological. If a client has Stuck Points about "doing it wrong" (grieving too little, too long, or too much), a therapist may find the handout called Examples of Stuck Points about Grief and Mourning (Handout 13.4) helpful. The therapist and client can go through the handout and see whether the client believes any of the statements, which can then be added to the Stuck Point Log.

Trauma in Adolescence and Its Effects on Other Developmental Periods

One of the only studies to be published on CPT with adolescents was conducted with incarcerated male adolescents (Ahrens & Rexford, 2002). This small study (with 19 participants in each group) compared a compressed (8-session) form of group CPT+A to a wait-list condition. Ahrens and Rexford shortened the protocol by excluding the Impact Statements and combining the five themes. In spite of the small sample and shortened protocol, PTSD self-report scores dropped by 50% in the treatment group, whereas they were unchanged in the wait-list group. There was a significant interaction between group and time on both PTSD and depression.

Taking the opposite approach, and following the tendency in Germany for PTSD treatment to be funded for 24–45 sessions, Matulis, Resick, Rosner, and Steil (2014) designed an adolescent adaptation that could be more easily disseminated into the German mental health system. They pilot-tested a 30-session therapy that not only included the 12 sessions of CPT+A, but also included 4 weeks of preparation and planning (therapy contract, emergency plan goals), 4 weeks of emotion regulation training, and (after CPT+A), three sessions on developmental tasks. They conducted the pilot study with 12 adolescent patients (10 females, 2 males) who had PTSD as a result of childhood sexual or physical abuse. The findings were quite promising: There were large effect sizes from pre- to posttreatment and follow-up on PTSD scores, as well as medium to large effect sizes on depression, dissociation, and emotion dysregulation. Two clients dropped out of treatment. There were no exacerbations of PTSD symptoms. The authors are currently conducting an RCT with adolescents.

Matulis et al. (2014) point out that adolescents have unique developmental tasks, which include individuation, educational/career-related decisions, and the development of intimate relationships. All of these developmental tasks may put them at risk not only for revictimization (which is more frequent among adolescents than adults), but also for PTSD or exacerbation of preexisting PTSD. However, every developmental period can be affected by PTSD, and so developmental stages should always be taken into account in CPT.

Clients in their 20s (or even older clients) may behave like adolescents and push away from their therapists if they were in fact traumatized during adolescence. They may try to pick fights with their therapists or try to cast them in the role of disapproving parents. They may test the therapists by refusing to do practice assignments or engaging in mind reading. Individuals in their 20s and 30s should typically be working on careers, starting families of their own, and beginning to reconcile with their parents (rather than assuming them to be "idiots," as they may have done in adolescence). They should also have a clear sense of identity, and after the age of 25 should have achieved full brain development (particularly in the prefrontal cortex and amygdala) and reasonably mature executive functions. When trauma in adolescence has disrupted clients' development in these areas, the task of CPT is not only to relieve the PTSD symptoms, but to help the clients regain a typical developmental trajectory.

There is likely to be a gap in time between the time of the trauma and the time when a client presents for treatment. The therapist should not assume that the client's cognitive, emotional, or social development has continued, or that the client's skills in these areas are congruent with his or her chronological age. Development may be quite spotty or completely stopped at the age of the earliest traumas. The client may display either–or categorical thinking, reflecting the development level of a small child. In spite of these effects of trauma, some clients may be able to compartmentalize and throw themselves into their education or work, but may have poor social skills or relationship success. The clients may act out and have the equivalent of temper tantrums if their emotional growth has been stunted.

For some Vietnam veterans who are now in their 60s or 70s, but who don't know what their identity is without their PTSD because it has been so much a part of their lives, we have introduced the concept of "retiring from PTSD." They have the same developmental task as other people their age without PTSD: deciding what they are going to do and who they are going to be without their "work" identity. In fact, even among those who have been holding down jobs and keeping extremely busy as a high-functioning form of avoidance, PTSD symptoms may reemerge upon retirement.

Among the elderly, PTSD symptoms may resurface as their age mates die off and they go through the process of life review. We have seen World War II veterans seek out treatment for PTSD that has been suppressed or ineffectively managed for 70 years or so. Because they may have difficulty learning new ways to think as dementia starts to emerge, CPT therapists may need to assign them to reread their successful worksheets every day, or to write their more balanced self-statements on cards or notes. They can keep the cards or notes with them and use these to help them remember the new thoughts with which they want to replace the long-term guilt cognitions or other Stuck Points. The modified or simplified worksheets discussed earlier may be useful as well.

Modified Challenging Questions Worksheet

Date: _____   Client: _____

Below is a list of questions to be used in helping you challenge your Stuck Points or problematic beliefs/Stuck Points. Not all questions will be appropriate for the belief you choose to challenge. Answer as many as questions you can for the belief you have chosen to challenge below.

Belief:

What is the evidence for and against this stuck point?

For:

Against:

Now choose one of the next three questions:

In what ways is your Stuck Point not including all of the information?

In what way is your Stuck Point focused on just one piece of the story?

(continued)

In what ways is this Stuck Point focused on unrelated parts of the story?

Now choose three of the following questions (the three you understand best):

Is your Stuck Point a habit or based on facts?

Does your Stuck Point include all-or-none terms?

Does the Stuck Point include words or phrases that are extreme or exaggerated (such as "always," "forever," "never," "need," "should," "must," "can't," and "every time")?

Where did this Stuck Point come from? Is this a dependable source of information on this Stuck Point?

How is your Stuck Point confusing something that is possible with something that is likely?

In what ways is your Stuck Point based on feelings rather than facts?

Modified Challenging Beliefs Worksheet

Date: _____   Client: _____

A. Situation	B. Thought/Stuck Point	D. Challenging Thoughts	E. Problematic Patterns	F. Alternative Thought(s)
Describe the event, thought, or belief leading to the unpleasant emotion(s).	Write thought/Stuck Point related to situation in section A. (How much do you believe this thought?) Rate your belief in this thought/Stuck Point from 0 to 100%.	Use **Challenging Questions** to examine your automatic thought from section B. Consider whether the thought is balanced and factual, or extreme.	Use the **Patterns of Problematic Thinking Worksheet** to decide whether this is one of your problematic patterns of thinking.	What else can I say instead of the thought in section B? How else can I interpret the event instead of this thought? Rate your belief in the alternative thought(s) from 0 to 100%.
	C. Emotion(s) Specify your emotion(s) (sad, angry, etc.), and rate how strongly you feel each emotion from 0 to 100%.	Evidence for? Evidence against? **One of the next three questions:** Not including all information? Not including all information? Focused on just one piece? Focused on unrelated parts? **Any three of the following questions:** Habit or fact? All-or-none? Extreme or exaggerated? Source dependable? Confusing possible with likely? Based on feelings or facts?	Jumping to conclusions: Exaggerating or minimizing: Ignoring important parts: Oversimplifying: Overgeneralizing: Mind reading: Emotional reasoning:	**G. Re-Rate Old Thought/ Stuck Point** Re-rate how much you now believe the thought/Stuck Point in section B, from 0 to 100%. **H. Emotion(s)** Now what do you feel? Rate it from 0 to 100%.

Simplified Challenging Beliefs Worksheet

Date: _____   Client: _____

Stuck Point	Challenging Questions	New Belief
List one of your Stuck Points here, and rate how much you believe it (from 0 to 100%).	Use these five questions to challenge your Stuck Point.	What can you tell yourself in the future, and how much do you believe it (from 0 to 100%)?
____%	Evidence for the Stuck Point? Evidence against the Stuck Point? Is the Stuck Point not including all the information? Is the Stuck Point extreme or exaggerated? Is the Stuck Point based on feelings rather than all the facts?	____%

Examples of Stuck Points about Grief and Mourning

1. Because grief and mourning decrease steadily over time, there is something wrong with me.

2. If I stop having flashbacks or nightmares, I will forget the person who died.

3. All losses should result in the same type of grief and mourning.

4. If I hang on to my guilt or anger, I won't have to accept that the person has died and feel sad.

5. The best way to recover from the death of someone is to get on with life and not think about the person.

6. Grief will affect the mourner emotionally, but should not interfere in other ways.

7. If I don't feel intensely about the person's death, this means I am not grieving right.

8. If I stop thinking about the deaths of the people I've lost, this means that they died for nothing, or that I and other people will forget them.

9. Continuing to grieve honors a person's death.

10. Losing someone to a sudden, unexpected, or violent death is the same as losing someone to an expected death.

11. Grief is over in a year.

12. Time heals all wounds.

14

Diversity and Cross-Cultural Adaptations

"Culture" includes the group or groups one identifies with and the values those groups espouse. We are born into particular cultures (based on our families' race/ethnicity, region/country, and religious views) or may move into or out of cultures (e.g., the military culture, different religions or sects within a religion). Some cultures are flexible in their beliefs, and some are very rigid. However, most cultures have changed over time with modernization, the effects of other groups, and even the advent of the Internet. When a client is strongly identified with a particular culture's beliefs, the culture may have positive or negative effects on recovery from trauma, depending on how that culture treats trauma survivors and on its beliefs about why people have traumatic experiences. However, it must be kept in mind that, like other beliefs, the beliefs of a particular culture or subculture can be distorted and then interfere with trauma recovery. Because earlier chapters have discussed the military culture and gender differences, this chapter focuses on race/ethnicity, sexual orientation/identity, and religion/spirituality, and particularly on adaptations of CPT for other languages and cultures.

Therapists should not avoid discussing topics related to racial/ethnic groups, sexual orientations, or religions that are not their own. These very topics may play an important role in why a traumatic event happened, or how a client reacted to the traumatic event and what Stuck Points developed. It is incumbent upon therapists to develop cultural competence through reading, workshops, ongoing coursework, and so forth. The fact that particular clients from particular cultures or subcultures say something does not make it true for those entire groups. The best approach is to deal with these issues in a very straightforward fashion and to ask clarifying questions.

For example, therapists do not need to be in the military in order to treat military members or veterans. Therapists just need to ask about military culture, what military or veteran clients were trained to believe, and what the usual protocols or rules of engagement were at the time of the clients' traumatic events. Likewise, therapists should ask about specific religious/moral belief structures, even if it is assumed that these are shared with some clients. Different clients have various levels of orthodoxy, which may or may not be consistent with general statements about their religious orientation or the practice of their clinicians. It may even be an advantage for a therapist *not* to have had the same experiences, because the therapist needs to ask more clarifying questions and does not make assumptions about how things "should" go. At the beginning of any therapy, the therapist should ask whether the client is comfortable working with them if cultural differences are obvious. The therapist should also ask for corrections if he or she misunderstands something, and should attempt to develop open dialogue on any topic.

Racial/Ethnic and Sexual Orientation Diversity

There is very little research on diversity in the use of CPT at this time with regard to race/ethnicity or sexual orientation. Although there is a bit more research on cross-cultural adaptations (discussed later in this chapter), it is a small amount in comparison to the studies conducted within the Western culture in which CPT was developed. Lester, Artz, Resick, and Young-Xu (2010) examined dropout and outcomes among female European American and African American clients across the Resick et al. (2002, 2008) studies combined; these authors found that while African American clients were more likely to drop out of treatment, they did equally well in the intention-to-treat analyses and improved more than European Americans who dropped out of treatment. The authors speculated that cultural messages and stigma against receiving therapy may have motivated the African American clients to achieve as much as possible in the shortest time possible.

With regard to sexual orientation, only one case study has been published to date with the use of CPT (Kaysen et al., 2005). This case involved the assault of a gay man that included homophobic slurs and a clear relationship between the event and his sexual orientation. He came to therapy very soon after the event and was diagnosed as having acute stress disorder. The therapist implemented CPT+A, and the client's fear of writing the accounts brought up additional Stuck Points regarding fear of censure by the therapist. His Stuck Points were generally typical assault-related Stuck Points (e.g., "All strangers are dangerous"), but they also included self-blame directed to the fact that he was gay (i.e., "All gay men are promiscuous," "I deserved it because I am gay"). The client's PTSD symptoms improved; by the end of treatment, he no longer met criteria for acute stress disorder or PTSD, and his functioning had improved as well. Follow-up assessments indicated sustained improvement.

Religion and Morality

Some therapists are reluctant to incorporate religious and moral issues into the therapeutic process. We do not believe that PTSD therapists can avoid these topics, however, because traumatic events often provoke large existential issues and may prove to be at the core of many clients' PTSD. Even if therapists have a different set of religious beliefs from those of clients (or are agnostics or atheists treating religious clients), they can stay client-focused in order to promote recovery. We consider religion a part of the larger set of cultural beliefs to be considered in CPT, and religion may be an important part of many clients' cultures. A client will not bring up religion as an issue in therapy unless there is some conflict or Stuck Point about it. Clients who derive comfort and support from their religion or their congregation may mention it in passing, but in these cases it will not typically be a process issue in therapy.

There are several ways that religion and morality may intersect with the beliefs leading to nonrecovery following traumatization. For those with PTSD who are religious, assimilated Stuck Points are often entangled in the just-world belief (e.g., "Why me?" or "Why not me?" or "Why did my friend/relative die?")—a belief that is taught directly by some religions. Even if the just-world belief is not directly taught by particular religious groups, the client may implicitly adhere to it. In addition to assimilated Stuck Points in the religious/moral realm, some clients have overaccommodated Stuck Points in this realm as a result of traumatization. For example, as a result of a traumatic event, a client may come to ask, "How could God let this happen?" or even come to disavow their religious beliefs. Even if a client does not ascribe to a particular religion or is even an atheist, a traumatic event can be construed as a violation of the client's preexisting moral or ethical code—a violation that some commentators have described as "moral injury" (e.g., "I killed while in the line of duty; therefore I'm a murderer"). Religious and moral issues can also involve the client's or others' trying to force forgiveness of the client or the perpetrator.

The just-world belief is taught not just by religious groups, but also by parents, teachers, the criminal justice system, and other persons or groups in authority. Indeed, as humans, we like to believe that if people follow the rules, good things will happen, and if people break the rules, they will be punished. There are societal benefits to the teaching of this belief. Unfortunately, some people fail to make their thinking sufficiently complex and nuanced to realize that the world is not perfectly just or orderly, or they revert to this simpler explanation in the face of traumatic events. Justice, in reality, is more accurately described as aspirational and as a probability (e.g., "If I follow the rules, it decreases my risk that something bad will happen"). If people adhere strongly to the just-world belief, they are likely to engage in backward reasoning. That is, they may well conclude that if something bad happened to them, they are being punished for doing something bad (or, in some cases, they may believe they were born bad). If they cannot determine what they did wrong, they may end up railing at the unfairness of the situation or of a higher being.

Few, if any, religions actually guarantee that good behavior will *always* be rewarded and bad behavior punished (at least in this lifetime). Clients who believe this either may have distorted views of their religion or may have been taught this by mistaken parents or religious leaders. As in any profession, there is variability in the extent to which religious leaders are educated in or adherent to the tenets of their religions. Therapists must make sure to differentiate a religion itself from an individual practitioner's interpretation of it when they discuss these issues with clients. It may be possible for therapists to check on the tenets of the religion through their own research or through consultation with clergy. A key principle here is that there are levels of orthodoxy in every religious sect.

When someone cannot understand how a higher power could let an event happen that involves the malicious actions of another (e.g., rape, assault, combat), the concept of "free will" may be very helpful. Most Western religions adhere to the concept of free will, or the choice to behave or misbehave. If a higher power gives an individual free will to make choices, then it does not follow that the free will of another person was taken away in order to punish a client. The perpetrator also had free will to fire a gun or to commit assault or rape. Free will implies that a higher power does not step in and stop the behavior of others, any more than this power forces the client to behave or misbehave. Furthermore, even when another person's behaviors and choices are not involved, it does not take a great deal of inspection of the world to find evidence that any higher power is not using natural events, accidents, or illnesses only to punish bad people. When we see these events happening to infants or children, or to people we know to be wonderful, caring individuals, one thing we may fall back on at that point is the idea that "God moves in a mysterious way." However, it could also be the case that God does not intervene in day-to-day lives and that the concept of God should be used for comfort, community, and moral guidance.

If clients believe in predetermination and are convinced that they have no free will, then their therapists may wonder with the clients why the clients have PTSD if their traumatic events were predetermined to occur. There should be no conflict between the occurrence of the traumatic events and the clients' prescribed destiny. This raises the question about other lurking beliefs that may be causing the clients' trouble in accepting their fate. Alternatively, these clients may need to experience the natural emotions that are predestined to occur after a traumatic event.

Clients will sometimes raise the notions of self- or other-forgiveness in the course of therapy. If these issues have been comforting or comfortable concepts for clients, they are unlikely to raise them. Instead, they are typically mentioned because there is some discomfort with, or conflict over, the notions of forgiveness. With regard to self-forgiveness, it is crucial first to determine the details of a traumatic event's context, to determine whether a client has anything for which to seek forgiveness. Because it is almost axiomatic that those with PTSD will blame themselves for traumatic events, it does not mean that they intended the outcome. Therefore, blame and guilt may be misplaced. People who are crime victims are just that: victims. There is nothing they could have done that would justify what happened to them. Even if they feel "dirty" or "violated," this does not mean that they did anything wrong that needs forgiveness. This would be an example of emotional reasoning. Similarly, killing someone in war is not the same as murdering someone. The person may have had no other options than what occurred at the time, so the Socratic dialogue needs to establish intent, available options at the time, and so forth.

There may be a place for self-forgiveness or self-compassion when it has been established, after clarification of the trauma context, that a client intended harm against an innocent person, had other available options at the time, and willfully chose this course of action. Killing a civilian by accident (e.g., someone caught in crossfire) in a war is just that: an accident. Committing an atrocity (e.g., raping women or children, torturing people) is clearly intended harm. In this case, guilt is an appropriate response to committing an atrocity or a crime, and the client may well need to accept the fact for what it is, be repentant, and seek self-forgiveness (or, if the client is religious, forgiveness within the church or other place of worship). Even then, clinicians should pose questions in Socratic dialogue that help such clients contextualize who they were then and what their values are now, to help the clients realize that people are capable of change. It may be helpful to remind these clients that truly psychopathic people are unlikely to have PTSD, because they experience no tension between intentional, harmful acts and their self-identity. Once all this has been thoroughly processed, some form of behavioral action in the form of restitution or community service may assist these clients in moving beyond the sense of a self-inflicted life sentence of self-flagellation.

Clients sometimes raise the notion of forgiving others who perpetrated traumatic events when the idea of forgiveness is premature or is forced by others. Part of successfully accommodating the concept that a traumatic event is not a client's fault involves recognition that the perpetrator intended harm and is to blame for the event. To foreclose on natural, righteous anger before letting it run its course may bring comfort to a family or institution, but this creates the same problem for a client as avoiding natural emotions that emanate from the traumatic event. It may be helpful to ask the client whether the perpetrator has asked for forgiveness. Most religions do not confer forgiveness on the unrepentant. If the perpetrator has not asked for forgiveness, there is nothing for the client to forgive. Even if the perpetrator of a traumatic event has asked for forgiveness, the client is not obliged to give it. Understanding why someone did something is not the same as excusing the person, and may be the preferable path for some trauma survivors. In such cases, clinicians might suggest that their clients refer the perpetrators to other sources of forgiveness (e.g., the larger community affected by the perpetrators' acts, or members of the clergy). In summary, the purpose of clients' granting forgiveness should not be enabling the perpetrators or others to feel relief, but only giving the clients some peace of mind. If forgiveness is being coerced by others, it will only bring frustration and guilt to the clients, and ultimately will not work. Forgiveness is not a requirement for recovery from PTSD.

Adaptations of CPT for Other Languages/Cultures

The original CPT manual (or parts of it) has been translated into 12 languages. Some of these translations are published, and some are available online.

Published

Finnish (Ylikomi & Verta, 2008)

German (König, Resick, Karl, & Rosner, 2012)

Hebrew (Resick & Derby, 2012)

Japanese (patient self-help only) (Ito, Kashimura, & Horikoshi, 2012)

Unpublished (available at www.guilford.com/cpt-ptsd)

Arabic

Chinese, both traditional and simplified characters

French

Icelandic (worksheet forms only)

Iraqi manual (in English, simplified and made culturally appropriate, with an emphasis on torture)

Japanese

Kurdish

Spanish

When we were first writing this book, we contacted colleagues from other countries, as well as U.S. therapists/researchers who have conducted CPT in both Westernized countries and developing nations. Most of them said that the major modifications that were needed were in translations of specific words or concepts, because literal translations did not always make sense. Indeed, modifications in some developing nations have had to go well beyond written translations. The most striking example of this was in the Democratic Republic of Congo, in which an RCT, reported in Chapter 2, was conducted (Bass et al., 2013). The concepts from the worksheets had to be simplified, taught orally, and memorized because of complete illiteracy and lack of paper for the participants living in a war-torn country. Moreover, because of the lack of mental health professionals in Congo, the therapists trained for the RCT had as little as a junior high school education and had to be taught therapy skills as well as CPT. The researchers found that the training took 2 weeks, and that it was most helpful to role-play and practice every single concept.

In Cambodia, the term "Stuck Points" became "Kut Caraeun," which means "thinking too much" (Clemens, personal communication, January 2016). In Iraq, the concept of esteem had to be changed to "respect" and intimacy to "caring," because the former terms do not exist in Kurdish (Kaysen et al., 2013). Pictures and more simplified language were used in countries in which illiteracy rates were high. However, colleagues in Germany, Denmark, Iceland, Hong Kong, Israel, and Japan either kept the protocol nearly identical to the original protocol or made only minor changes. For example, several of our colleagues in Japan said that providing more examples in the practice assignments, especially for adolescent clients, were important. So far, with the first 30 pilot cases in Japan, the participants like doing the practice assignments and like to write their accounts. There has been only one dropout so far (Horishaki, personal communication, July 2015).

In Israel, clients were encouraged to write their trauma accounts in the clinic, in which they had privacy and felt safe (Derby, personal communication, January 2016). In preparing for an RCT in Israel, our team has found cultural differences with regard to Israel being a more collectivistic culture than the United States and having various levels of religious orthodoxy. Both projects in Israel have taken into account ongoing terrorism, which affects both the culture and the treatment. Derby said that Israeli patients were not good about completing practice assignments, which was not the case with Russian immigrants. Overall, the basic message from these and other researchers is that the "heart" of CPT has been maintained, but that adaptations to language and cultural differences, usually through simplifications of the concepts and worksheets, have been common.

A few articles have been written about the process of adapting CPT to other cultures. Kaysen et al. (2013) described the iterative process of adapting CPT for both untrained therapists and clients in Iraq. The most frequent type of trauma being treated was torture. Although the CPT protocol did not need to be modified except for language differences, the therapists needed a great deal more practice with each of the steps of therapy. In the Bolton et al. (2014) study comparing BATD and CPT for depression and PTSD in Kurdistan (see Chapter 2), the major cultural impediment mentioned was that the stigma of mental health treatment might affect the community's perceptions of families' reputations and the clients' marriageability. Also, as in the study conducted by the same group in Congo, illiteracy was widespread and there were few trained therapists, so the protocol needed to be adapted for the population.

Schulz, Huber, et al. (2006) wrote about the adaptation of CPT for Bosnian and Afghanistan refugees in the United States as part of the War Trauma Recovery Project. They also discussed issues in conducting therapy through interpreters. It was important that the interpreters translate what the therapists were saying, without trying to intervene as therapists themselves. The therapists looked at the clients, not the interpreters, and the therapists debriefed the interpreters after the sessions. The therapy took place in the clients' homes because they were too afraid to travel to attend therapy. The home-based treatment was effective; however, it often included tea ceremonies that might have served as culturally appropriate social events, but in the context of this therapy could have also served as avoidance. All of the participants had multiple traumas, and most had had family members killed.

Marques et al. (2016) conducted a study in which they compared dysfunctional thinking (Stuck Points) in the Impact Statements of Latino and non-Latino clients. They found that although the themes were for the most part similar, there were many comments by Latinos that appeared to minimize family violence, discussed family role obligations, and emphasized religion. The Latinos generated fewer Stuck Points than the non-Latinos, so this study may indicate that therapists will need to do more work with Latino clients to help them understand the concept, and to use the Stuck Point Help Sheet (Handout 6.4) and the Stuck Point guide for therapists (Figure 6.1) for examples.

Another important point is that therapists need to be aware of the beliefs within any given culture that may be keeping clients stuck. The basic scaffolding of CPT appears to be hardy, but cognitions, Stuck Points, and basic assumptions are different from place to place and from culture to culture. Socratic dialogue has been used successfully to challenge clients in even the most rigid cultures, and therapists need to keep in mind that cultures change over time or that cultural beliefs may be overgeneralized as Stuck Points. Local experts should be used to determine whether the Stuck Points the clients attribute to their culture are actually strong cultural beliefs or distortions that have been taught by family members or assumed by the clients themselves. Cultural Stuck Points may be core beliefs; as such, some careful Socratic dialogue and perhaps multiple worksheets may be needed to examine these viewpoints from different perspectives. However, we have heard therapists say that they can't do anything about a particular belief because it is part of a client's culture. This may be a therapist Stuck Point, rather than anything fixed about the culture.

Sometimes therapists working with clients from different cultures think that they need to change the CPT protocol before they have even tried it as it was developed. Again, this may be an assumption (or Stuck Point) on the part of these therapists; in any case, as soon as they change the protocol, CPT is no longer an evidence-based treatment. Our advice to therapists and researchers who are planning to use CPT for a different culture is to try the protocol as it was developed first. Then, when they have had time to develop their skills and see the results, they can decide whether to change the wording of the worksheets or the instructions. For example, perhaps clients can be instructed to read the corrected Challenging Beliefs Worksheets every day to incorporate the new, more balanced thoughts. Consultation with local stakeholders is also important, in order to determine how PTSD is regarded in the community and whether there is a belief in the recovery model. The first step may be to educate the community that PTSD is a normal reaction to an abnormal situation, and that people can recover from this disorder. Removing shame and stigma may be an important first step toward engaging people in treatment.

References

Ahrens, J., & Rexford, L. (2002). Cognitive processing therapy for incarcerated adolescents with PTSD. *Journal of Aggression, Maltreatment and Trauma, 6,* 201–216.

American Psychiatric Association. (1980). *Diagnostic and statistical manual of mental disorders* (3rd ed.). Washington, DC: Author.

American Psychiatric Association. (2000). *Diagnostic and statistical manual of mental disorders* (4th ed., text rev.). Washington, DC: Author.

American Psychiatric Association. (2013). *Diagnostic and statistical manual of mental disorders* (5th ed.). Arlington, VA: Author.

Anderson, H., & Goolishian, H. (1992). The client is the expert: A not-knowing approach to therapy. In S. McNamee & K. J. Gergen (Eds.), *Therapy as social construction* (pp. 25–39). London: Sage.

Asamsama, H. O., Dickstein, B. D., & Chard, K. M. (2015). Do scores on the Beck Depression Inventory–II predict outcome in cognitive processing therapy? *Psychological Trauma: Theory, Research, Practice and Policy, 7,* 437–441.

Barlow, D. H., & Craske, M. G. (1994). *Mastery of your anxiety and panic: II.* Albany, NY: Graywind.

Bass, J. K., Annan, J., McIvor Murray, S., Kaysen, D., Griffiths, S., Cetinoglu, T., . . . Bolton, P. A. (2013). Controlled trial of psychotherapy for Congolese survivors of sexual violence. *New England Journal of Medicine, 368*(23), 2182–2191.

Beck, A. T., & Greenberg, R. L. (1984). *Cognitive therapy in the treatment of depression.* New York: Springer.

Beck, A. T., Rush, A. J., Shaw, B. F., & Emery, G. (1979). *Cognitive therapy of depression.* New York: Guilford Press.

Beck, A. T., Steer, R. A., & Brown, G. K. (1996). *Beck Depression Inventory–II.* San Antonio, TX: Psychological Corporation.

Bishop, W., & Fish, J. M. (1999). Questions as interventions: Perceptions of Socratic, solution focused, and diagnostic questioning styles. *Journal of Rational-Emotive and Cognitive-Behavior Therapy, 12*(2), 115–140.

Bohus, M., & Steil, R. (in progress). *RELEASE study.* Grant funded by the German Federal Ministry of Education and Research (No. 01KR1303B).

Bolten, H. (2001). Reason in practice. *Philosophy of Management, 3*(1), 21–34.

Bolton, P., Bass, J. K., Zangana, G. A. S, Kamal, T., Murray, S. M., Kaysen, D., . . . Rosenblum, M. (2014). A randomized controlled trial of mental health interventions for survivors of systematic violence in Kurdistan, Northern Iraq. *BMC Psychiatry, 14,* 2–15.

Briere, J. (1995). *The Trauma Symptom Inventory (TSI): Professional manual.* Odessa, FL: Psychological Assessment Resources.

Brownmiller, S. (1975). *Against our will.* New York: Simon & Schuster.

Bryan, C. J., Clemans, T. A., Hernandez, A. M., Mintz, J., Peterson, A. L., Yarvis, J. S., . . . STRONG STAR Consortium. (2016). Evaluating potential iatrogenic suicide risk in trauma-focused group cognitive behavioral therapy for the treatment of PTSD in active duty military personnel. *Depression and Anxiety, 33*(6), 549–557.

Bryant, R. A., Mastrodomenico, J., Felmingham, K. L., Hopwood, S., Kenny, L., Kandris, E., Cahill, C., & Creamer, M. (2008). Treatment of acute stress disorder: A randomized controlled trial. *Archives of General Psychiatry, 65,* 659–667.

Burgess, A. W., & Holmstrom, L. L. (1976). Coping behavior of the rape victim. *American Journal of Psychiatry, 133,* 413–418.

Butollo, W., Karl, R., König, J., & Rosner, R. (2015). A randomized controlled clinical trial of dialogical exposure therapy vs. cognitive processing therapy for adult outpatients suffering from PTSD after type I trauma in adulthood. *Psychotherapy and Psychosomatics, 85,* 16–26.

Chard, K. M. (2005). An evaluation of cognitive processing therapy for the treatment of post-traumatic stress disorder related to childhood sexual abuse. *Journal of Consulting and Clinical Psychology, 73*(5), 965–971.

Chard, K. M., Ricksecker, E. G., Healy, E. T., Karlin, B. E., & Resick, P. A. (2012). Dissemination and experience with cognitive processing therapy. *Journal of Rehabilitation Research and Development, 49*(5), 667–678.

Chard, K. M., Schumm, J. A., Owens, G. P., & Cottingham, S. M. (2010). A comparison of OEF and OIF veterans and Vietnam veterans receiving cognitive processing therapy. *Journal of Traumatic Stress, 23*(1), 25–32.

Chard, K. M., Schuster, J. L., & Resick, P. A. (2012). Cognitive processing therapy. In J. G. Beck & D. M. Sloan (Eds.), *The Oxford handbook of traumatic stress disorders* (pp. 439–448). New York: Oxford University Press.

Clark, L. A. (1993). *SNAP—Schedule for Nonadaptive and Adaptive Personality: Manual for administration, scoring, and interpretation.* Minneapolis: University of Minnesota Press.

Clarke, S. B., Rizvi, S. L., & Resick, P. A. (2008). Borderline personality characteristics and treatment outcome in cognitive-behavioral treatments for PTSD in female rape victims. *Behavior Therapy, 39,* 72–78.

Derogatis, L. R. (1977). *SCL-90-R: Administration, scoring and procedures manual–II.* Towson, MD: Clinical Psychometric Research.

Dickstein, B. D., Walter, K. H., Schumm, J. A., & Chard, K. M. (2013). Comparing response to cognitive processing therapy in military veterans with subthreshold and threshold post-traumatic stress disorder. *Journal of Traumatic Stress, 26,* 703–709.

Dondanville, K. A., Blankenship, A. E., Molino, A., Resick, P. A., Wachen, J. S., Mintz, J., . . . STRONG STAR Consortium. (2016). Qualitative examination of cognitive change during PTSD treatment for active duty service members. *Behaviour Research and Therapy, 79,* 1–6.

Edinger, J., & Carney, C. (2008). *Overcoming insomnia: A cognitive-behavioral therapy approach therapist guide.* Oxford, UK: Oxford University Press.

Elder, L., & Paul, R. (1998). The role of Socratic questioning in thinking, teaching, and learning. *The Clearing House, 71,* 297–301.

Falsetti, S. A., Resnick, H. S., & Davis, J. L. (2008). Multiple channel exposure therapy for women with PTSD and comorbid panic attacks. *Cognitive Behaviour Therapy, 37,* 117–130.

Foa, E. B., Cashman, L., Jaycox, L., & Perry, K. (1997). The validation of a self-report measure of posttraumatic stress disorder: The Posttraumatic Diagnostic Scale. *Psychological Assessment, 9*(4), 445–451.

Foa, E. B., Hearst-Ikeda, D., & Perry, K. J. (1995). Evaluation of a brief cognitive-behavioral program for the prevention of chronic PTSD in recent assault victims. *Journal of Consulting and Clinical Psychology, 63,* 948–955.

Foa, E. B., & Kozak, M. J. (1986). Emotional processing of fear: Exposure to corrective information. *Psychological Bulletin, 99,* 2–35.

Foa, E. B., Rothbaum, B., Riggs, D., & Murdock, T. (1991). Treatment of posttraumatic stress disorder in rape victims: A comparison between cognitive-behavioral procedures and counseling. *Journal of Consulting and Clinical Psychology, 59*(5), 715–723.

Foa, E. B., Zoellner, L. A., & Feeny, N. C. (2006). An evaluation of three brief programs for facilitating recovery after assault. *Journal of Traumatic Stress, 19,* 29–43.

Forbes, D., Lloyd, D., Nixon, R. D., Elliott, P., Varker, T., Perry, D., . . . Creamer, M. (2012). A multisite randomized controlled effectiveness trial of cognitive processing therapy for military-related posttraumatic stress disorder. *Journal of Anxiety Disorders, 26*(3), 442–452.

Gallagher, M., & Resick, P. A. (2012). Mechanisms of change in cognitive processing therapy and prolonged exposure therapy for posttraumatic stress disorder: Preliminary evidence for the differential effects of hopelessness and habituation. *Cognitive Therapy and Research, 36*(6), 750–755.

Galovski, T. E., Blain, L. M., Chappuis, C., & Fletcher, T. (2013). Sex differences in recovery from PTSD in male and female interpersonal assault survivors. *Behaviour Research and Therapy, 51*(6), 247–255.

Galovski, T. E., Blain, L. M., Mott, J. M., Elwood, L., & Houle, T. (2012). Manualized therapy for PTSD: Flexing the structure of cognitive processing therapy. *Journal of Consulting and Clinical Psychology, 80,* 968–981.

Galovski, T. E., Harik, J. M., Blain, L. M., Elwood, L., Gloth, C., & Fletcher, T. (2016). Augmenting CPT to improve sleep impairment in PTSD: A randomized clinical trial. *Journal of Consulting and Clinical Psychology, 84*(2), 167–177.

Galovski, T. E., Monson, C., Bruce, S. E., & Resick, P. A. (2009). Does cognitive-behavioral therapy for PTSD improve perceived health and sleep impairment? *Journal of Traumatic Stress, 22*(3), 197–204.

Galovski, T. E., & Resick, P. A. (2008). Cognitive processing therapy for posttraumatic stress disorder secondary to a motor vehicle accident: A single-subject report. *Cognitive and Behavioral Practice, 15,* 287–295.

Galovski, T. E., Sobel, A., Phipps, K., & Resick, P. A. (2005). Trauma recovery: Beyond the treatment of symptoms of PTSD and other Axis I psychopathology. In T. A. Corales (Ed.), *Trends in posttraumatic stress disorder research* (pp. 207–227). Hauppauge, NY: Nova Science.

Garner, D. M. (1991). *Eating Disorder Inventory–2: Professional manual.* Odessa, FL: Psychological Assessment Resources.

Gilman, R., Schumm, J. A., & Chard, K. M. (2011). Hope as a change mechanism in the treatment of posttraumatic stress disorder. *Psychological Trauma: Theory, Research, Practice, and Policy, 4,* 270–277.

Gradus, J. L., Suvak, M. K., Wisco, B. E., Marx, B. P., & Resick, P. A. (2013). Treatment of posttraumatic stress disorder reduces suicidal ideation. *Depression and Anxiety, 30,* 1046–1053.

Grady, D. (2013, June 5). Therapy for rape victims shows promise in Congo. Retrieved from *www.nytimes.com/2013/06/06/health/therapy-for-rape-victims-shows-promise.html*

Griffin, M. G., Resick, P. A., & Galovski, T. (2012). Does physiologic response to loud tones change following cognitive-behavioral treatment for posttraumatic stress disorder? *Journal of Traumatic Stress, 25,* 25–32.

Haagen, J. F. G., Smid, G. E., Knipscheer, J. W., & Kleber, R. J. (2015). The efficacy of recommended treatments for veterans with PTSD: A metaregression analysis. *Clinical Psychology Review, 40,* 184–194.

Haines, S. (1999). *The survivor's guide to sex: How to have an empowered sex life after child sexual abuse.* San Francisco: Cleis Press.

Hariri, A. R., Bookheimer, S. Y., & Mazziotta, J. C. (2000). Modulating emotional responses: Effects of a neocortical network on the limbic system. *NeuroReport, 11*(1), 43–48.

Hariri, A. R., Mattay, V. S., Tessitore, A., Fera, F., & Weinberger, D. R. (2003). Neocortical modulation of the amygdala response to fearful stimuli. *Biological Psychiatry, 53*(6), 494–501.

Hinton, D. E., Pham, T., Tran, M., Safren, S. A., Otto, M. W., & Pollack, M. H. (2004). CBT for Vietnam refugees with treatment-resistant PTSD and panic attacks: A pilot study. *Journal of Traumatic Stress, 17,* 429–433.

Hollon, S. D., & Garber, J. (1988). Cognitive therapy. In L. Y Abramson (Ed.), *Social cognition and clinical psychology: A synthesis* (pp. 204–253). New York: Guilford Press.

Horowitz, M. D., Wilner, N., & Alvarez, W. (1979). Impact of Event Scale: A measure of subjective stress. *Psychosomatic Medicine, 41,* 209–218.

Ito, M., Kashimura, M., & Horikoshi, M. (2012). 伊藤正哉 . 樫村正美 . 堀越勝、2012、こころを癒すノート：トラウマの認知処理療法自習帳、創元社 (*The healing notebook for a wounded heart: Cognitive processing therapy workbook for trauma survivors*). Osaka, Japan: Sogensha.

Iverson, K. M., Gradus, J. L., Resick, P. A., Suvak, M. K., Smith, K. F., & Monson, C. M. (2011). Cognitive-behavioral therapy for PTSD and depression symptoms reduces risk for future intimate partner violence among interpersonal trauma survivors. *Journal of Consulting and Clinical Psychology, 79,* 193–202.

Iverson, K. M., King, M. W., Cunningham, K. C., & Resick, P. A. (2015). Rape survivors' trauma-related beliefs before and after cognitive processing therapy: Associations with PTSD and depression symptoms. *Behaviour Research and Therapy, 66,* 49–55.

Janoff-Bulman, R. (1989). Assumptive worlds and the stress of traumatic events: Applications of the schema construct. *Social Cognition, 7,* 113–136.

Janoff-Bulman, R. (1992). *Shattered assumptions: Towards a new psychology of trauma.* New York: Free Press.

Jayawickreme, N., Cahill, S. P., Riggs, D. S., Rauch, S. A. M., Resick, P. A., Rothbaum, B. O., & Foa, E. B. (2014). Primum non nocere (first do no harm): Symptom worsening and improvement in female assault victims after prolonged exposure for PTSD. *Depression and Anxiety, 31*(5), 412–419.

Johnson, S. B., Blum, R. W., & Giedd, J. N. (2009) Adolescent maturity and the brain: The promise and pitfalls of neuroscience research in adolescent health policy. *Journal of Adolescent Health, 45,* 216–221.

Kaysen, D., Lindgren, K., Zangana, G. A. S., Murray, L., Bass, J., & Bolton, P. (2013). Adaptation of cognitive processing therapy for treatment of torture victims: Experience in Kurdistan, Iraq. *Psychological Trauma: Theory, Research, Practice, and Policy, 5*(2), 184–192.

Kaysen, D., Lostutter, T. W., & Goines, M. A. (2005). Cognitive processing therapy for acute stress disorder resulting from an anti-gay assault. *Cognitive and Behavioral Practice, 12*(3), 278–289.

Kaysen, D., Schumm, J., Petersen, E. R., Seim, R. W., Bedard-Gilligan, M., & Chard, K. (2014). Cognitive processing therapy for veterans with comorbid PTSD and alcohol use disorders. *Addictive Behaviors, 39*(2), 420–427.

Kennerley, H. (1996). Cognitive therapy of dissociative symptoms associated with trauma. *British Journal of Clinical Psychology, 35,* 325–340.

Kessler, R. C., Sonnega, A., Bromet, E., Hughes, M., & Nelson, C. B. (1995). Posttraumatic stress disorder in the National Comorbidity Survey. *Archives of General Psychiatry, 52,* 1048–1060.

Kilpatrick, D. G., Resick, P. A., & Veronen, L. J. (1981). Effects of a rape experience: A longitudinal study. *Journal of Social Issues, 37,* 105–122.

Kilpatrick, D. G., Veronen, L. J., & Resick, P. A. (1979). Assessment of the aftermath of rape: Changing patterns of fear. *Journal of Behavioral Assessment, 1,* 133–147.

Kilpatrick, D. G., Veronen, L. J., & Resick, P. A. (1982). Psychological sequelae to rape: Assessment and treatment strategies. In D. M. Doleys, R. L. Meredith, & A. R. Ciminero (Eds.), *Behavioral medicine: Assessment and treatment strategies* (pp. 473–497). New York: Plenum Press.

König, J., Resick, P. A., Karl, R., & Rosner, R (2012). *Posttraumatische belastungsstörung: Ein manual zur cognitive processing therapy.* Gottingen, Germany: Hogrefe.

Kroenke, K., Spitzer, R. L., & Williams, J. B. (2001). The PHQ-9: Validity of a brief depression severity measure. *Journal of General Internal Medicine, 16,* 606–613.

Lang, P. J. (1977). Imagery in therapy: An information processing analysis of fear. *Behavior Therapy, 8,* 862–886.

Lejuez, C. W., Hopko, D. R., Acierno, R., Daughters, S. B., & Pagoto, S. L. (2011). Ten year revision of the brief behavioral activation treatment for depression: Revised treatment manual. *Behavior Modification, 35,* 111–161.

Lejuez, C. W., Hopko, D. R., & Hopko, S. D. (2001). A brief behavioral activation treatment for depression: Treatment manual. *Behavior Modification, 25,* 255–286.

Lerner, M. J. (1980). *The belief in a just world: A fundamental delusion.* New York: Plenum Press.

Lester, K., Artz, C., Resick, P. A., & Young-Xu, Y. (2010). Impact of race on early treatment termination and outcomes in posttraumatic stress disorder treatment. *Journal of Consulting and Clinical Psychology, 78*(4), 480–489.

Lewinsohn, P. M. (1974). Clinical and theoretical aspects of depression. In K. S. Calhoun, H. E. Adams, & K. M. Mitchell (Eds.), *Innovative treatment methods in psychopathology* (pp. 63–120). New York: Wiley.

Liberzon, I., & Sripada, C. S. (2008). The functional neuroanatomy of PTSD: A critical review. *Progress in Brain Research, 167,* 151–169.

Lloyd, D., Couineau, A.-L., Hawkins, K., Kartal, D., Nixon, R. D. V., & Forbes, D. P. (2015). Preliminary outcomes of implementing cognitive processing therapy for posttraumatic stress disorder across a national veterans' treatment service. *Journal of Clinical Psychiatry, 76*(11), e1405–e1409.

Mahoney, M. J. (1981). Psychotherapy and the human change process. In J. H. Harvey & M. M. Parks (Eds.), *Psychotherapy research and behavior change* (pp. 73–122). Washington, DC: American Psychological Association.

Mahoney, M. J., & Lyddon, W. J. (1988) Recent developments in cognitive approaches to counseling and psychotherapy. *Counseling Psychologist, 16,* 190–234.

Maieritsch, K. P., Smith, T. L., Hessinger, J. D., Ahearn, E. P., Eickhoff, J. C., & Zhao, Q. (2016). Randomized controlled equivalence trial comparing videoconference and in person delivery of cognitive processing therapy for PTSD. *Journal of Telemedicine and Telecare, 22*(4), 238–243.

Marques, L., Eustis, E. H., Dixon, L., Valentine, S. E., Borba, C. P. C., Simon, N., . . . Wiltsey-Stirman, S. (2016). Delivering cognitive processing therapy in a community health setting:

The Influence of Latino culture and community violence on posttraumatic cognitions. *Psychological Trauma: Theory, Research, Practice, and Policy, 8*(1), 98–106.

Matulis, S., Resick, P. A., Rosner, R., & Steil, R. (2014). Developmentally adapted cognitive processing therapy for adolescents suffering from posttraumatic stress disorder after childhood sexual or physical abuse: A pilot study. *Clinical Child Family Psycholological Review, 17,* 173–190.

McCann, I. L., & Pearlman, L. A. (1990). *Psychological trauma and the adult survivor: Theory, therapy, and transformation.* New York: Brunner/Mazel.

McCann, I. L., Sakheim, D. K., & Abrahamson, D. J. (1988). Trauma and victimization: A model of psychological adaptation. *Counseling Psychologist, 16,* 531–594.

Meichenbaum, D., & Cameron, R. (1983). Stress inoculation training: Toward a general paradigm for training coping skills. In D. Meichenbaum & M. E. Jare (Eds.), *Stress reduction and prevention* (pp. 115–154). New York: Plenum Press.

Milad, M. R., Pitman, R. K., Ellis, C. B., Gold, A. L., Shin, L. M., Sasko, N. B., . . . Rauch, S. L. (2009). Neurobiological basis of failure to recall extinction memory in posttraumatic stress disorder. *Biological Psychiatry, 66,* 1075–1082.

Mitchell, K. S., Wells, S. Y., Mendes, A., & Resick, P. A. (2012). Treatment improves symptoms shared by PTSD and disordered eating. *Journal of Traumatic Stress, 25,* 535–542.

Monson, C. M., & Friedman, S. J. (2012). *Cognitive-behavioral conjoint therapy for PTSD: Harnessing the healing power of relationships.* New York: Guilford Press.

Monson, C. M., Friedman, M. J., & La Bash, H. A. J. (2014). A psychological history of PTSD. In M. J. Friedman, T. M. Keane, & P. A. Resick (Eds.), *Handbook of PTSD: Science and practice* (2nd ed., pp. 60–78). New York: Guilford Press.

Monson, C. M., Macdonald, A., Vorstenbosch, V., Shnaider, P., Goldstein, E. S. R., Ferrier-Auerbach, A. G., & Mocciola, K. E. (2012). Changes in social adjustment with cognitive processing therapy: Effects of treatment and association with PTSD symptom change. *Journal of Traumatic Stress, 25*(5), 519–526.

Monson, C. M., Rodriguez, B. F., & Warner, R. (2005). Cognitive-behavioral therapy for PTSD in the real world: Do interpersonal relationships make a real difference? *Journal of Clinical Psychology, 61,* 751–761.

Monson, C. M. & Shnaider, P. (2014). *Treating PTSD with cognitive-behavioral therapies: Interventions that work.* Washington, DC: American Psychological Association.

Monson, C. M., Schnurr, P. P., Resick, P. A., Friedman, M. J., Young-Xu, Y., & Stevens, S. P. (2006). Cognitive processing therapy for veterans with military-related posttraumatic stress disorder. *Journal of Consulting and Clinical Psychology, 74*(5), 898–907.

Morland, L. A., Hynes, A. K., Mackintosh, M., Resick, P. A., & Chard, K. M. (2011). Group cognitive processing therapy delivered to veterans via telehealth: A pilot cohort. *Journal of Traumatic Stress, 24*(4), 465–469.

Morland, L. A., Mackintosh, M. A., Rosen, C. S., Willis, E., Resick, P. A., Chard, K. M., & Frueh, B. C. (2015). Telemedicine versus in-person delivery of cognitive processing therapy for women with posttraumatic stress disorder: A randomized noninferiority trial. *Depression and Anxiety, 32*(11), 811–820.

Mowrer, O. H. (1960). *Learning theory and behavior.* New York: Wiley.

Nixon, R. D. (2012). Cognitive processing therapy versus supportive counseling for acute stress disorder following assault: A randomized pilot trial. *Behavior Therapy, 43*(4), 825–836.

O'Donnell, M. L., Alkemade, N., Nickerson, A., Creamer, M., McFarlane, A. C., Silove, D., . . . Forbes, D. (2014). Impact of the diagnostic changes to post-traumatic stress disorder for DSM-5 and the proposed changes to ICD-11. *British Journal of Psychiatry, 205*(3), 230–235.

Owens, G. P., Pike, J. L., & Chard, K. M. (2001). Treatment effects of cognitive processing therapy on cognitive distortions of female child sexual abuse survivors. *Behavior Therapy, 32,* 413–424.

Padesky, C. A. (1996). *Guided discovery using Socratic dialogue.* Newport Beach, CA: Center for Cognitive Therapy.

Paul, R., & Elder, E. (2006). *The thinker's guide to the art of Socratic questioning.* Dillon Beach, CA: Foundation for Critical Thinking Press.

Paykel, E. S. (1974). Recent life events and clinical depression. In E. K. Gunderson & R. H. Babe (Eds.), *Life stress and illness.* Springfield, IL: Charles C Thomas.

Piaget, J. (1971). *Psychology and epistemology; Towards a theory of knowledge.* New York: Viking Press.

Price, J. L., MacDonald, H. Z., Adair, K. C., Koerner, N., & Monson, C. M. (2016). Changing beliefs about trauma: A qualitative study of cognitive processing therapy. *Behavioural and Cognitive Psychotherapy, 44*(2), 156–167.

Price, M., Gros, D. F., Strachan, M., Ruggiero, K. J., & Acierno, R. (2013). The role of social support in exposure therapy for Operation Iraqi Freedom/Operation Enduring Freedom veterans: A preliminary investigation. *Psychological Trauma: Theory, Research, Practice, and Policy, 5,* 93–100.

Pruiksma, K. E., Molino, A., Taylor, D. J., Resick, P. A., & Peterson, A. L. (2016). Case study of cognitive behavioral therapy for comorbid PTSD, insomnia, and nightmares. In C. Martin, V. R. Preedy, & V. B. Patel (Eds.), *Comprehensive guide to post-traumatic stress disorders* (pp. 2249–2258). New York: Springer.

Pruiksma, K. E., Taylor, D. J., Wachen, J. S., Mintz, J., Young-McCaughan, S., Peterson, A., . . . STRONG STAR Consortium. (in press). Residual sleep disturbances following PTSD treatment active duty military personnel. *Psychological Trauma: Theory, Research, and Practice.*

Rauch, S. L., Whalen, P. J., Shin, L. M., McInerney, S. C., Macklin, M. L., Lasko, N. B., . . . Pitman, R. K. (2000). Exaggerated amygdala response to masked facial stimuli in posttraumatic stress disorder: A functional MRI study. *Biological Psychiatry, 47,* 769–776.

Resick, P. A. (2001). *Cognitive processing therapy: Generic version.* Unpublished manuscript, University of Missouri, Saint Louis, MO.

Resick, P. A., Bovin, M. J., Calloway, A. L., Dick, A., King, M. W., Mitchell, K. S., . . . Wolf, E. J. (2012). A critical evaluation of the complex PTSD literature: Implications for DSM-5. *Journal of Traumatic Stress, 25,* 241–251.

Resick, P. A., & Derby, D. S. (2012). טיפול מיתסתנ טוסס סופ תנומסתב לופיט – םישדח םיקפוא עיבוד בהרזת גוניטיבי [*New horizons: Treating post traumatic stress disorder using cognitive processing therapy*]. Tel Aviv: Galil Press.

Resick, P. A., Galovski, T. E., Uhlmansiek, M. O., Scher, C. D., Clum, G., & Young-Xu, Y. (2008). A randomized clinical trial to dismantle components of cognitive processing therapy for posttraumatic stress disorder in female victims of interpersonal violence. *Journal of Consulting and Clinical Psychology, 76*(2), 243–258.

Resick, P. A., Jordan, C. G., Girelli, S. A., Hutter, C. K., & Marhoeder-Dvorak, S. (1988). A comparative outcome study of group behavior therapy for sexual assault victims. *Behavior Therapy, 19,* 385–401.

Resick, P. A., Monson, C. M., & Chard, K. M. (2007). *Cognitive processing therapy, veteran/ military version: Therapist's manual.* Washington, DC: Department of Veterans Affairs. (Revised in 2008, 2010, 2014)

Resick, P. A., Monson, C. M., & Rizvi, S. L. (2013). Posttraumatic stress disorder. In W. E. Craighead, D. J. Miklowitz, & L. W. Craighead (Eds.), *Psychopathology: History, diagnosis, and empirical foundations* (2nd ed., pp. 244–284). Hoboken, NJ: Wiley.

Resick, P. A., Nishith, P., Weaver, T. L., Astin, M. C., & Feuer, C. A. (2002). A comparison of cognitive processing therapy, prolonged exposure and a waiting condition for the treatment of posttraumatic stress disorder in female rape victims. *Journal of Consulting and Clinical Psychology, 70*(4), 867–879.

Resick, P. A., & Schnicke, M. K. (1992). Cognitive processing therapy for sexual assault victims. *Journal of Consulting and Clinical Psychology, 60*(5), 748–756.

Resick, P. A., & Schnicke, M. K. (1993). *Cognitive processing therapy for rape victims: A treatment manual.* Newbury Park, CA: Sage.

Resick, P. A., Schnicke, M. K., & Markway, B. G. (1991, November). *Personal Beliefs and Reactions Scale: The relation between cognitive content and posttraumatic stress disorder.* Paper presented at the 25th Annual Convention of the Association for Advancement of Behavior Therapy, New York.

Resick, P. A., Suvak, M. K., Johnides, B. D., Mitchell, K. S., & Iverson, K. M. (2012). The impact of dissociation on PTSD treatment with cognitive processing therapy. *Depression and Anxiety, 29*(8), 718–730.

Resick, P. A., Suvak, M. K., & Wells, S. Y. (2014). The impact of childhood abuse among women with assault-related PTSD receiving short-term cognitive-behavioral therapy. *Journal of Traumatic Stress, 27*, 558–567.

Resick, P. A., Wachen, J. S., Mintz, J., Young-McCaughan, S., Roache, J. D., Borah, A. M., . . . Peterson, A. L. (2015). A randomized clinical trial of group cognitive processing therapy compared with group present-centered therapy for PTSD among active duty military personnel. *Journal of Consulting and Clinical Psychology, 83*(6), 1058–1068.

Resick, P. A., Wachen, J. S., & Peterson, A. L. (in progress). *Variable length cognitive processing therapy for combat-related PTSD.* Grant funded by the Department of Defense (Nos. W81XWH-13-2-0012 and W81XWH-13-2-0014).

Resick, P. A., Williams, L. F., Suvak, M. K., Monson, C. M., & Gradus, J. L. (2012). Long-term outcomes of cognitive-behavioral treatments for posttraumatic stress disorder among female rape survivors. *Journal of Consulting and Clinical Psychology, 80*(2), 201–210.

Rutter, J. G., Friedberg, R. D., VandeCreek, L., & Jackson, T. L. (1999). *Innovations in clinical practice: A source book.* Sarasota, FL: Professional Resource Press.

Schnurr, P. P., Friedman, M. J., Engel, C. C., Foa, E. B., Shea, T., Chow, B. K., . . . Bernardy, N. (2007). Cognitive-behavioral therapy for posttraumatic stress disorder in women: A randomized controlled trial. *Journal of the American Medical Association, 297*, 820–830.

Schulz, P. M., Huber, L. C., & Resick, P. A. (2006). Practical adaptations of cognitive processing therapy with Bosnian refugees: Implications for adapting practice to a multicultural clientele. *Cognitive and Behavioral Practice, 13*(4), 310–321.

Schulz, P. M., Resick, P. A., Huber, L. C., & Griffin, M. G. (2006). The effectiveness of cognitive processing therapy for PTSD with refugees in a community setting. *Cognitive and Behavioral Practice, 13*, 322–331.

Schumm, J. A., Dickstein, B. D., Walter, K. H., Owens, G. P., & Chard, K. M. (2015). Changes in posttraumatic cognitions predict changes in posttraumatic stress disorder symptoms during cognitive processing therapy. *Journal of Consulting and Clinical Psychology, 83*, 1161–1166.

Seligman, M. E. P. (1971). Phobias and preparedness. *Behavior Therapy, 2*, 307–321.

Shalev, A. Y., Ankri, Y., Israeli-Shalev Y., Peleg, T., Adessky, R., & Freedman, S. (2012). Prevention of posttraumatic stress disorder by early treatment: Results from the Jerusalem trauma outreach and prevention study. *Archives of General Psychiatry, 69*, 166–176.

Shin, L. M., Orr, S. P., Carson, M. A., Rauch, S. L., Macklin, M. L., Lasko, N. B., . . . Pitman, R. K. (2004). Regional cerebral blood flow in the amygdala and medial prefrontal cortex during traumatic imagery in male and female Vietnam veterans with PTSD. *Archives of General Psychiatry, 61*(2), 168–176.

Shin, L. M., Rauch, S. L., & Pitman, R. K. (2006). Amygdala, medial prefrontal cortex, and hippocampal function in PTSD. *Annals of the New York Academy of Sciences, 1071,* 67–79.

Shin, L. M., Whalen, P. J., Pitman, R. K., Bush, G., Macklin, M. L., Lasko, N. B., . . . Rauch, S. L. (2001). An fMRI study of anterior cingulate function in posttraumatic stress disorder. *Biological Psychiatry, 50,* 932–942.

Shnaider, P., Vorrstenbosch, V., Macdonald, A., Wells, S. Y., Monson, C. M., & Resick, P. A. (2014). Associations between functioning and PTSD symptom clusters in a dismantling trial of cognitive processing therapy in female interpersonal violence survivors. *Journal of Traumatic Stress, 27,* 526–534.

Sobel, A. A., Resick, P. A., & Rabalais, A. E. (2009). The effect of cognitive processing therapy on cognitions: Impact Statement coding. *Journal of Traumatic Stress. 22,* 205–211.

Stein, D. J., Koenen, K. C., Friedman, M. J., Hill, E., McLaughlin, K. A., Petukhova, M., . . . Kessler, R. C. (2013). Dissociation in posttraumatic stress disorder: Evidence from the World Mental Health Surveys. *Biological Psychiatry, 73,* 302–312.

Suris, A., Link-Malcolm, J., Chard, K., Ahn, C., & North, C. (2013). A randomized clinical trial of cognitive processing therapy for veterans with PTSD related to military sexual trauma. *Journal of Traumatic Stress, 26*(1), 28–37.

Tarrier, N., Sommerfield, C., & Pilgrim, H. (1999). Relatives' expressed emotion (EE) and PTSD treatment outcome. *Psychological Medicine, 29,* 801–811.

Taylor, D. J., & Pruiksma, K. E. (2014). Cognitive and behavioural therapy for insomnia (CBT-I) in psychiatric populations: A systematic review. *International Review of Psychiatry, 26,* 205–213.

Thase, M. E., & Beck, A. T. (1993). An overview of cognitive therapy. In J. H. Wright, M. E. Thase, A. T. Beck, & J. W. Ludgate (Eds.), *Cognitive therapy with inpatients: Developing a cognitive milieu* (pp. 3–34). New York: Guilford Press.

Thrasher, S., Power, M., Morant, N., Marks, I., & Dalgleish, T. (2010). Social support moderates outcomes in a randomized controlled trial of exposure therapy and (or) cognitive restructuring for chronic posttraumatic stress disorder. *Canadian Journal of Psychiatry/ Revue Canadienne de Psychiatrie, 55,* 187–190.

Voelkel, E., Pukay-Martin, N. D., Walter, K. H., & Chard, K. M. (2015). Effectiveness of cognitive processing therapy for male and female U.S. veterans with and without military sexual trauma. *Journal of Traumatic Stress, 28,* 174–182.

Wachen, J. S., Dondanville, K. A., Pruiksma, K. A., Molino, A., Carson, C. S., Blankenship, A. E., . . . Resick, P. A. (2016). Implementing cognitive processing therapy for posttraumatic stress disorder with active duty U.S. military personnel: Special considerations and case examples. *Cognitive and Behavioral Practice, 23*(2), 133–147.

Wachen, J. S., Jimenez, S., Smith, K., & Resick, P. A. (2014). Long-term functional outcomes of women receiving cognitive processing therapy and prolonged exposure. *Psychological Trauma: Theory, Research, Practice and Policy, 27,* 526–534.

Walter, K. H., Bolte, T. A., Owens, G. P., & Chard, K. M. (2012). The impact of personality disorders on treatment outcome for veterans in a posttraumatic stress disorder residential treatment program. *Cognitive Therapy and Research, 36,* 576–584.

Walter, K. H., Buckley, A. B., Simpson, J. M., & Chard, K. M. (2014). Residential PTSD treatment for female veterans with military sexual trauma: Does a history of childhood sexual abuse influence outcome? *Journal of Interpersonal Violence, 6,* 971–986.

Walter, K. H., Dickstein, B. D., Barnes, S. M., & Chard, K. M. (2014). Comparing effectiveness of CPT to CPT-C among U.S. veterans in an interdisciplinary residential PTSD/TBI treatment program. *Journal of Traumatic Stress, 27,* 438–445.

Watts, B. V., Schnurr, P. P., Mayo, L., Young-Xu, Y., Weeks, W. B., & Friedman, M. J. (2013).

Meta-analysis of the efficacy of treatments for posttraumatic stress disorder. *Journal of Clinical Psychiatry, 74,* 541–550.

Weathers, F. W., Litz, B. T., Herman, D. S., Huska, J. A., & Keane, T. M. (1993, October). *The PTSD Checklist (PCL): Reliability, validity, and diagnostic utility.* Paper presented at the the International Society for Traumatic Stress Studies, San Antonio, TX.

Weathers, F. W., Litz, B. T., Keane, T. M., Palmieri, P. A., Marx, B. P., & Schnurr, P. P. (2013). *The PTSD Checklist for DSM-5 (PCL-5).* Available from the National Center for PTSD at *www.ptsd.va.gov*

Weathers, F. W., Marx, B. P., Friedman, M. J., & Schnurr, P. P. (2014). Posttraumatic stress disorder in DSM-5: New criteria, new measures, and implications for assessment. *Psychological Injury and Law, 7,* 93–107.

Weissman, M. M., & Paykel, C. S. (1974). *The depressed woman: A study of social relationships.* Chicago: University of Chicago Press.

World Health Organization. (1992). *ICD-10 classifications of mental and behavioural disorders: Clinical descriptions and diagnostic guidelines.* Geneva: Author.

Wright, J. H., Basco, M. R., & Thase, M. E. (2006). *Learning cognitive behavioral therapy: An illustrated guide.* Washington, DC: American Psychiatric Publishing.

Ylikomi, R., & Virta, V. (2008). *Raiskaustrauman Hoito: Opas CPT-Menetelmän Käyttöön.* Jyväskylä, Finland: PS-Kustannus.

Index

Note: *f* following a page number indicates a figure.